# Dancing with Yin and Yang

## John Chitty

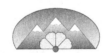

**Polarity Press**
**Boulder, Colorado**

**Disclaimer:**

The information in this book is intended for general inquiry and informational purposes only and should not be considered a substitute for medical advice, diagnosis, or treatment. If you think you, or those under your care, are ill or in need of health care, please seek immediate medical attention. Always consult a doctor or other competent licensed clinical professional for specific advice about medical treatments for yourself or those under your care. Any use of, or reliance in any way upon, the information contained in this book is solely at your own risk.


*Cover Art: Dani Burke*

# Dancing with Yin and Yang

## Ancient Wisdom, Modern Psychotherapy and Randolph Stone's Polarity Therapy

John Chitty

# Praise for *Dancing with Yin and Yang*

*Dancing with Yin and Yang* provides a passionate, articulate, and eclectic vision of how an appreciation of ancient insights, alternative strategies of treatment, and contemporary neuroscience can co-exist and be mutually explanatory in understanding the human experience and in facilitating mental and physical health.

**Stephen Porges, PhD**
**Author, *Polyvagal Theory***

I had the great good fortune, as a young psychiatrist in the 1960s and 1970s, to experience apprenticeships with Fritz Perls and Ida Rolf at Esalen Institute, followed by three years of study with Randolph Stone in India and the United States. Those close relationships with such legendary teachers have defined and shaped my somatic psychotherapeutic work, and my many years of teaching Buddha Dharma, up unto the present time.

Now, much to my delight and amazement, John Chitty has produced THE much-awaited book that summarizes, accurately categorizes, and artfully blends the wisdom that flowed from my old teachers in those magical times. *Dancing with Yin and Yang* is a major accomplishment, a breakthrough interpretation of ancient teachings into modern somatic psychology. Fritz Perls and Randolph Stone never met in person, but John Chitty has introduced them to us as icons of their time and prophets of the future.

**Robert K. Hall, MD**
**Author, *Out of Nowhere***

John's new book is a wonderful expression of his ability to integrate concepts from many disciplines into a cohesive and dynamic whole. He shines a light on familiar ideas and makes interesting new connections, effectively simplifying complex interdisciplinary ideas. His inquiry is respectful of both wisdom traditions and modern neuroscience. This book is a significant addition to integrative knowledge and mind-body healing. I can wholeheartedly recommend it to all!

**Franklyn Sills, RCST, UKCP**
**Author, *Foundations of Craniosacral Biodynamics,***
**_The Polarity Process,_ and *Being and Becoming***

*Dancing with Yin and Yang* is a very stimulating, thought-provoking book, packed with valuable and unique insights. One of the most intriguing (and fresh) perspectives it offers is how it revives and expands the old two-chair process (Fritz Perls, ca. 1970), incorporating current findings from the ever-growing field of trauma resolution; I myself have experimented with the approach described here, and found it remarkably effective. I also appreciated reading the author's original viewpoint, suggesting how ancient wisdom can be positively integrated in present-day neuroscience and psychotherapy methods. John Chitty draws from many diverse sources, merging them into a comprehensive synthesis that significantly contributes to the literature in this field. I highly recommend this innovative book for those seeking an alternative, big-picture understanding of mind-body wellness.

**Diane Heller, PhD,**
**Author, *Crash Course***

John Chitty is one of the premier Polarity Therapy teachers in the world today and with the book *Dancing with Yin and Yang* he has done an enormous service to the whole

Polarity Therapy community by bringing the unique psychological aspects of the work of Randolph Stone, ND, DO, DC into clear focus. He artfully expresses the underlying Polarity theories on the role of consciousness and its interaction with the nervous system, and weaves a unique therapeutic approach which draws deeply on the ancient oriental philosophy of yin and yang, updated for the modern world, as well as blending in the unique work of Fritz Perls the renowned founder of Gestalt psychotherapy. Any bodywork therapist interested in exploring the psychology of their clients with a view to enabling a deeper level of healing will benefit enormously from the theories, concepts and practical methods outlined within.

**Phil Young, PTP**
**Author,** *Pranotherapy: The Evolution of Polarity Therapy*
*and European Neuromuscular Technique*
*The Art of Polarity Therapy, A Practitioner's Perspective*

More than developing a synthesis of modalities, John Chitty has generated a new paradigm of healing. *Dancing with Yin and Yang* clearly matches clients' needs with gentleness, kindness and respect. His approach reduces fear and promotes a deeper and more profound healing process.

**Michael Shea, PhD, BCST**
**Author,** *Biodynamic Craniosacral Therapy, Volumes 1-5*

# Grateful Acknowledgments
*in approximate chronological order*

**Anna Chitty** has taught Polarity Therapy and biodynamic craniosacral therapy since 1981. Her instructional approach emphasizes experiential learning, reflecting Randolph Stone's guidance: "Ability and skill are developed by effort and experience, not by talk."[1] She is a major source for material throughout this book. In addition to being my work partner, she is also my partner in life, since 1972.

**Alive Polarity Teachers** introduced me to Polarity Therapy.

**Franklyn Sills** expertly describes the intersection of topics covered in this book; he has been inspirational as mentor and colleague.

**Ray Castellino** revealed the super-sentient world of babies, both in the womb, during birthing and thereafter.

**Peter Levine**, developer of Somatic Experiencing®, illuminated the field of trauma resolution, transforming my view of healing.

**Stephen Porges** revolutionized my understanding of the all-important autonomic nervous system through his Polyvagal Theory, and graciously reviewed materials for this book.

**Jaap van der Wal** showed how the embryo's process is a super-focused microcosm of the whole human story.

**Zhi Gang Sha** was extraordinarily generous, kind and inspiring with support at an important time, and greatly expanded my understanding of the esoteric knowledge of his Tao lineage.

I am also grateful for the support of my children Haley and Elizabeth, and my siblings Ben, Em and Nathan.

Thanks to Anna Chitty, Phil Young, Em Chitty, Kim Haroche, Elizabeth Chitty, Ann Hazen, Zach Malone, Sam Yates, Ben Chitty, Nadene Pettry, Barry Ryan, Deb Kloor, Elise Martin and Sam Galler for editorial help.

Thanks to Lori Olcott and David Harel for their dedicated work on www.DigitalDrStone.org, which greatly helped this project.

This book was facilitated by support from an anonymous benefactor to whom I am profoundly grateful. You know who you are!

Finally, I am especially appreciative of the inspiration arising from my students and clients, for whom I hope this project is helpful.

---

[1] R. Stone, *Health Building*. CRCS, 1986. p. 26.

# Table of Contents

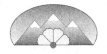

# Preface

As I was organizing materials for this book, an unexpected resource arrived at my door, the latest issue of *Scientific American Mind*. "Sharpen Your Focus" proclaimed the cover. "How the science of mindfulness can improve attention and lift your mood," continued the subtitle. I thought, *"Science* of *mindfulness*, what an auspicious message!" "Science" implies objective, cerebral, western PhDs. "Mindfulness" implies tranquil meditators immersed in inner subjective awareness. The effect was completed with a full-page close-up image of the perfectly symmetrical face and intense direct gaze of a beautiful female model, informing me that the magazine's designers were aware of the subtle workings of the autonomic nervous system. "This is it!" I thought, "All I have to do is explain this cover."

Wisdom traditions of the East and psychology studies of the West have both examined human wellness, but from different angles: one from the inside-out and the other from the outside-in. The resulting findings have been preserved and embellished in separate departments of our universities. However, given that psychology, philosophy and spirituality books are in different parts of the library, and additionally often written in different styles, the chances of effective cross-pollination stay pretty low. Now the separation of disciplines is declining, a much-appreciated side effect of globalization.

When I wrote my undergraduate senior thesis about Marshall McLuhan over 40 years ago, it was about how perception and meaning are molded by information processing.[2] New electronic media were transforming how we thought and behaved; studies were showing that television led to questioning of authority, in contrast to how print seemed to lead to acceptance of authority. At the time the whole line of thinking was partly an attempt to comprehend the culture-quaking sixties. Today, McLuhan seems to be even more validated than he already was in my mind back then: the internet is repeating the same kind of shift, a fourth major transformation (the others being radio, movies and television, all following print) in less than a century and this time on a faster-paced, global scale. We are on a consciousness roller coaster, so perhaps the time is right for a new synthesis.

As an undergraduate student in college, I was curious about states of consciousness and the science of personal and social behavior. However I was too squeamish for psychology because of the seemingly cruel treatment of the test animals. I chose to major in sociology instead; at that time it had more wiggle room for a misfit like myself.

After college, my attention was drawn to the Himalayan wisdom traditions. Initially this was just part of the counter-culture trend of the times, but my interest deepened steadily as I learned more about the depth and value of Asia's ancient knowledge, particularly the pervasive theme of Yin and Yang and the reality of mind-body wholeness. In time, the circle was completed for me, as I combined my new fascination with Eastern body-centered health care systems with my previous explorations in Western psychology and sociology. "Alternative" health care became my focus, providing a mixing bowl for my curiosity as well as a career that has been endlessly fascinating.

---

[2] Marshall McLuhan, *The Gutenberg Galaxy*. University of Toronto Press, 2011. First published in 1962.

The niche for my interests seems to be increasing. My clients are often those for whom regular treatment has not worked. My students are often veteran health-care professionals looking for a deeper explanation of suffering, as well as relief from some of the more frustrating limitations in allopathic medicine. I also see a lot of young people who suspect that there must be more to life than materialism. I continue to seek new information (including that subscription to *Scientific American Mind* and similar publications) but after all these years, the Yin and Yang model continues to confirm itself every day, one session or class at a time as well as in my personal life. Experience has made me confident. Try some of the methods offered here, and see for yourself. As Tao Master Zhi Gang Sha says, "If you want to know if the pear is sweet, taste it!"[3]

Abundant neuroscience research confirms the value of the ancient wisdom traditions in resolving mental-emotional suffering.[4] A wealth of clinical experience produces applications that can be readily tested. This book is an attempt to blend theory and practice together, with a firm belief that the resulting approach can be universally helpful.

Perhaps the title needs explanation. "Dancing" refers to the art of graceful appropriate movement that blends spontaneity and structure in a rhythmic give-and-take of complementary expressive action. In due course I will argue that the flow of dancing is a useful metaphor for all health, mental as well as physical.

"Yin and Yang" refers to the universal observation that the world exists in a great dualistic interplay of polarized complementary phenomena. Attraction and repulsion,

---

[3] See www.drsha.com.

[4] The Dalai Lama, *Destructive Emotions: How Can We Overcome Them?*. Bantam, 2003. Narrated by Daniel Goleman.

expansion and contraction, light and dark, fast and slow, hot and cold; these polarities form the basis of our reality. Everything demonstrates the same principles. The dualistic arrangement can be found in the western sciences, the wisdom traditions of the East, in consciousness studies, and everywhere else.

This book is about how the same theme is observable in human experience, particularly psychology: mind and body, male and female, parent and child, old and young, boss and employee, anxiety and depression are the ever-present polarities of our inner reality of thoughts and feelings. Furthermore, understanding how these dualities work offers a key to better health. If we can learn how the game of life is played, "when to hold and when to fold," we can achieve higher states of wellness, increased equanimity and fulfillment, and better mental-emotional health.

## *What This Book Is...*

• **Theory:** This includes general principles of Yin and Yang, along with supportive ideas such as a guiding cosmology, a general understanding of the healing process and a set of priorities for personal and professional use.

• **Treatment:** Here we will explore how to use Yin and Yang theory to efficiently address many psychological and emotional conditions.

• **Prevention:** A Yin and Yang approach places a high value on living an orderly life that is more likely to avoid common mental-emotional upsets.

These three strands are presented separately at the start but gradually mixed together as we proceed.

## *...And What This Book Is Not*

• I am not claiming that the Yin and Yang model is any kind of Utopian magic wand that solves all mental, emotional or physical distress. My intention is modest, seeking to support other psychotherapy models and health care systems.

- Similarly this book is not a spiritual path or guide to enlightenment. The quest for spiritual experience and psychotherapy do overlap to some degree, with the latter supporting the former. Perhaps a Yin and Yang understanding can help build a relatively safe, stable

## Polarity Therapy and Randolph Stone

Polarity Therapy combines esoteric and scientific principles to create a comprehensive health care vision. Drawn from ancient and modern sources, representing both East and West, Polarity has a unique position as an inclusive umbrella spanning and unifying many health care ideas.

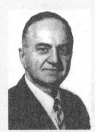

**Randolph Stone**
**DO, DC, ND**
**1890-1981**

Polarity's creator, Randolph Stone, conducted a thorough investigation of "energy in the healing arts" during his 60-year medical career. Surveying all the sources available to him, he observed that many philosophies and religions held similar basic beliefs, and that many health care systems also had significant common ground.

Putting his surveys into practice, Stone experientially confirmed the ancient idea of a Human Energy Field, and showed that it is affected by touch, diet, movement, sound, attitudes, relationships and life experiences. He applied these findings in his Chicago medical practice with excellent results, and published seven books to describe his methods.

He chose the term "Polarity" as a reference to a bar magnet or electromagnetic field that has charged north and south poles of attraction and repulsion. Modern science confirms Stone's findings with its essential theme of energetic relationship (for example, atomic particles' attraction and repulsion) as the basis of electrochemical bonding and material form. Polarity applies this understanding to health care.

Polarity methods include touch, diet, exercise and counseling and draw upon many health care systems (including Osteopathy, Chiropractic, Naturopathy, Oriental Medicine and Ayurveda) as well as multiple spiritual teachings. Stone was liberal and eclectic in his quest to find the best practices from around the world, and to make them popularly available for the general public.

foundation for spiritual pursuits, but the intention here is mainly about worldly wellness.

• This is not a description of trauma resolution therapy, although hopefully it can add some value to the material in that field. For the complete explication of trauma therapy theory and methods, I recommend Peter Levine's *In An Unspoken Voice* as well as numerous other resources that are arising constantly.

• This book is not intended to be a treatise on Christianity, Yoga, Taoism, Ayurveda, Buddhism or any other wisdom tradition. These all have vast bodies of knowledge of their own, far beyond my scope or expertise.

• This book is also not attempting to describe all of Polarity Therapy; this is just about its counseling applications. For Polarity information, I urge readers to use Franklyn Sills' *The Polarity Process*, as well as Dr. Randolph Stone's writings and the many other Polarity Therapy books available. This book is not even an authoritative treatment of Polarity; it is just a field report from a branch of Stone's family tree that specialized in psychological applications.

• This book is also not an over-simplification of gender dynamics. The Yin and Yang approach is firmly opposed to chauvinism in any form. I see chauvinism (supposed superiority of one culture or persons over others) as a Yang dysfunction that is so omnipresent in modern culture that we simply take it for granted. For me, Yin and Yang understanding is an antidote to chauvinism, not a cause of it.

### Basic Initial Agreements

**Terminology:** "Yin" and "Yang" are well-established in the popular mind. Other terms could also have been used, such as *Tamas-Rajas* or *Kapha-Pitta*, corresponding terms from India. However these are far less well-known. "Energy" could be another candidate to describe the theory and methods presented here, but the term has drawbacks relating to its use in New Age jargon, multiple technical definitions in science and an indefinite meaning in popular culture. "Polarity" is another candidate, but it lacks sufficient recognition and could mean one particular modality. So the terms "Yin" and "Yang" have been chosen, not least for their rich heritage and wealth of resources. If these terms seem foreign, please give them a chance and perhaps they will grow on you. If you have other terms that make more sense, please substitute freely. The meaning is what is important, more than the terminology.

**Religion:** I intend to separate Yin and Yang from any particular religion. Most (if not all) of the world's spiritual belief systems explore the dualistic concept, but using any one system limits its availability to people of different cultures. I have tried to bring in diverse sources to support my arguments. Even the words "Yin" and "Yang," arising from Taoism and related traditions of the Far East, are obviously identified with a particular culture and therefore perhaps not as appealing to a Western audience. However, my desire is to proceed independently of any one religion, medical system or culture.

**Polarity:** Next it will be helpful to have a beginning point, where some of the groundwork has already been done. This needs to be well-proven in practical health care effectiveness, with substantial psychological underpinnings. Randolph Stone's Polarity Therapy offers a body of knowledge to meet these needs: it already combines the essential information in a package that is not overly identified with any one specialized modality, and it has stood the test of time as being effective for a wide range of applications.[5]

---

[5] Stone's biography may be viewed at www.energyschool.com.

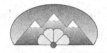

# Part One: Theory

## Chapter 1

# General Principles

Our starting points are simple:

• All phenomena, including human behavior and psychological wellness, reflect the dynamic interdependence of universal complementary processes that we will be calling Yin and Yang. Graceful balance and flow between these two leads to a natural emergence of order and harmony.

• Losing balance between these processes often leads to health problems on physical, emotional and/or mental levels.

• Understanding how these dualistic forces operate in practical life can add value to many psychotherapy methods, consistently enhancing clinical results without interfering with other systems' contributions.

Making a case for this feels a little like doing a large jigsaw puzzle. First we need to do the outer border, then we can figure out the major features, and finally we can clean up the details. The defining edge is about Yin and Yang and how these ideas fit in to a big picture (known as a *cosmology*, discussed in Chapter 2). Luckily we have the box top so we know what we are looking for. Turning all the pieces over on the table, we find all the ones with flat edges, and we sort these by color to figure out the top, bottom and sides.

*Introducing Yang*

Yang is the creative, centrifugal,[6] outgoing, expansive, warming part of the universal cycle. It is a forceful pulsation from the dense hot core toward the spacious cool edge, comparable to the sun's streaming radiation into the solar system.

Yang is experienced in every moment of our lives. In the body it manifests in processes such as inhalation of breath, "getting involved" in the physical world. Yang also manifests as arterial blood flow (away from the heart), motor nerve action including muscular contraction, mobilization and excitation chemistry. Yang has the perspective of a witness, a stance of objectivity or separateness. Its bodily direction is downward, starting as a mental process in the head and moving toward physicalization in the body.

*Introducing Yin*

Yin is a powerful, subtle, paradoxical, ever-changing counter-force to Yang. It is centripetal in that its action is a gravitational return flow of information back to the center or source. Its flow carries the findings of experience from the busy spacious periphery back to the restful dense core. Yin is represented by the moon's cyclic reflection of the sun as the moon waxes and wanes, affecting the ocean tides.

Yin is also experienced in every moment of our lives. It is the exhalation phase of breath, "letting go" of engagement with the material world. It is the venous part of blood

--------

[6] Categorization of Yin and Yang as centrifugal or centripetal can be argued either way, with authoritative sources expressing both positions. The seeming contradiction can be explained as a question of perspective and process, whether we are talking about the source or destination. The same issue can be seen in allocating triangles to exemplify Yin and Yang; different sources point up or down for either. For our purposes, these language variations are just curiosities; the essential meanings are what is most important.

circulation, returning to the core at the heart. Yin is the sensory nerves carrying field information back to headquarters. Its orientation is subjective or inward-looking, and its perceptual base is that of a participant more than an observer. Its bodily direction is upward, from the physical processes toward the more subtle emotional and mental processes.

Yin is expressed in the metabolic churning of the body's basic functioning, including digestion, respiration and elimination, which generally happen without conscious intervention. Yin is also represented in the restorative action of dreamtime when we digest the experiences of our waking hours.

### Yin and Yang Together

Yin and Yang are always in dynamic interplay with one another, without exception. If one moves up, the other must move down, like the seats on a playground seesaw. In the body, high blood pressure implies that Yang is somewhat excessive and therefore Yin will be correspondingly imbalanced.

Totally one-sided processes do not exist. There is no "pure" Yin or Yang, they always exist in relative measure. Generally the terms need to be preceded by the comparative words "more" or "less." Additionally, "in the fullness of one is the seed of the other," as one leads inevitably to its complement. Night follows day and winter follows summer as the natural cycles ebb and flow in all phenomena.

The universality of Yin and Yang principles is observable in physics, biology and human experience; everywhere we look, we see cycles of action and rest, pushing forward and falling back. In our busy modern world, we go on vacations or out in nature to experience the un-busy side of the process, and we return invigorated for the next phase of action. When one is more than the other, or when we become fixated in one and lose contact with the other, problems begin. The reciprocal balance effect is relatively obvious in the physical world, represented by Isaac Newton's

## Three Principles Summary

|  | YANG | YIN | NEUTRAL |
|---|---|---|---|
| **Subatomic particle & charge** | Proton (+) | Electron (-) | Neutron (0) |
| **System action** | Core to periphery | Periphery to core | Reversal, stillness |
| **Worldly focus** | Getting involved | Letting go | Flexibility for either |
| **Cell parts** | Nucleus | Membrane | Cytoplasm |
| **Drama** | Beginning | Climax | Dénouement (resolution) |
| **Embryonic germ layers** | Ectoderm, external interface | Endoderm, internal interface | Meso- cells, blood, fascia, muscle, bone |
| **Government** | Executive | Legislative | Judicial |
| **Hegel's Dialectics** | Thesis | Antithesis | Synthesis |
| **Sentiments** | Antipathy, Dispassion | Sympathy, Impassioned | Empathy, Compassion |
| **Muscle action** | Flexion | Extension | Rest |
| **Primary Colors** | Red, warm | Blue, cool | Yellow, temperate |
| **Scientific Inquiry** | Rationalism | Empiricism | Skepticism |
| **Solving Crimes** | Motive | Means | Opportunity |
| **Solving Math** | Pre-rigorous (intuitive) | Rigorous (precision) | Post-rigorous (refinement) |
| **Spatial Dimensions** | Front-Back (depth) | Top-Bottom (height) | Side-to-side (width) |
| **Astrology** | Cardinal | Fixed | Mutable |
| **Taoism** | Yang | Yin | Tao |
| **Christianity** | Father | Son | Holy Spirit |
| **Ayurveda** | *Rajas* or *Pitta* | *Tamas* or *Kapha* | *Satva* or *Vata* |
| **Hinduism** | Brahma | Vishnu | Shiva |

third law of motion ("for every action there is an equal and opposite reaction"); this book explains how the same principle applies in the more subtle world of psychology.

## Introducing Neutral

Yin and Yang are the cycles of attraction and repulsion or expansion and contraction, but there are three nodes in this model. Yin and Yang refer to the polar opposites, but there is always a balance point between the two extremes, as in the action of neutrons relative to protons and electrons. The Neutral principle also represents the transitional reversal of activity that is always present in any system. Between the increasing light of spring (Yang) and the decreasing light of fall (Yin) are transitory phases of reversal, and in their midpoints are moments of balance. Pre-Christian cultures celebrated the three-day solstice as a magical neutral time of resurrection and transformation.[7] Similarly, a brief moment of stillness exists between the outgoing flow of the arteries and incoming flow of the veins in a reversal point in the capillaries and the heart. A neutral reversal is also experienced between breathing in and breathing out. Even on day one, immediately after conception, a neutral stillness is observed for about twenty-four hours before growth begins.

Yin and Yang are the *two* well-known names for the whole concept, but really it is always about *three*. As the table above shows, the Three Principles can be speculatively identified in almost any field of study.

## Introducing the Five Elements

Following the Three Principles are the *Five Elements*. While the Three Principles describe the overall big-picture progression of events, the Five Elements give a closer, more detailed perspective. Originating in ancient times (Babylonia,

---

[7] Peter Joseph, *Zeitgeist: The Movie.* DVD, 2007.

Egypt, Greece, India and China), the Five Elements are a very useful subsection in the Yin and Yang system.

Wisdom tradition philosophies recognize progressions of all manifestation, transitioning from very subtle to very dense. In the Five Elements model, these are:

- Ether   *So light as to be immaterial*
- Air     *Minimal density, but perceptible*
- Fire    *Obvious action but no actual weight*
- Water   *More dense than Fire, but still no fixed structure*
- Earth   *Fully densified*

We cannot connect the immaterial ("spirit") and the fully dense ("matter") directly; intermediate steps are needed. For example, a hydroelectric dam is the source of electricity for a home, but along the way are a series of transformers and smaller gauge wires. The delivery process begins with massive turbines and ends in the delicate filament of a light

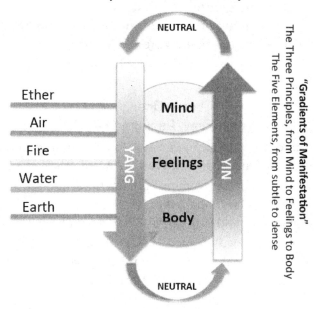

*Spirit: "Father Sky"*

*Matter: "Mother Earth"*

bulb. Connecting the dam's turbines directly to the bulb would not work. Polarity Therapy is based on an understanding of this two-layered Principles/Elements cosmology.

Newcomers often need time to comprehend the difference between the Principles and the Elements. The Principles of Yin, Yang and Neutral are the primary foundation of the whole system. Within the Principles, the Elements are stages of development, providing detailed information about how life unfolds, including many useful specifics about the body, emotions and mind.

### Five Themes for Yin and Yang Psychotherapy

With Yin and Yang as a foundation for a psychotherapy, the next step is to define guiding themes to explore the possibilities. Here we follow the lead of modalities such as Hakomi and Macrobiotics, which also have "guiding themes." I propose five main themes for this approach:

1. **Increasing flow, reducing fixation**
2. **Being gentle and gradual**
3. **Focusing on the present, through the body**
4. **Knowing that awareness heals**
5. **Using the full therapeutic spectrum**

## Theme One:
## Increasing Flow, Reducing Fixation

Yin and Yang therapy is based on the understanding that health arises from movement and that disease accompanies fixation. Movement is the natural state, whereas fixation is an unnatural adaptation. In the presence of threat, we brace ourselves and normal flow is reduced. Just as body therapies are designed to increase circulation and range of motion in the physical body, Yin and Yang psycho-emotional strategies seek to increase movement in the realm of thoughts and feelings. The goal is reducing stasis, congestion and fixation while increasing a sense of flow, choice and new options. Stone's adage, "Running water clears itself,"[8] can be applied to psycho-emotional states. The theme applies to emotional binds, compulsive behaviors, post-traumatic stress, anxiety, depression, stuck attitudes, unrealistic expectations, feelings of no choice and relationship problems. When mental or emotional fixation is relieved, conditions improve.

In this approach, there are two main priorities:

- **Treatment**: Recognizing fixation and restoring movement on mental, emotional and physical levels.

- **Prevention**: Changing or avoiding behaviors that are likely to lead to fixation, ideally before the fixations happen.

### All Behaviors Are a Search for Safety and Equilibrium

A significant step toward reducing fixation in clients is to "de-pathologize" their conditions. De-pathologizing means recognizing that all conditions and behavioral states are based on physiologically intelligent efforts to survive and flourish, even if the strategy is degenerative or dangerous.

The principle of de-pathologizing is a psychological application of a well-established theme of physical medicine. The founder of osteopathy, Andrew Taylor Still, taught his students, "To find health should be the object of the doctor. Anyone can find disease."[9] Seeing all behaviors as attempts to maintain equilibrium means focusing on the health.

At one of the simplest levels, we can see the principle in cellular biology. Biologist Bruce Lipton describes how the cell membrane has two basic decision-making categories: opening

---

[8] Stone, *Polarity Therapy, Vol. 1.* CRCS, 1986. Book 1, p. 60.

[9] A. T. Still, *Philosophy of Osteopathy.* Forgotten Books, 2012. First published in 1899.

toward nourishment or closing against threat.[10] Either gesture is essentially intelligent when viewed in context. Human behavior is the same, although vastly more complex. We have basic needs, and we adapt constantly to our experiences of these needs being fulfilled or denied.

Being diagnosed with a particular condition, particularly one with major negative implications, can contribute to further deepening of the state. Depressed clients may feel even more depressed after learning that their condition is "depression." I have met many clients with cyclic anxiety and depression who mournfully announce that they have been diagnosed as "bipolar," only to discover that the situation is much more nuanced and ultimately much more hopeful. Moving away from pathological labeling helps restore the possibility for movement instead of fixation.

For a Yin and Yang approach, we view clients from the basic curiosity that an inherent goodness and health is present in all behaviors. Even immobilization caused by shock, which is an expression of a fixated state, is actually an intelligent response to conditions. The behavior may be problematic or even life-threatening, but we can assume that there were preceding conditions that justified the response. Severe dysfunctions arise in a person's desperate attempts to adapt to trauma, but even the distortions can be seen as authentic attempts to find equilibrium.

"De-pathologizing" has been advocated by many thoughtful counselors. For example, British psychiatrist R.D. Laing's comment that "insanity is a sane reaction to an insane situation" supports shifting away from pathology labels.[11]

---

[10] B. Lipton, *The Biology of Belief*. Hay House, 2008.

[11] R.D. Laing, *The Politics of Experience*. Pantheon, 1967. For a more recent application: Jaydean Morrison, *I'm not sick. Society is!: ADD/ADHD is an adaptation to society - not an illness*. AuthorHouse, 2006.

## De-Pathologizing on a Grand Scale

Modern western psychology arose from a landscape of pervasive trauma; European history is a tale of continuous war and exploitation. With so much suffering, some psychology pioneers justifiably concluded that evil must be inherent in humanness. Religion's "original sin" described a desperate, perpetual struggle to overcome innate destructive tendencies. Darwin seemed to confirm this view with the competitive "survival of the fittest" (the predator-prey "law of the jungle") as a primary basis for behavior.

As psychology progressed, the effects of trauma were increasingly appreciated. Beginning with extreme events that were clearly "not normal," such as "shell shock" in war veterans, the definition of trauma widened steadily. The more trauma was understood, the more psychology developed a new paradigm: human nature is essentially good, but that it is susceptible to damage by events and circumstances, as the massive "Adverse Childhood Events" study famously showed.*

The difference between the early and later outlooks is enormous. Mental wellness becomes "normalized" and expected as a natural property of humanness. In theory, people living in "good enough" conditions will have health more than disturbances. Daily life will inevitably present challenges, but people will be able to cope under normal conditions.

There are few untraumatized populations to study to test the new view definitively; anthropological studies of peaceful uncivilized indigenous tribes** are perhaps the closest candidates for such research. War, racism, chauvinism, abuse, exploitation, deprivation, financial pressure, environmental issues and flawed belief systems are too widespread to find out what would happen in their relative absence. It was only in the last century or two that the morality of invading, conquering and exploiting a foreign people even began to be questioned by more than a liberal fringe of society.

This new emphasis on fundamental goodness does not mean that negative tendencies and emotions are insignificant in human experience. In the wisdom traditions negativity is inevitable (Buddhism's opening statement is, "There is Suffering") and negative emotions even have an esoteric explanation (see Chapter 12). The emphasis relates to the healing process: a bias toward innate goodness provides significant therapeutic advantages. I respond more favorably to appreciation than criticism, and I know that prevention (elevating the good) can be much more cost-effective than treatment (reducing the bad).

* See www.acestudy.org **See www.peacefulsocieties.org

Research finding that a high proportion of criminals were abused as children supports this idea.[12] Even some of history's worst villains have been found to be victims of traumatic childhoods.[13]

Similarly, psychiatrist Thomas Szasz also wrote eloquently about the dark side of pathologizing, differentiating between "diseases" and "behaviors."[14] Diseases are labels and categories that individuals are classified by, for various institutional purposes, but the category is never really fully descriptive of the whole person. In contrast, behaviors are much more about the actual people, in the full context of their lives. The difference is enormous.

Rollin Becker, DO, makes the point well:

> The patient is guessing as to a diagnosis, the doctor is scientifically guessing as to a diagnosis, while the patient's body knows the problem and is manifesting it through the tissues.[15]

Becker is reminding us that our seemingly objective diagnoses are actually secondary to the inner reality of the client, which is as unique as personality itself.

A few years ago I experienced the pathologizing problem personally when I developed a major medical condition. One doctor pronounced my diagnostic definition and from then on, in his mind, I was a category rather than my actual experience. In theory, all I had to do was look up the outcomes for the category and find out the result. In the doctor's mind, the case was closed and all that was left to do

---

[12] National Data Archive on Child Abuse and Neglect http://www.ndacan.cornell.edu.

[13] Alice Miller, *For Your Own Good: Hidden Cruelty in Child-Rearing and the Roots of Violence*. FSG, 1983.

[14] Thomas Szasz, *The Second Sin*. Doubleday, 1973.

[15] Rollin Becker, *Life In Motion*, Stillness Press, 2001. p. 142.

was follow the prescribed category's officially accepted (and rather bleak) action plan. A subtle shift had taken place; my individuality was no longer in the foreground, and my resources for healing were underestimated. This was no fun for me, and it could have been disastrous if I happened to be highly suggestible as a hypnosis subject. I might have subconsciously believed the categorical references more than my own experience.

De-pathologizing a client's condition can have significant and immediate benefits. A teenage client had spontaneous panic attacks and thought she was becoming mentally ill. She was being prescribed medications and special education in high school, throwing her whole progression toward college into disarray. When she discovered that her panic attacks were her autonomic nervous system responding intelligently to something in the environment, she felt immediate relief and the attacks began to subside. From a calmer state of mind she was able to identify the source of the disturbance, change the problematic conditions in her home, practice self-awareness of autonomic states ("mindfulness"), and get her life back on track. Later she commented that the worst part of the experience was being labeled as learning-disabled by authorities, and fearing that her life might be over. Getting distance from the label, de-pathologizing both her and her condition, had significant value even before other therapeutic methods were used.

De-pathologizing does not mean trivializing the seriousness of any condition. Obviously, health problems can bring enormous suffering, and dysfunctional behavior can be extremely painful for oneself and for others. Major interventions may be necessary. However, having a belief that all states are expressions of an underlying search for balance enables clients to regain a measure of stability and creates a better foundation for healing. This is true even for people experiencing fatal diseases, severe mental illnesses or criminal behaviors.

## *Examining the Present as Well as the Past*

Psychotherapy often focuses on the past, for good reasons. Obviously traumatic events, faulty beliefs from childhood and developmental deficiencies are all significant factors in suffering.

However, what is happening in the present is sometimes overlooked. In psychological teachings, this idea is supported by the "social materialist" school articulated by British psychologist David Smail.[16] Some clients may have inadvertently made an error that goes against the grain of natural order (in Yin and Yang terms, they managed to somehow become fixated, or habitually too much or too little of one or the other), and now they are experiencing the inevitable consequences. This is different from having a deep instinctual character flaw from the distant forgotten past, and it is easier to address.

For example, a scientist with marital problems, father of two young children, asked for sessions seeking relief from acute anger. In the first interview, he attributed his problems to the imperfections of his childhood, derived from his dysfunctional parents. He knew enough about psychology to already have received and believed the opinion that he had an "Avoidant" attachment style with "Narcissistic tendencies." The pursuit of a solution down this path could have been quite complex because the origins would be shrouded in ancestral mists. Having a busy life and young family, he did not have the time or money for a long excavation project.

---

[16] David Smail, *Power, Interest and Psychology - Elements of a Social Materialist Understanding of Distress*. PCCS Books, 2005.

Probing further, we also discovered that the fundamental Yin and Yang dynamics of his home had become compromised due to a common pitfall observed in many parents of young children, which I call "husband lost in space" (Chapter 10). In addition to supporting a softening of his attachment style (Chapter 9), we explored a direct correction for the imbalance in his relationship with his wife in their new-parent circumstances. I explained the "lost in space" syndrome and suggested a remedy that he could practice on his own. A week later he said that the whole situation had improved and he felt better. The problem was partly that he and his partner had no "Yin and Yang Operator's Manual" for being new parents. His anger subsided "on time and under budget," as his fellow engineers might say.

I like a "pebble-in-my-shoe" analogy. Perhaps a client has a limp, and our curiosity could easily be drawn to exploring possible vertebral, hip, or knee "causes." But perhaps there is just a pebble in the shoe, an unrecognized current behavior that goes against Yin and Yang principles in their natural operation. When the pebble is removed, the limp is reduced and the related body parts naturally self-correct.

Our inquiry into circumstances can include conditions of the past, with a question such as, "What was happening in the months prior to the appearance of the first symptoms?" From a Yin and Yang perspective, illnesses do not happen in isolation; they interact with the totality of life's experiences.

It may sound unrealistic to think that conscious actions can be effective when the symptoms are being generated by the subconscious intelligence. Stone understood this, saying, "Merely telling a patient to relax is useless."[17] However, we

---

[17] R. Stone, *Polarity Therapy, Vol. 1*. CRCS, 1986. Book 1, p. 85. Stone called his advice a "Dutch Uncle Talk."

can definitely speak certain phrases, make healthful adjustments and solve interpersonal puzzles through negotiated agreement based on mutually held values. The angry husband found relief for an involuntary emotion by intentionally shifting behaviors in the present, even though part of the anger was due to much earlier events. Voluntary actions such as repetitively performing a particular practice can shift the involuntary stress responses. Repeated conscious actions can actually change the brain.[18] Consciously applying the guidelines arising from Yin and Yang understanding can help re-establish movement in a system. That movement can then loosen the binds contributing to the painful condition. Taking pebbles out of our shoes is a voluntary act, but it can correct involuntary problems such as posture and gait.

## Theme Two:
## Being Gentle and Gradual

*All real growth is slow and gentle, almost imperceptible, like in Nature. We don't see the grass grow but we know that it needs cutting regularly.*[19]

In nature, flow and circulation arise gracefully. When water moves downhill, the current meanders and swirls as it makes its way through the path of least resistance and establishes a watercourse. Flow volume gradually increases. Pulse diagnosis practitioners take the subtle pulse of their clients to detect flow changes before and after treatment, but they do not expect pulsation to just appear abruptly: there is a delay while it builds and reorganizes.

---

[18] Daniel Siegel, *Mindsight: The New Science of Personal Transformation*. Bantam, 2011. Also: Daniel Amen: *Change Your Brain, Change Your Life*. Three Rivers Press, 1998, and Rick Hanson, *Buddha's Brain: The Practical Neuroscience of Happiness, Love and Wisdom*. New Harbinger, 2009.

[19] R. Stone, *Mystic Bible*. RSSB, 1956. p. 302.

Similarly, in psychology, enduring change does not usually happen suddenly. Slow and steady wins the race. Gradual change is more likely to be stable and lasting. Health arises at the pace of nature, not as a forced march but rather as a gradual organic process. In a Yin and Yang approach, there is less catharsis and more repeated body-centered awareness. This approach enables clients to take stable, progressive steps back to optimum function instead of trying to jump ahead all at once. Trying to go too fast can lead to chaos.

A slower pace can be transformational in life as well as psychology. For example, when I drive through my neighborhood on my way home from work, I see people in their yards but don't interact, other than an occasional wave. If I ride my bike, I will definitely wave and probably say hello as I whiz by. But if I walk, I will notice details such as textures and smells, and buy lemonade at the six-year-old neighbor girl's stand across the street, chat with her parents and enjoy observing how her 3-year-old brother studiously serves as her assistant.

Cathartic and reenactment therapies may have counter-productive side effects, inhibiting movement instead of promoting it. As Peter Levine says, "...there is a good chance... that the cathartic reliving of an experience can be traumatizing rather than healing."[20] The re-living of a trauma may invoke a fresh wave of overwhelming emotions, thereby causing renewed compartmentalization and fixation. For some, intense emotional therapy may seem to provide a form of immunity due to familiarization, but for others the trauma echoes are driven even deeper into the system; a problem is that it can be hard to tell the difference because the immobilization effect of shock can resemble tranquility.

---

[20] Peter Levine, *Waking the Tiger.* North Atlantic, 1998.

Gentle and gradual therapies take a step-by-step approach. First, safe emotional support is developed, then practical life skills are expanded, then later the release of emotions can be integrated safely, without becoming overwhelming. Firm interventions and strong emotional processes are still used, but with caution and discretion, and they are not the primary foundation for the method.

## Theme Three:
## Healing Occurs In the Present and in the Body

Yin and Yang therapy is largely about current-time awareness, focusing on physical sensation in the body as a method to arrive and stay in the present. This method borrows heavily from "body-centered psychotherapy" systems, which will be discussed below.

Stone clearly called for a psychology that included physiological dimensions:

> Our research in Psychiatry would benefit greatly if we could reduce this jumble of man's mental-emotional impulses to an exact science of mental-emotional anatomy, coordinated with the physical one. Then a sound Psycho-physiology [Somatic Psychology] and even a Pathology of these finer energy fields [Yin, Yang and Neutral] could be established. This would be a great step forward in the science of understanding the mystery of man's complex being, which defies all present man-made rules and findings.[21]

### The Value of Body-Centered Approaches

Different psychological methods can be categorized based on whether they are more centered on the processes of thinking (analysis), feeling (emotionality) or the physical

---

[21] R. Stone, *Polarity Therapy, Vol. 1.* CRCS, 1986. Book 3, p. 13.

body (sensations). All three have potential value; the Yin and Yang approach emphasizes the third.

We all have these three processing systems: in the presence of a disturbing event, we can think about the problem (*mental*), respond with expressions of emotions (*feelings*) and/or use sensations, gestures and shapes (*physical*) as ways to manage and digest the event.

Mental and emotional-level processing can be limited because the possibilities are so vast. On a mental level, we can imagine being anywhere, instantaneously, past or future and all around the universe. The options are endless, and confusion can arise easily. Analysis often leads to such complexity that we lose track of practical meaning, hence the term "psychobabble."

In turn, feelings are so potent and compelling that we can cycle into an emotional vortex from which there seems to be no escape.[22] Emotional therapy can be dramatic but also stressful; the client may enter the session with one measure of unhappy feelings and exit with two, if re-traumatizing happens. Plus, emotions are also likely to be about the past or future, instead of the present, where the problem is.

Physical body processing, also known as somatic psychotherapy, is in-the-moment and much less likely to be overwhelming.[23]

The difference is between a "bottom-up" approach and a "top-down" approach.[24] "Bottom-up" means a body-to-mind process, which would be a more Yin treatment, whereas "top-down" works from mind-to-body, a more Yang

---

[22] Chapter 10 will describe a reliable way out of this common problem.

[23] Susan Aposhyan, *Body-Mind Psychotherapy: Principles, Techniques, and Practical Applications.* Norton, 2004.

[24] Pat Ogden, Kikuni Minton, Clare Pain, *Trauma and the Body: A Sensorimotor Approach to Psychotherapy.* Norton, 2008.

approach. Each has enormous potential individually; when combined, the effects are greatly magnified. Our quest in this book is to elevate a Yin (bottom-up) method to equality with Yang's top-down.

Body-centered therapies are still not fully accepted in mainstream psychology, despite an abundance of evidence indicating their effectiveness. For war veterans with post-traumatic stress disorder (PTSD), the current primary strategies are pharmacotherapy, exposure therapy and cognitive restructuring.[25] Regrettably, body-centered psychotherapy has not yet made the government-approved list for this important population. The situation exemplifies a problem found in many other areas of science, the common delay between a definitive research finding and institutional acceptance. As Nobel Prize-winning physicist Max Planck has been paraphrased, "Science progresses one funeral at a time."

## Problems with Causation

Many therapy systems have focused on identifying and resolving what is thought to be the "root cause" of a problem. I often hear clients express a desire to "get to the bottom" of their issue, once and for all. The Yin and Yang approach softens the urgency of this quest because the search for causality often is an oversimplification of the real story; the process can be shifted into an abstract mental dimension as an unintended effect. Doctor and author Deepak Chopra describes it directly:

> Modern medicine is still dominated by the notion that disease is caused by objective agents. A

---

[25] For an excellent, comprehensive article about veteran's care, see www.ptsd.va.gov/professional/pages/treatment-iraq-vets.asp. For a body-centered example, see Peter Levine's DVD, *Ray: Iraq War Vet with Severe PTSD/TBI*. FHE, 2009.

sophisticated analysis shows that this is only partly true.[26]

In reality, every traumatic event also has pre-existing conditions, stretching back to earlier times. For example, we commonly hear that particular mental-emotional symptoms are because of maternal bonding problems or a specific traumatic event. These statements are not incorrect, because such events do have high impact. However they are also not entirely comprehensive, because the mother no doubt had other issues or the trauma may have happened in a particular context with other factors. In either case, it is also likely that later events also compounded the effect.

Therefore I am a little suspicious when supposedly definitive cause-and-effect explanations are offered for a particular condition, because I know from experience that there is more to the story. In the Yin and Yang approach, the primary focus is on present-tense states and how to optimize the client's experience within the current context. Working with causes is still interesting and useful, but less pressing because it will not necessarily have a clear resolution.

Even if a "cause" *is* found and supposedly solved, it is likely to re-surface when the appropriate stimuli are applied again. For example, a blank sheet of paper, once crumpled, will move back into the same fold lines when new pressure is applied, even if it has been smoothed out in the interim. The relevant phrase in a Yin and Yang approach is to "play the cards that are on the table," and use less time figuring out how those cards arrived in the first place.

This is true for even basic seemingly straightforward physical problems. We might hear that whiplash neck pain was "caused" by a recent car accident; however, the accident itself probably had preceding conditions, such as the driver

---

[26] Deepak Chopra, *Quantum Healing.* Bantam, 1990. p. 211.

being distracted or the neck being already weakened by earlier events. Similarly, exposure to wet, cold weather could be said to "cause" the flu; however, the sick person's immune system may have been predisposed to illness due to earlier stress or lifestyle factors. Two people experiencing the same sequence of stressors will probably have quite different responses and outcomes. What is true for physical problems is likely to also be true for subtle psychological problems.

Stone discusses this and adds an interesting twist, that an accident may have had some balancing effect:

> Locked-up mental conditions usually precede accidents, because the mind is more in the field of unawareness, or occupied with its "pet peeve," instead of constructive thinking. Failure to be alert causes many accidents. The resulting shock and pain usually break up the mental, pent-up pattern that caused the trouble in the field of lines of force. Cause and effect balance each other.[27]

Stone's last comment here prompts further consideration. If "cause and effect balance each other," and the effect is observed in the totality of the client's life, the cause probably also represents the totality of the client's life at the time when the trouble started. A maternal bonding deficiency or traumatic incident are important parts of that totality, but certainly not all of it.

In addition, a client often has a "secondary gain" (when there is a benefit to an otherwise problematic condition) that deserves close attention.[28] A secondary gain adds another variable to the equation, further complicating the supposed value of an identified "cause."

---

[27] R. Stone, *Polarity Therapy, Vol. 1*. CRCS, 1986. Book 1, p. 56.
[28] See http://www.ncbi.nlm.nih.gov/pubmed/10172109

The causality problem in psychology has analogues elsewhere in science. Science has a deep desire for objective materialistic simplicity, and an ongoing problem with anomalous data.[29] Physicist Werner Heisenberg's 1925 demonstration of the Uncertainty Principle in physics, showing that matter was not so objectively fixed as previously thought, posed doubts about scientific materialism; quantum physics has only increased the questions. Even the "Big Bang Theory," supposedly a cornerstone of modern science, has been unable to fully resolve the preceding conditions issue.[30] Yin and Yang's softening of causation-focus can serve a similar purpose for "psychological materialism."

Fortunately, full resolution of the past is not necessary. The healing process can often be simplified by using methods that are primarily focused on the present. Yin and Yang offers just such a model, as do many other body-centered trauma resolution systems.

Moving away from causality can be a great relief for clients, who may feel that they have been dealt a life sentence of suffering due to some disastrous past event that they may not even remember on a conscious level. It can also be a great relief for practitioners, because the difficult detective skills of definitively solving a psychological "whodunnit" become secondary compared to the real-time present-tense improvement of current life experience.

Focusing on causation is so prevalent in the health care field that it is largely invisible. Shifting away from this way of thinking has the potential to transform many specialties and applications. Even the venerable organization Alcoholics

---

[29] Rupert Sheldrake, *The Science Delusion.* Coronet, 2012.

[30] William Mitchell, *Bye Bye Big Bang, Hello Reality.* Cosmic Sense Books, 2002, p. 52. Also, Eric Lerner, *The Big Bang Never Happened.* Vintage, 1992.

Anonymous partially fails to appreciate the problems inherent in focusing too much on causation. The personal greeting to the group in a meeting, "I am an alcoholic..." is questionable in this perspective, since in the present it is not the full truth. While the statement guards against denial, a worthy goal, it is incomplete as a statement of identity for a person who has been sober for a long time, and it can actually be a self-hypnotic reinforcement of the disease. An alternative approach under the new paradigm of reduced causality and de-pathologizing would focus on re-connecting clients with their inherent health, and acknowledge how the substance abuse probably had a strategic value in the context of their original circumstances. Now that the strategy is obsolete, perhaps it can be replaced.

### Problems with the Verb "To Be"

To take this a step further, it has been pointed out that the English language is seriously flawed by its central usage of the verb "to be," which can never be fully accurate. Reality is better described by shades of gray, not black and white. Any use of "I am" or "I am not" is an oversimplification.[31] A more accurate phrasing would use other verbs that acknowledge the relativity of the situation. "Your body believes every word you say" sounds an important message of caution.[32] The mind can be a master hypnotist and the body can become even more of the state being named. Fixation can be reduced by avoiding common language such as "I am sick," or "I am tired." Instead we could say, "I am noticing these symptoms of illness or fatigue." This kind of

---

[31] Robert Anton Wilson, *Quantum Psychology: How Brain Software Programs You and Your World.* New Falcon, 1990. p. 97. Also useful on this topic is *Psychosemantic Parenthetics* by James Russell. IHTR, 1988.

[32] Barbara Hoberman Levine, *Your Body Believes Every Word You Say.* Aslan, 1991.

attention to phrasing has been proven to create significant, beneficial changes.[33]

Developed in the 1920s by Alfred Korzybski, "General Semantics" was a systematic study of the subtle effects of language. Changing word choices was used effectively in the treatment of World War I trauma patients. The method did not catch on, perhaps (ironically) because the descriptions of it were so complex, as suggested by the daunting title of the founder's primary book on the subject.[34] Only an elite specialist can readily decipher Korzybski's book title.

### Autonomic Nervous System Focus

Yin and Yang counseling focuses strongly on the mechanisms involved in the stress response, particularly the autonomic nervous system (ANS),[35] discussed in Chapter 6.

Generally the ANS is the set of nerves and nerve functions that are primarily involuntary. The ANS is at work when little or no conscious control is being exerted. This includes bodily activities that are just taken for granted, such as breathing, heartbeat and digestion. Similarly, it includes mental and emotional phenomena that arise without conscious intention. In threatening situations, our ANS springs into action to protect us through mental, emotional and physical responses, driven by complex neurochemistry.

---

[33] Among many psychology teachings on the subject of semantics, see Virginia Satir, *The New Peoplemaking*. Science and Behavior Books, 1988.

[34] Alfred Korzybski, *Science and Sanity: An Introduction to Non-Aristotelian Systems and General Semantics*. IGS, 1996; first published in 1933. See also: Wendell Johnson, *People in Quandaries: The Semantics of Personal Adjustment*. IGS, 1995.

[35] The ANS is often under-appreciated in psychoanalytic models, but is growing in "psychobiological" approaches such as Peter Levine (1998, 2010), Marion Soloman and Stan Tatkin (2011), and Dan Siegel (2011).

It is increasingly clear that the ANS is the major playing field for most medical problems, including psycho-emotional conditions. As osteopathic physician James Jealous states, "eighty percent or more of all health conditions are autonomic nervous system events."[36] Similarly, Bruce Lipton writes: "..stress is the primary cause of illness and is responsible for up to ninety percent of all doctor visits."[37] Randolph Stone was far ahead of his time in 1948 when he identified ANS function as the cornerstone of health and taught specific methods for ANS-based therapy.

All the causes discussed above, from maternal bonding problems to traumatic events, find their expression in the ANS. By focusing on the ANS, we can focus on the common ground rather than the details, which are not definitively knowable anyway.

Autonomic responses happen in real time, in the present, as the system seeks optimum equilibrium for survival in ever-changing conditions. The presence of this constant adjustment of the ANS is more evidence that the original programming for balance is always on duty, even if it is obscured or seemingly working against the client, as in autoimmune disorders.

The ANS is arguably our most important anatomical system, but it is also the least understood and protected. The reason for this unrecognized status is probably due to its relative subtlety. It is operating in the background and its anatomical components are not as tangibly obvious as an organ system. Full appreciation of the workings of the ANS would lead to highly beneficial transformations throughout

---

[36] James Jealous, Audio CD Lecture, 2004.

[37] Bruce Lipton, *The Honeymoon Effect*. Hay House, 2013. p. 50, citing Miller and Smith, *The Stress Solution*. Pocket Books, 1995. p. 12.

health care, including birthing practices, emergency response methods, childhood education and other institutions.

In a Yin and Yang approach, clients are educated about the ANS and taught methods to self-regulate in the present so that ANS states like anxiety or depression do not become so fixated. The second half of this book is mainly about how to do this safely and effectively. By shifting our attention to body awareness, the ANS can be retrained back into rhythmic movement using repeated voluntary exercises that affect involuntary processes. With practice, many ANS disturbances can be reduced or eliminated entirely.

## Theme Four:
## Awareness Heals

The phrase, "awareness is curative" originated in Buddhist tradition and is used in Core Process psychotherapy.[38] This theme emphasizes the value of increasing self-awareness and expanding our capacity to identify our own various states of being. Self-awareness, also known as mindfulness, helps us have greater choice and less tendency for fixation when dealing with life's common stumbling blocks. As doctor, author and neuroscientist Daniel Siegel puts it, "Name it to tame it."[39] Although a person's history will always be a part of the process, it is no longer always on center stage.

In Yin and Yang counseling, we focus on the ANS states that precede behaviors. Most clients do not know that they have an autonomic nervous system, much less how to identify and manage its various states. We want to increase our ability to recognize and regulate our own ANS states.

---

[38] Franklyn Sills, *Being and Becoming: Psychodynamics, Buddhism and the Origins of Selfhood.* North Atlantic, 2009.

[39] *Daniel Siegel, Mindsight: The New Science of Personal Transformation.* Bantam, 2011.

The capacity for change of state begins with accurate recognition. Stone's comments show the way:

> "That is the key to psychiatry. Can we direct our attention and concentrate on that which is really worth while, and which we want, or are we merely attracted by the glitter of sensation and show or craving?... Can we make the best of adversity, and forge ahead by perseverance and concentration? Proper attitude is the key to psychology.[40]

To support this principle, we need to cultivate the skill of recognition, as discussed in "Practitioner Skills" (Chapter 7). Clients constantly express and act out their subtle attitudes and expectations; part of the practitioner's job is to serve as a neutral, well-informed mirror to help them become more self-aware. We help name the gestures and states, and clients gradually begin to have a better understanding of their own processes.

An analogy is the common practice of having a mirror near the front door so that it is easy to quickly check our appearance before going out. Seeing the reflection facilitates a change, for example if our hair needs combing. With the mirror, it is easy to see the problem and self-correct; without the mirror we are oblivious.

Along with general awareness of states, clients can also benefit by learning to differentiate between positive and negative states. "Positive" means feelings of success, self-worth and safety; when these are present a health-enhancing neurochemical cascade nourishes the whole system. "Negative" means feelings of failure, low self-esteem and fear. We are often are so immersed in our states that we cannot name which side of the balance is in operation.

---

[40] R. Stone, *Polarity Therapy, Vol. 1.* CRCS, 1986. Book 1, p. 41

In addition, states can become a fixed identity, instead of a moving object of curiosity. Stone commented,

> Negative thoughts and fears make grooves in the mind as negative energy waves of despondency and hopelessness... We must assert the positive, and maintain a positive pattern of thinking and acting as our ideal.[41]

> Now we come to the psychological aspects of disease, where the emotions and mind are great factors. What a patient fears, believes or thinks affects his health and can create energy blocks in the emotional field... We will become that which we contemplate... We cannot think negative thoughts and reap positive results.[42]

Similarly, we can educate clients about Yin and Yang. Gaining this awareness can have a big effect on behavior, helping clients sort out their life experiences with a reliable frame of reference. Without a clear sense of what works, life is just a perpetual trial-and-error experiment; many of the errors are costly, and some are irreversible.

Many people experience their states at face value, without much self-awareness. By naming states such as fear or anger and understanding experiences based on a larger frame of reference, we gain the gift of self-understanding. In his *1971 Notes*, Stone stated repeatedly: "I am not these elements. I see them. I am a witness to them,"[43] a clear call to awareness as a key to health. When a state is recognized and named, it is no longer all-encompassing and undifferentiated. We are not swallowed up in the experience, but rather have the perspective of a witness and thereby gain more capacity for objectivity and self-awareness.

---

[41] R. Stone, *Health-Building*. CRCS, 1986. p. 4.

[42] *ibid.* pp. 10, 12, 13.

[43] R. Stone, *Polarity Therapy, Vol. 2*, CRCS, 1986. Book 6, Chart 24.

The phrase "awareness heals" also suggests the limits of the approach. The Yin and Yang vision of health care is most likely usable by clients who have sufficient resources to actually use their minds to manage their lives. Stone wrote, "Suffering makes the mind small,"[44] and a glance at the news will remind us that many people have passed the tipping point for using awareness to self-heal. Those who suffer most will at least need extra support in using Yin and Yang methods. Mindfulness programs for incarcerated criminals are an admirable application, and offer a glimpse of the steep learning curve and desperate need for a truly disadvantaged population.[45]

Needless to say, the enormity of suffering in the world is vast. Stone recognized that some people would not have the capacity to really take ownership of their health, but he also called for a shifting of professional and societal priorities:

> May this work reach the seekers who are looking for a deeper perspective of a common denominator in the healing art, to push it along in keeping with all the other atomic discoveries of today. The health and well-being of the people should not be neglected. It should really be the first concern of the scientists, doctors and educators. Without health and happiness, all our modern conveniences are of little comfort to us.[46]

## Theme Five:
## Use the Full Therapeutic Spectrum

Most health care strategies can be located on a spectrum that ranges from "outside-in" to "inside-out." Outside-in refers to corrections coming from an external source, whereas

---

[44] R. Stone, *Polarity Therapy, Vol. 1*, CRCS, 1986. Book 3, p. 107.

[45] For example: http://www.prisonyoga.org

[46] R. Stone, *Polarity Therapy Vol. 2*, CRCS, 1986. p. 77.

inside-out refers to healing from within. Both approaches have great value. A Yin and Yang approach elevates the Yin side of the spectrum to a status equal to the Yang side. Bringing Yin up to its rightful place would mean a transformation of health care. To paraphrase John Lennon: "All we are saying, is give Yin a chance!"

The outside-in, direct Yang approach views the client as a relatively passive recipient of treatment, and the practitioner as the external deliverer of remedies. This is the

## The Health Care Spectrum

| Quality | DIRECT • YANG | INDIRECT • YIN |
|---|---|---|
| Guiding Vision | *"Contraria contrariis curantur."* [Curing by opposites] –Hippocrates | *"Similia similibus curantur."* [Curing by similars] – Paracelsus |
| Healing | Top Down | Bottom Up |
| Power source | Centralized (core) | Distributed (periphery) |
| Correction | From the Outside In | From the Inside Out |
| Focus | Symptom focus | Whole person focus |
| Resources | Emphasis on outer resources | Emphasis on inner resources |
| Funding | Well-developed & funded | Less-developed & funded |
| Method | Drugs and Surgery | Self-awareness, personal growth |
| Treatment | Researched Treatment Protocols | "Inherent Treatment Plan" |
| Belief | Belief in Cause and Effect | Belief in Complexity |
| System | Individual singularity | Interconnectedness |
| Perception | Objectification "Antipathy" | Subjectification "Sympathy" |
| Attitude | Diagnose and Fix | Nurture and Support |
| Process | Treatment | Prevention |

familiar realm of pharmaceuticals, surgery and allopathic medicine. It is a huge industry in the modern world, and valid for many situations: for arterial bleeding or acute appendicitis, a direct method is clearly essential.

The complement to this, the inside-out Yin approach, is growing rapidly but still lags far behind Yang methods. Of course, ultimately, all healing comes from the inside: the doctor may stitch up a cut and apply an antiseptic, but the actual cellular changes and immune responses are coming from the inside, especially from the ANS and its partners.

CHART NO. 2. OPPOSITES POLARIZED. DIAGRAM OF THE PATTERN OF LIFE FORCE AND THE TISSUE CELL.

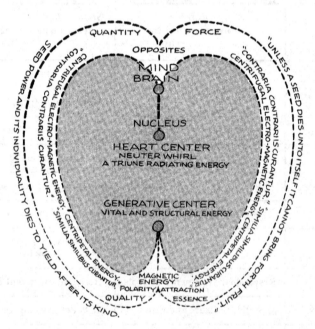

*Randolph Stone's diagram shows the theoretical basis for full-spectrum health care.* Direct methods are appropriate at the north end, where a fountain (Yang) flows out from the center, and Indirect methods are appropriate at the south end, where a vortex (Yin) carries information from the periphery back to the core. The apple or doughnut shape is called a *tube torus* and in physics is considered to be a basis for all form.

An eloquent definition of the indirect philosophy is offered by osteopath Paul Lee:

> The purpose of the treatment is to arouse the body physiology of the patient to evaluate its own health patterns and to treat its own traumatic or disease conditions with the resources of its anatomic-physiological mechanisms. [47]

The same spectrum is also found in psychology, with different terminology. Psychologist and author Scott Kellogg describes the two paradigms as Facilitating (Indirect) and Modifying (Direct). He quotes representatives of the two branches, beginning with an indirect approach:

> [In Gestalt] the therapist rejects any kind of authority position toward the person with whom he is working. The therapist does not lead, guide, advise, or in other ways take away the person's responsibility for himself or herself. Rather, each person knows best what he needs for himself and how to get it; even when he is stuck, he is more capable of finding his solutions than anyone else. [48]

In contrast, a direct psychology school describes the benefits of the opposite approach:

> In Redecision Therapy, the client is the star and the drama is carefully plotted to end victoriously... The therapist is the director of the drama, writer of some of the lines, and occasionally interpreter... We do not

---

47 Paul Lee, *Interface*. Stillness Press, 2003. p. 103.

48 J.A. Greenwald, *The Ground Rules in Gestalt Therapy*, in *The Handbook of Gestalt Therapy*, by Hatcher and Himmelstein (Eds.). Aronson, 1976. pp. 267-280. Cited in Scott Kellogg, *Dialogical Encounters: Contemporary Perspectives on "Chairwork" in Psychotherapy*. Psychotherapy: Theory, Research, Practice, Training, 2004, Vol. 41, No. 3, pp. 310-320.

want to produce tragedies– we are interested in happy endings.[49]

It is important to appreciate one side of the spectrum without negating the other. Frequently advocates of one group, science "skeptics" or "alternative" enthusiasts, feel compelled to mock those at the other end of the spectrum. Ridicule has no proper place in science and health care.[50] Both approaches have real merit and valid applications.

Stone recognized the value of both outside-in and inside-out therapies, and used both successfully. With his interest in Eastern methods, he was probably an easy target for the skeptics of his day, despite his effectiveness with his patients.[51] He called for a truce:

> In such a confusion, conscientious minds of thinkers and researchers will naturally look for an answer that could do justice to all and shed light on a dark road of misunderstanding and persecution of one group by another.[52]

An outside-in Yang strategy involves the therapist's direct intervention, advice, firm contact and education about the archetypes. An inside-out Yin strategy involves building

---

[49] Goulding and Goulding, *Changing Lives through Redecision Therapy*. Grove Press, 1997. Cited in Scott Kellogg, above.

[50] Sniping between factions has been a problem for centuries. From Galileo to Wilhelm Reich, too many people have been persecuted for their ideas. Perhaps the saddest example is Ignaz Semmelweis, MD (1818-1865), who stated that doctors in birthing hospitals should wash their hands between patients. His career and life were ruined by the outraged medical scientists of his era. His main error was in being just slightly ahead of his time, for his ideas were accepted just a decade later when Joseph Lister and Louis Pasteur proved their validity.

[51] According to legend, for decades Stone advertised his practice to other Chicago-area doctors with the bold phrase, "Send me your hopeless cases." He was disappointed that so few of his colleagues followed up to find out how his good results were obtained.

[52] R. Stone, *Polarity Therapy, Vol. 1.* CRCS, 1986. Book 3, p. 1.

up the client's inner strength, increasing self-awareness of autonomic states, letting clients find their own solutions, and gently reflecting instead of intervening.

The two approaches complement each other, and they do not have to be contradictory. In a health care scenario in which the two approaches are equally available, a trip to the emergency room could include encounters with the Yang action team administering medicines and stitching up the injury while Yin caregivers support ANS balance and build inner resources. If Yin is elevated, clients will be pulled gently toward taking more responsibility for their conditions and prevention will become equal to treatment. Additionally the full-spectrum therapy process will promote better preventive practices and enable faster recovery times. A full spectrum approach would be more cost-effective for everyone involved.

## Yin and Yang in Psychotherapy Traditions

To bring Yin and Yang principles into counseling, we first survey the field and identify methods that support the above principles. Then we extract relevant practices and adapt them as needed. The intended result is an inclusive, open-ended synthesis of effective ideas and methods. The following criteria help identify which psychotherapy traditions might be included in a Yin and Yang system:

The combined method will have at least some of these traits. It will...

- ...refer to the Three Principles/Five Elements model.
- ...induce movement and reduce fixation.
- ...clearly link physical phenomena with emotional and mental experience.
- ...have a body-centered and experiential style, as opposed to primarily analytical or interpretive.

- ...seek to elevate the client's will power and determination for self-regulation. Is there a clearly stated intention of client empowerment and autonomy?

- ...engage in inquiry about the "journey of the soul," life energy, the purpose of life, the role of spirit in wellness, the existence of an invisible world and related esoteric material.

- ...provide "life coaching" and guidance about common life experiences such as relationships, lifestyle choices and diet.

- ...integrate smoothly with touch therapies, in recognition of the inseparable nature of the body-mind unity of human experience.

Surveying the current field of psychotherapy, several schools of thought seem to meet parts of these criteria:

• **Body-Centered Trauma Resolution systems** such as the body-awareness practices developed by Eugene Gendlin, Peter Levine, Diane Heller, Susan Aposhyan, Pat Ogden and others involve guiding the client to focus on physical sensation and using the attention to oscillate between sites of distress and non-distress.

Levine gives a good summary, while also acknowledging Stone as an influence:

...The two polarities, just like in Polarity Therapy, are expansion and contraction. The two results of polarization are expansion and contraction, so you have a wave undulation between the expansive quality of the energy movement and its contraction. That's the normal response of that universe: expansion-contraction, expansion-contraction.

As you go into the trauma vortex you could call that the compression vortex or the constriction vortex. As you move out of that into the inner vortex, then the experience is one of expansion. Again, they have to be linked together, because from a physics point of view, singularities are notoriously unstable. If you have something that's just one polarity, either expansion or contraction, it will eventually go into an unstable explosion or annihilation, either rigidity or fragmentation.

You have to have this pulsing back and forth. This is the key that we come to over and over, really the fundamental essence phenomenologically of this approach [Somatic Experiencing]. The movement between expansion and contraction is the normal process of self-regulation, the energetic basis of self-regulation.

As I talk about this, I really see how deeply I was influenced by Stone [in 1970]. I had not thought about it for years, but being here I can really see how he got me to start thinking in these terms, how he helped me start to put these thoughts together, as did many others mentioned in the book [*Waking the Tiger* (1998)] acknowledgements...[53]

• **Neurobiology research** is leading to a new therapeutic model based on understanding the autonomic nervous system and recognizing how subconscious impulses manifest in actual behavior. Innovative authors such as Daniel Seigel, Jon Kabat-Zinn, Allan Schore, Paul Ekman, Stan Tatkin, Bonnie Badenoch, Richard Davidson and Rick Hanson have contributed to this growing area. Knowledge of attachment styles, autonomic display cues and micro-movements can be very beneficial for any body-centered therapy, especially Yin and Yang counseling.

---

[53] Peter Levine, audio recording, June 1997 American Polarity Therapy Association Annual Conference, Toronto, Ontario. For Somatic Experiencing information, see www.traumahealing.org.

• **Two-Chair technique**, adapted from its original sources by Fritz Perls and modified by Perls' Polarity Therapy students, offers a similar embodiment of Yin and Yang principles. Changing chairs represents a physical oscillation between two points of view, facilitating increased movement and reduced fixation. The two-chair process described in Chapter 10 is an adaptation of Perls' two-chair method.

• **Communication therapies**, for which there are many advocates and methods, can be included because successful communication requires effective listening and talking, which can be seen as a flow between two people. Nonviolent Communication (NVC), as taught by Marshall Rosenburg is a prime example of communication skills that effectively increase circulation.[54]

• **Attachment theory** proposes that the ability to fully and gracefully oscillate between awareness of Self and awareness of Other is a key indicator of mental-emotional health. Well-attached people have equal skill and ease with self-care and care for others.

• **Codependence therapies** propose a dynamic tension between two personalities in which problems arise when one becomes over-functioning and the other becomes under-functioning, or co-dependent and anti-dependent. This whole body of work can be said to employ Yin and Yang Principles by creating a dualistic context for interpreting fixated behavior patterns.

Within the whole of Codependence Therapy, the work of Pia Mellody is of particular interest because she created an elegant five-layered psychological model that fits with the psycho-emotional dimensions of the Three Principles ("Too

---

[54] Marshall Rosenberg, *Nonviolent Communication*. Puddledancer Press, 2003.

Much, Too Little, and Good Enough") and Five Elements (the "Five Inalienable Rights of the Child") bases of Yin and Yang.[55] Mellody's ideas are discussed in Chapter 12.

• **Attachment Repatterning,** developed by Diane Heller and her colleagues, effectively combines body-centered processing with research on attachment styles.

As a companion to Attachment Theory, Object Relations theory is also of interest from a Yin and Yang perspective. Object relations theory notes that a young child forms images of the nature of self and others based on interactions with the mother and other significant caregivers. The child then projects that image as an attitude and expectation on self and others throughout life, whether or not it is valid, realistic or rewarding. The "attachment styles" originate in these early-childhood images and projections, which can effectively create a form of hypnotic trance that lasts throughout life unless a successful intervention brings a change. The study of projected reality fits with the Yin and Yang model in their mutual emphasis on the interaction between subtle programing and gross manifestation.

• **Pre- and peri-natal psychology** offers many rich insights for Yin and Yang counseling. Understanding that the prenate and infant are sentient (even super-sentient) beings is a revelation with enormous implications for birthing procedures and pediatric medicine. The reality of the phenomenon has been thoroughly documented by David Chamberlain[56] and others, and therapeutic applications have

---

55 Pia Mellody and Lawrence S. Freundlich, *The Intimacy Factor.* HarperOne, 2003.

56 David Chamberlain, *The Mind of Your Newborn Baby.* North Atlantic, 1998.

been well-developed by practitioners such as Ray Castellino, [57] William Emerson [58] and Franklyn Sills.

• **Hakomi Therapy,** which originated with Ron Kurtz and his colleagues, has founding principles that are very compatible with the themes and methods described here. [59]

• **Sensorimotor Psychotherapy**, developed by Pat Ogden and her colleagues, has strong links to Hakomi Therapy and Somatic Experiencing.

• Stephen Porges' **Polyvagal theory**, while not a psychotherapy discipline, has great relevance because it proposes a tremendous advance in understanding the autonomic nervous system. [60]

• **Reichian psychology** (Wilhelm Reich) and its derivative **BioEnergetics** (Alexander Lowen) are partly compatible with Yin and Yang ideas. Reich's ideas about a universal energy that he called "orgone" has some similarities to nineteenth century western ideas of "Vitalism" and the eastern concepts of *Chi* in China and *Prana* in India. Both Reich and Lowen placed a strong emphasis on the value of body-centered work within psychotherapy.

*Other Non-Psychology Systems*

• **Biodynamic Craniosacral Therapy** as developed by Franklyn Sills arises from early twentieth-century osteopathic observations of a polyrhythmic expansion-contraction

---

[57] Castellino (www.raycastellino.com) deserves special acknowledgement in this field; he studied with Stone in person.

[58] For Emerson information, see http://emersonbirthrx.com

[59] Ron Kurtz, *Body-Centered Psychotherapy: The Hakomi Method: The Integrated Use of Mindfulness, Nonviolence and the Body.* LifeRhythm, 1990.

[60] Stephen Porges, *The Polyvagal Theory: Neurophysiological Foundations of Emotions, Attachment, Communication, and Self-Regulation.* Norton, 2011.

micro-movement in the body. The biodynamic approach greatly informs and enriches the indirect Yin perspective.[61]

• **Hatha yoga** offers exercises to increase range of motion, reduce fixation and quiet the mind. Many psychotherapeutic applications have been developed.[62] Stone used yoga principles in his "Polarity Yoga."[63]

• **Heart rate variability** (HRV) research finds that the range of motion of the heart's electromagnetic wave-form, seen in systolic (Yang, peak pressure) and diastolic (Yin, least pressure) cycles, is a signature of health. Of particular interest as exhibiting recognizable Yin and Yang principles is the work of Irving Dardik, Dan Winter, Bob Whitehouse and HeartMath Institute. HRV biofeedback applications meet several important criteria including empowerment of clients to self-regulate their own health care.

Yin and Yang unifies and illuminates many aspects of these therapy models, and many more. I am not attempting to represent these systems, I am just hoping to add additional resources for everyone's benefit.

---

[61] John Chitty, *Gifts: How Polarity and Craniosacral Complement Each Other.* www.energyschool.com, 2008.

[62] Swami Rama, *Swami Ajaya, Rudolph Ballentine, Yoga and Psychotherapy: The Evolution of Consciousness.* Himalayan Institute, 1976.

[63] John Chitty and Mary Louise Muller, *Energy Exercises*, Polarity Press, 1990.

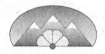

# Chapter 2

# Yin and Yang Cosmology

*At the very core of the search for true health lies the essential question of what life is for.*[64]

Randolph Stone offered a comprehensive world-view, or cosmology,[65] as the basis for his health care vision. Drawing his inspiration from ancient wisdom sources, he started from an understanding of the big picture and built his practical strategies from there. As a result, theory and treatment intersect: what supports inner coherence also leads to clear thinking and relief from symptoms on any level. Stone's approach unifies science and philosophy.

Indigenous peoples and ancient cultures viewed health conditions as inseparable from the mysteries of life and human experience. The health-care provider might also be the shaman or priest. Illnesses of the body were often interpreted as indicators of problems in other dimensions. While some of these associations may be discarded as fable or superstition, others have real merit and lead to effective treatments.

Stone did not invent his cosmology; he learned it from the wisdom traditions that he studied avidly starting in the

---

[64] R. Stone, *Health Building*. CRCS, 1986. p. 4.

[65] Here the term "cosmology" is used in its philosophical meaning, not as it is used in physics. "a: A branch of metaphysics that deals with the nature of the universe; b: a theory or doctrine describing the natural order of the universe." (Merriam-Webster Dictionary), not "the science of the origin and development of the universe." (Google Dictionary)

1920s. Beginning with Bible study, he went on to explore philosophies such as Vitalism, Mysticism, Ayurveda, Buddhism, Hinduism, Taoism and Sufism, and saw that they had significant common ground. Stone's Polarity Therapy is a synthesis of esoteric content from all these sources, an astounding achievement considering the era, when most of these were unknown in America.[66]

*Analogy: A Traveler Makes a New Home*

An effective analogy for Stone's cosmology is imagining the experience of a traveler who is moving to a new place such as an uninhabited island. Upon arrival, the first order of business is to create a dwelling; human anatomy is not designed for withstanding the elements. The process begins with a design phase. First the traveler decides on a location and size, and begins to create a plan. Everything that happens subsequently will come from this blueprint. At this early stage, changes are easy to make and are far-reaching in their effect. For example, the building could be quickly moved or changed, adding a window or door, with just a few seconds' work with an eraser and pencil.

When the blueprint is sufficiently developed, the second phase begins. Here the blueprint is brought into physical expression. The builder gathers materials and goes into action, beginning with the earthy foundation and progressing to the airy roof, and then all the interior finishing. Changes from the original design may still be created, but now they take longer. To add a window or door now, there may have to be some deconstruction.

---

[66] For an illustrated summary of Stone's sources, see http://www.energyschool.com/CSES_Home/Resources.html. Several books detail the links between Polarity Therapy to different wisdom traditions including Franklyn Sills' *Polarity Process* (Buddhism), Bruce Burger's *Esoteric Anatomy* (Hinduism) and Katarina Werhli's *The Why in the Road* (Yogananda and Self-Realization Fellowship).

After construction, the travelers can move in. The new owners bring their possessions and decorations, and personalize the dwelling with their own unique preferences and life events. Now changes are increasingly difficult because they will disturb the interior finish and intrude on daily life. The progression is from pure idea to fluid blueprint to increasingly finished structure, from easily changed to increasingly "set in stone."

The dynamic process of habitation is never really finished. By living in the house, the owners acquire feedback about the blueprint. Perhaps a door is slightly inconvenient for the traffic pattern, or a window could have been placed better to frame a particular view. Only by living in the house do the inhabitants gain experience to really evaluate the value of the plan. In time they may decide to remodel and correct aspects of the original design that later proved to be less than optimum for their purposes. When a building is purchased by new owners, they invariably do something to put their personal stamp on their new home as a gesture of linking their mental and physical levels of experience.

This cycle of design, experience and review is an example of a *recurrent feedback loop*, an important concept in science. Information flows from the blueprint through the construction to the habitation, then a return signal is generated and carried back to the blueprint. As Stone put it, "Mind patterns are expressed in the body, and the body returns the compliment by impressing itself on the mind." [67] The process continues as long as we are in the house, as we constantly try out different possibilities and adapt to new circumstances.

In our Yin and Yang cosmology, this analogy describes the human story. The traveler/homeowner is the *soul*, a "unit

---

[67] R. Stone, *Polarity Therapy, Vol. 2.* CRCS, 1986. Book 5, Chart 7.

of consciousness from another sphere," needing a suitable dwelling (the body) to exist on earth.[68] The journey to a new place is *incarnation*, a mysterious transit from an invisible dimension to the familiar, visible world. The three phases (blueprint, construction, habitation) of housebuilding reflect the three phases of being: mind, feelings, and body.

The flow of information from blueprint to form (in the diagram below, the downward arrow) is the Yang aspect of life experience; Stone used the term *involution* to describe this part of the process. The return flow of information from body

---

### About Recurrent Feedback Loops

The recurrent feedback loop is an important concept in biology and many other fields of science; it means a flow of information inducing adaptation, where one factor affects another and the second then affects or "informs" the first, often in a progressive way.

Therapies based on biofeedback provide a useful example. Technology has been created to make visible the subtle workings of body processes that are generally not perceptible, such as heart rate. By watching the information flow from the machine, the subject can learn to self-regulate far beyond the normal reach of the conscious mind. As the heart rate is brought into optimum variability range, other parts of the system respond favorably.

Interpersonally, when one person gives a signal of appreciation to another, the second person feels warmth and may shift to more authentic communication; this deeper level of information may then inspire the first person to new insights, and the second person may then have a completely new idea that was previously unavailable. The progressive creation of something new resulting from an effective recurrent feedback loop is known as *synergy*, in which the sum is more than the parts. Ideally the mind and body can produce a synergistic expansion of consciousness that would be unavailable to either one acting in hypothetical isolation.

---

[68] Stone, *Polarity Therapy, Vol. 1*. CRCS, 1986. Book 1, p. 9.

back to mind (the upward arrow) is the Yin aspect, also known as *evolution*.

## The Purpose of Life

The purpose of the whole cyclic process is to create a dwelling for the soul and to constantly refine it, based on learning through the recurrent feedback loop process. In Stone's words, "The purpose of life... is the fulfillment of consciousness."[69] Health counselor Edgar Cayce noted, "Each soul has a definite job to do; you alone can find and do that

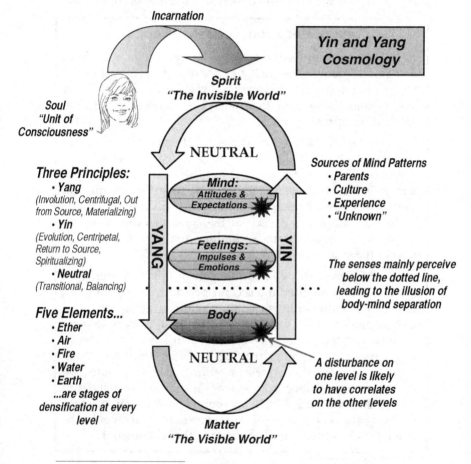

69 R. Stone, *Polarity Therapy, Vol. 1*, CRCS, 1986. Book 3, p. 11.

job."[70] Through trial and error over many lifetimes (Stone noted that many ancient wisdom traditions agreed about the reality of reincarnation and karma), souls gradually learn more about their purpose and increase their self-awareness. "Fulfillment of consciousness" means increased understanding and awareness, ultimately revolving around the capacity to give and receive love with self and others.

A psychological system based on a profound understanding of the purpose of life is revolutionary. Stone pondered the situation eloquently:

> Most of our psychology and psychiatry is derived from the Greeks, who understood the travel of the soul and mind, the various patterns and fields of expressions and perversions of searching externally in order to find satisfactions. The story of Psyche and her Pandora Box; the many myths and stories of the gods, as internal powers of energies and their universal supply and reactions; the story of Narcissus, self-seeking; the Oedipus complex, and many others which explain the cross currents of energies in the mind and its external travel of experiences.

> Our modern psychiatrists are using all these stories for want of better ones; for nowhere have we a complete picture of the travel of the soul. We know the path of the planets outside much better than we know the orbit of our own soul, mind, or senses in their functions. That is too close to home, so we go on seeking and suffering in strange lands and fields of energy, ever outward, expending our precious heritage, as all prodigals do.[71]

---

[70] Edgar Cayce Reading #2823-1. www.edgarcayce.org.

[71] R. Stone, *Polarity Therapy, Vol. 1.* CRCS, 1986. Book 1, p. 29.

Author Barbara Brennan linked health and purpose succinctly, "Health is about attunement with purpose."[72] Similarly, psychology pioneer William Sheldon wrote:

> Deeper and more fundamental than sexuality, or deeper than the craving for social power, deeper even than the desire for possessions, there is a still more generalized and more universal craving in the human make-up. It is the craving for knowledge of the right direction or orientation. Above all, we seem to always want to know in what direction we are going.[73]

Few people today can give a simple, direct response to the question, "What is the purpose of your life," much less organize their attitudes and expectations around the answer. We often can't see the forest for the trees, busying ourselves with minutiae but not contemplating the large questions of life. Stone advocated elevating philosophical questions to a higher position, so that smaller issues could be viewed from a basis in life understanding.

Modern science has also confirmed the importance of having a sense of purpose. In some studies, having *any* purpose seems to be as important as *which* purpose is being used; others have found that a more noble purpose has a stronger immune system benefit.[74] In either case, the link between having a sense of purpose and health is indisputable. Well-documented benefits include:[75]

---

[72] Barbara Brennan, *Hands of Light*. Bantam, 1988.

[73] William Sheldon, "Psychology and the Promethean Will," quoted in Dorothy Berkley's *The Choice is Always Ours*. Quest Books, 1974, p. 33.

[74] Barbara Fredrickson, *A functional genomic perspective on well-being*. Proceedings of the NAS-USA, July 29, 2013.

[75] *Health Benefits of Having a Sense of Purpose*. Archives of General Psychiatry, March 2, 2010.

- Lower risk of Alzheimer's disease (50%) and other cognitive impairment
- Lower risk of heart attack (30%)
- Lower levels of cortisol and inflammatory hormones
- Better levels of HDL ("good cholesterol")
- Positive correlation with better waist-hip ratio (a fitness marker implicated in heart conditions)
- Increased longevity

Imagine the scenario when a medical intake form of the future includes "Please describe the purpose of your life," along with asking for height, weight and allergies.

### Pre-Actualization: The traveler and the journey

The next level of discussion is to explore the three levels of mind, feelings and body in more depth, first by naming and defining the parts. The preceding diagram (page 52, above) can be reviewed to keep track of the discussion of the next few pages.

### Soul, Reincarnation and Karma

As described in the previous pages, "soul" refers to the consciousness that exists beyond physicality. Use of the term inevitably leads to companion terms, *reincarnation* and *karma*.

These words can be problematic because of their religious associations. Most religions have some form of belief about what happens after death. Some of these are quite complicated, such as that depicted in Dante's *Inferno*. Here we seek to de-mystify the terms. For our purpose, reincarnation means continuation of consciousness between lifetimes, and karma means cause and effect, with additive information somehow conserved in both short and long terms.

These ideas are indigestible for materialistic science because the effects are subtle, not measurable by normal investigation and conflicting with popular dogma. However, there is thoroughly-documented evidence that the "survival of consciousness" exists.[76] Many of our normal assumptions about time and space have to be amended to describe what happens and how, but we don't need to pursue those topics for our purposes here. Some form of continuation of consciousness is actually the simplest and most workable explanation for the data.[77] When considered with an open mind, on face value, the evidence is substantial. Chopra's excellent book on the topic has an astonishing 48 laudatory endorsements by other best-selling health experts, reflecting the quality of the data and analysis. The concepts are embraced by many psychologists privately, while publicly they remain unmentionable and taboo. Yin and Yang psychotherapy invites reincarnation and karma to come out of the proverbial dogma-closet.

The idea of karma is actually not so foreign as we might initially think: the Biblical phrases that are readily meaningful for westerners include, "As you sow so shall you reap"[78] and "Do unto others as you would have them do unto you."[79] These both imply balance between action and reaction.

Acceptance of the notion of karma can have profound benefits for troubled clients, because it reduces the pressure of finding a cause and also adds a sense of direction for meeting many of life's challenges. The leverage of the concept is enormous; people who accept the idea of karma and

---

[76] Gary Schwartz, William Simon and Deepak Chopra, *The Afterlife Experiments: Breakthrough Scientific Evidence of Life After Death*. Atria, 2003.

[77] Deepak Chopra, *Life After Death: The Burden of Proof*. Harmony Books, 2006.

[78] In the Bible, see: Job 4:8 ("As I have observed, those who plow evil and those who sow trouble reap it."); Psalm 126:5 ("Those who sow in tears will reap with songs of joy."); Galatians 6:7 ("Be not deceived; God is not mocked: for whatsoever a man soweth, that shall he also reap.")

[79] In the Bible, see: Matthew 7:12, Luke 6:31. The first origin of the thought may be traceable to Confucius.

reincarnation are more likely to be mindful of their behavior due to a commonsense concern about consequences. On a shallow level, this could seem to be just a manipulative guilt-inducer, but more deeply the effect is profound. For a culture that embraces cause-and-effect, we have a remarkable blind spot about consequences, most evident in the environmental realm where our throw-away society cannot quite comprehend the reality that there is no "away."

Among many data sources for karma, near-death experience (NDE) testimonials support its experiential reality even if science cannot explain it yet. People who have "been to the other side" and come back are often kinder, calmer and more focused about the importance of giving love and service to others. The common NDE report of asking oneself "What have you done with your life?" is apparently quite impactful for the people who then return to the living.[80]

Soul, reincarnation and karma are embedded in Stone's philosophy, but these are not absolutely necessary to practice a Yin and Yang approach. Other parts and methods can still be used. These esoteric ideas just strengthen the whole system and enable the theory to more fully accommodate the data.

*Anomalies of Consciousness and Brain Research*

Since the existence of anything beyond the physical world is a problem for science, and this cosmology goes there quickly, it may be useful to remember the many well-verified anomalies relating to the workings of the mind. Some scientists would have us believe the "mind" is the same as the physical brain. However, there is clearly substantial evidence of non-physical processes, starting with the brain itself:

---

[80] Betty Eadie, *Embraced by the Light*. Bantam, 2002; first edition 1992); Dannion Brinkley, *Saved by the Light*. HarperOne, 2008; Eben Alexander, *Proof of Heaven: A Neurosurgeon's Journey into the Afterlife*. Simon & Schuster, 2012.

**Ten Unsolved Mysteries of the Brain:**[81]
- How is information coded in neural activity?
- How are memories stored and retrieved?
- What does the baseline activity in the brain represent?
- How do brains simulate the future?
- What are emotions?
- What is intelligence?
- How is time represented in the brain?
- Why do brains sleep and dream?
- How do the specialized systems of the brain integrate with one another?
- What is consciousness?

With a list like this, we wonder what exactly we *do* know! Neuroscience textbooks are full of details, but where is a comprehensive theory that actually addresses the unknown areas (above) and anomalies (below)?

To strengthen the idea of the existence of a non-physical reality, here are examples of thoroughly documented metaphysical information-processing phenomena that defy explanation using currently accepted neuroscience:

- **Phantom limb research** includes accounts in which the severed limb conveys verifiable sensory and other information to the body, without a physical connection.[82]

- **The memories of babies** seem to precede the maturity of the supposedly necessary brain areas.[83]

- **Savant Syndrome** literature has hundreds of documented cases of people who are capable of prodigious

---

[81] Dan Eagleman, *Ten Unsolved Mysteries of the Brain*. Discover Magazine, Aug. 2007.

[82] See V.S. Ramachandran, *Phantoms in the Brain: Probing the Mysteries of the Human Mind*. William Morrow Paperbacks, 1999.

[83] David Chamberlain is an excellent resource for this topic. See http://birthpsychology.com

mental feats, without the presence of an exceptional, identifiable brain mechanism.[84]

• **Heart and other organ transplant** recipients have taken on personality traits and specific memories of donors.[85]

• In some severe cases of **hydrocephalus**, the brain has been crowded by cerebrospinal fluid pressure from within the ventricles, but the people are full-functioning adults with normal intelligence even though there is less than 10% of the brain still present.[86]

• "The Sense of Being Stared At" describes systematic, thorough research project showing **non-local cognition** without an apparent mechanism.[87]

• **Autonomic nervous system pre-cognition** experiments verified that the ANS detects certain stimuli accurately before the events actually occur.[88]

Hopefully these examples are sufficient to loosen the binds of reductionist science and materialism on the study of the mind. The metaphysical cosmology deserves respect at

---

[84] Darold A.Treffert, *Extraordinary People: Understanding Savant Syndrome.* Backinprint, 2006.

[85] See Paul Pearsall, Gary Schwartz and Linda Russak, *Organ Transplants and Cellular Memories.* Nexus Magazine, April-May 2005. Also see http://www.namahjournal.com/doc/Actual/Memory-transference-in-organ -transplant-recipients-vol-19-iss-1.html.

[86] Roger Lewin, "Is your brain really necessary?" *Science*, Dec. 1980. The article describes the astonishing findings of British neurologist John Lorber at Children's Hospital in Sheffield England.

[87] Rupert Sheldrake has collected a wealth of data in this field. See http://www.sheldrake.org/Research/morphic/

[88] Rupert Sheldrake, *The Sense of Being Stared At; And Other Unexplained Powers of Human Minds.* Park Street Press, 2013. This contains a description of Dean Radin's often-duplicated experiments at the University of Nevada in 1997, in which ANS biofeedback accurately predicted the nature of stimuli microseconds before the stimulating event.

least because, unlike the prevailing model, it is a theory that can accommodate the actual evidence.

## The First Phase of Actualization: Creating a Design

The blueprint or mind can also be described as *attitudes and expectations*. To a large degree, experience is pre-formed and pre-exercised at this subtle level. Attitudes and expectations are extremely powerful, far beyond common comprehension and largely invisible to the casual observer. Attributes of attitudes and expectations have several origins, called "Sources of Mind Patterns" in the diagram. Most attitudes and expectations come from these four influences: Parents, Culture, Experience and "Unknown."

**Parents:** Most obvious are our parents and principal caregivers, and their life experiences. We learn our basic orientation toward life based on our formative experience of our parents. The imprint can manifest as both positive and negative expressions, with the parents being imitated or opposed. As infants we are basically in a hypnotic trance during the first years of life, imprinting their attitudes and expectations and making them our own.

**Culture:** The origin of attitudes and expectations can be expanded to include the second influence, our culture and its history. Parents who grew up in a particular region that experienced a major event, such as the Great Depression or World War II, will have attitudes and expectations about life that have qualities beyond just the familial imprint, and these are transferred to the next generation. The extent of echoes of past events being carried into the future has been broadened by recent discoveries in epigenetics, in which a famine experienced by grandparents was found to have physically changed genetic expression two and three generations later.[89]

---

[89] *The Ghost in Your Genes*, PBS video, 2008.

Both personal and social history are also "cultural" sources for attitudes and expectations. Early events mold later attitudes. Personal or societal trauma can create attitudes and expectations that last a lifetime.[90] People from a certain region exhibit a certain style, over and above their family or personal history. Similarly, a cultural subgroup, such as a religious, intellectual, linguistic or racial community, can have characteristic beliefs, attitudes and expectations that are perpetuated in subsequent generations.

**Life Experiences:** Attitudes and expectations are also constantly molded by life experiences. When traumatic events occur, we naturally guard against recurrence with specialized adaptations at the level of attitudes and expectations, if we touch a hot stove once, we will start to expect that all stoves are hot. The effect is true for remembered experience, but also for "pre-memory" experiences that happen before normal memory is formed. Many people have demonstrated the capacity to recall events of infancy and even pre-birth and pre-conception, casting yet another vote for the reality of reincarnation and karma.[91]

**"Unknown:"** The fourth source is the effect of karma. The reality of this source of attitudes and expectations is more justification for reducing the emphasis on finding the cause of a condition, since this part cannot be fully known. Health care systems such as doctor and Tao Master Zhi Gang Sha's "Soul Mind Body Medicine" achieve excellent results by emphasizing karma healing in their methods.[92]

---

[90] Bessel van der Kolk, *Traumatic Stress: The Effect of Overwhelming Experience on Mind, Body and Society.* Guilford, 2006.

[91] Michael Newton, *Journey of Souls.* Llewellyn, 1994.

[92] Zhi Gang Sha, *Soul Mind Body Medicine: A Complete Soul Healing System for Optimum Health and Vitality.* New World Library, 2006. Sha describes how metaphysicians can intervene for release from the effects of previous actions. The www.drsha.com website provides numerous impressive case studies.

Attitudes and expectations have a profound effect on everything that follows, just as the blueprint determines the later house. Despite this enormous leverage, the blueprint of our attitudes and expectations is often invisible, because we are so totally immersed in it. Being invisible to us, we are normally unable to make changes just out of choice. If we could choose to do so, lowering our expectations of ourselves and others might serve as a buffer against stress because we would be less likely to be disappointed. However, the effect might be reduced because we would miss some of the benefits of having an attitude of optimism and appreciation, which directly support the immune system.[93] In any case, studious exploration of attitudes and expectations can be a revelation in counseling, as we will explore later in the book.

### *The Second Phase of Actualization: Enacting the Blueprint*

Returning to the house-building analogy, we proceed into more detail about the second phase of construction. This phase represents feelings, in which the blueprint is brought into manifestation by a direct flow from attitudes to actions. Here the blueprint becomes somewhat more visible, especially if feelings are intense.

The terms "motives" and "impulses" can be useful for this feelings phase. Something drives us to make choices, decide courses of action, and become who we eventually become. We may think that major life decisions are rational outcomes of a clear mental process, but this is usually not correct. Asking people why they did their major actions such as choosing a life partner or career path, their answer is often vague. We usually act because somehow we "feel like it;" we have an impulse to act and the true origins are shrouded in a multi-faceted, complex attitude or expectation.

---

[93] B. Bower, *Science News*, "*Sniffle-busting personalities: positive mood guards against colds.*" Vol. 170. p. 387.

Furthermore, many major life decisions arise from what we choose *not* to do. Many decisions come about through a process of elimination, rather than a real choice. Actions based on "not that" are arising from an emotional basis that often turns out to leave us in surprising circumstances. For example, we may try to "choose" to marry someone who is *not* like one of our parents only to discover later that the same characteristics are present, just in a different "wrapping" that we did not initially recognize.

The feelings level includes emotional responses that derive significantly from expectations; therefore we have a direct link from the mind to the feelings. Risky activities that would be traumatic for one person, such as high speed driving in traffic, are not an issue for those who expect the experience, such as race-car drivers. Laboratory animals experience more symptoms of post-traumatic stress disorder if the stressor is unexpected. Events that are counter to expectations can be more traumatic. Betrayal trauma is so deeply distressing because the victim expected love and protection but received the opposite.[94]

### *The Third Phase of Actualization: Manifesting Form*

The third phase, the body, is most obvious and tangible. Here the blueprint has been converted into seemingly solid matter and made visible. The apparent solidity of the body leads to a common illusion, because it becomes easy to think of the body as separate from the rest. After all, the body is the only part that is tangible with our primary senses. The separation of mind and body originates partly just in the senses, which can only see, hear, taste, smell and touch within

---

[94] J. Corsi, *Healing From Trauma*. Marlowe & Co., 2007. pp. 2-4. Corsi references additional supportive sources including Scharff (2004) and Allen (1995). A similar resource Jennifer Freyd, *Betrayal Trauma*. Harvard, 1998.

limited ranges. We cannot see x-rays, hear a dog whistle or smell even a fraction of what an animal smells. A Yin and Yang approach directly confronts this error. As A. T. Still put it, "We look at the body in health as meaning perfection and harmony, not in one part, but in the whole." [95]

As science author Fritjof Capra describes, the matter of which we are made is not really as dense as it seems:

> Far from being the hard and solid particles they were believed to be since antiquity, the atoms turned out to consist of vast regions of space ... It is not easy to get a feeling for the... magnitude of atoms ...
>
> In order to visualize this diminutive size, imagine an orange blown up to the size of the Earth. The atoms of the orange will then have the size of cherries.... In our picture of cherry-sized atoms, the nucleus of an atom will be so small that we will not be able to see it... To see the nucleus, we would have to blow up the size of the atom (the cherry) to the size of the biggest dome in the world, the dome of St. Peter's in Rome (138 feet across)...
>
> In an atom of that size, the nucleus would have the size of a grain of salt! A grain of salt in the middle of the vast dome of St. Peter's, and specks of dust whirling around it in the vast space of the dome: this is how we can picture the nucleus and electrons of an atom. [96]

Author Deepak Chopra confirms this view and quantifies the spaciousness as he explains the situation:

> When you get to the level of atoms, the landscape is not one of solid objects moving around each other like a dance, following predictable steps. Subatomic

---

[95] A. T. Still, *Philosophy and Mechanical Principles of Osteopathy.* Forgotten Books, 2012. First published in 1902.

[96] F. Capra, *The Tao of Physics.* Shambhala, 1983. pp. 65-66.

particles are separated by huge gaps, making every atom more than 99.999 percent empty space.[97]

Our materialistic belief systems also derive from our childhood training. We all learned to spell and count. *Spell* could be interpreted to mean the casting of a spell, or being hypnotized into a linear, left-brain, alphabetic reality. *Count* could be developed as meaning a training in materialism through the medium of arithmetic: when something "counts," it really "matters" and the rules of arithmetic and geometry make the world seem supremely measurable in a way that is actually not accurate. The slippery nature of reality was revealed definitively long ago in 1803 by Thomas Young in his famous Double-Slit experiment, which showed that a photon could appear as either a wave or particle depending on the observer's presence. This contradicted Newtonian ideals and was not fully comprehended, much less explained to innocent first graders. Imagine if we told children on their first day of school, "There really is an invisible world, in addition to what you can see, and you exist here for an important purpose, the fulfillment of consciousness."

Instead, phenomena outside the predominant belief system are not noticed or are discounted. Shouldn't the files be updated every century or so? As the great American philosopher Yogi Berra said, "If I hadn't believed it, I wouldn't have seen it."

Yin and Yang is like a reset button for the whole system, taking a fresh look at all these kinds of basic reality questions. It embraces inquiries about the whole spectrum of human conditions, from visible to invisible. We constantly work to erase the perceptual line separating body from feelings and mind. The whole is not separated into parts; although we may be focused on a particular physical symptom, we are

---

[97] Deepak Chopra, *Quantum Healing.* Bantam, 1990. p. 96.

always holding a part of our perceptual process for the client's whole being. Conversely, mental problems can be expected to have physical correlates, to the point that we can observe the body's gestures for clues about the mind.

In this approach, anomalies are appreciated with curiosity instead of being dismissed, and there is a constant openness about the possibility of "miracles," surprises or unexplained happenings. In a Yin and Yang approach, we remember that a soul inhabits the multi-layered dwelling of our clients, and that the "Journey of the Soul" is always a sub-plot in every narrative.

### The Five Elements

Each level of the "traveler metaphor" cosmology can be sub-divided into the Five Elements.[98] Form coalesces in stages, from very subtle to very dense. The five elements of space (also known as "ether"), air, fire, water and earth are progressive densities that accomplish particular requirements. Space provides a container, air gives a connective medium with respiration's exchange of gases, fire enables digestive heat and metabolism, water provides fluidic continuity and circulation, and earth gives structure.

As an analogy, we experience the five elements when we pay the monthly bills (rent for space; electricity, phone and internet for air; furnace and air conditioning for fire; water supply and sewer for water; structure and trash for earth). Non-payment of any one, or lack of repairs, will mean reduced quality of life and eventual termination.

Having five elemental steps, not four or six, is a curiosity. The appearance of five digits on the hands and feet,

---

[98] Polarity Therapy is based on Indian tradition, but the Five Elements concept is equally sophisticated in Traditional Chinese Medicine. In *The Web That Has No Weaver*, Ted Kaptchuk links the two (India/China: Ether/Earth, Air/Wood, Fire/Fire, Water/Metal, Earth/Water).

and five appendages on the body (counting the neck and head as an appendage), is not accidental but rather an expression of nature's fundamental "laws of form." The ratio of three to five is the first and lowest numbered appearance of the Fibonacci series, a famous mathematical progression named for a 12th-century Italian mathematician. To create the series, start with 0 and 1; add the sum of these to the second number to create the progression: 0, 1, 1, 2, 3, 5, 8, 13, 21, 34....[99] The Fibonacci series is recognized as a basis for natural form, particularly the appearance of spirals in nature and the path of least resistance in plant growth and fluid flow.[100]

Together, three and five are the smallest numbers approximating the Golden Mean, or Phi Ratio, famous in art and architecture for being the most aesthetically pleasing visual proportions,[101] in mathematics for being the basis for fractals,[102] and in music for defining harmonious chords.[103]

Summarizing, again, the Yin and Yang cosmology offers two great layers: Three Principles and Five Elements. As Stone put it, "...the five aspects of matter in their three modes of motion."[104] Principles refer to the cyclic Yang movement from design into form, followed by a temporary equilibrium and reversal of flow (the Neutral Principle), and then a Yin return information flow to convey the lessons of experience

---

[99] http://www.youtube.com/watch?v=aBzAO72Nulc&feature=share

[100] Erik Andrulis, *Theory of the Origin, Evolution, and Nature of Life*. Life Journal, 2012. www.mdpi.com/journal/life.

[101] Robert Lawlor, *Sacred Geometry Theory and Practice*. Thames and Hudson, 1982.

[102] Michael Schneider, *A Beginner's Guide to Constructing the Universe: Mathematical Archetypes of Nature, Art, and Science*. HarperPerennial, 1995.

[103] John Beaulieu, *Human Tuning: Sound Healing with Tuning Forks*. Biosonic, 2010.

[104] R. Stone, *Polarity Therapy, Vol. 1*, CRCS, 1986. Book 3, p. 21.

back to the design function which can then make adjustments for the next phase of the process.

Within the large Three Principles movement of cyclic information flow, the discrete steps of the Five Elements can indicate precise detail about conditions. The Three Principles/Five Elements model provides a simple and effective basis for understanding conditions and giving treatment. In the presence of a health problem, we try to develop an hypothesis including a combination of which Principle and which Element is relevant in the condition, and create strategies based on that assessment. This topic will be developed further in Chapter 13.

## *The Journey of the Soul*

Stone's cosmology unifies the traditional concerns of the scientist and philosopher. The essential questions at the heart of philosophical inquiry are, "What is humanity?" "What is consciousness, and life?"

Stone's answers to these questions constitute "the Journey of the Soul." Here is a summary, in Stone's words:

> ...The soul which inhabits this body is a unit of consciousness from another sphere, of much finer essences... Each incarnating soul or entity brings with it a design of life, of its own, by which it differs from others...[105]

> The soul...steps down its energy and becomes a slave of the mind, and expresses itself through the senses. The senses relate to the mind as units to the whole ... seeking experience in multiplicity and outward expenditure of energy...

> In matter, it is action for the sake of action; namely, the sensations, the enjoyment of the senses, the reactions, the accumulation of things, and personal

---

[105] R. Stone, *Polarity Therapy, Vol. 1.* CRCS, 1986. Book 1, p. 9.

honor, pride and self-aggrandizement through possessions and power... [but] every pleasure in this world, indulged in as such, has its resulting sorrow, if not immediately, at some time in the future. The same principle is still active when a child insists on touching a hot stove; it must experience the sensation and the resulting pain.[106]

Our energies are constantly going outward, seeking in things the thrills and satisfactions which are not there. It is a mirage. Only the very highest universal source really has what we seek and crave. So, after maturity of years, after aeons of wanderings and sufferings, the soul finally is convinced of this fact and, like the 'Prodigal Son,' remembers his Father's house and all its abundance. He then rises up within himself, turns his energy and longings of the soul inwards, and comes back home to his Universal Source...[107]

Stone thus describes life as a school, with a centrifugal force propelling units of consciousness out from a primordial source, into the dense world of experience (involution), until through painful experience the deepest lessons are learned, providing the motivation for a centripetal return to the center (evolution).

The purpose is for the experience of souls embodied in forms and placed in outer space of matter and resistance in order to gain awareness through perception and action, for the fulfillment of consciousness.[108]

Man alone stands at the top of the ladder of all Creation. He alone is endowed with all the faculties necessary to understand his Source, his Being, and

---

[106] *ibid.*, p. 31.

[107] *ibid.*, p. 29.

[108] R. Stone, *Polarity Therapy, Vol. 1.* CRCS, 1986. Book 3, pp. 9, 11.

his relationship to Nature. Writings of the Ancients became sacred because they endeavored to reveal to man some hints about his Source, his marvelous pent-up energies and soul powers, and how to use them wisely in Nature, how to transcend the ego and thereby find his way to his REAL HOME.[109]

## The Meaning of Gender

Both genders have all Three Principles, or they could not function even at the very start, but there is a slight preponderance of Yang in males and Yin in females, or they would not have their anatomical differences. These manifest in a wide variety of forms throughout life, internally as hormone activity and procreation processes, and externally as societal experiences. Both genders are built of ecto-, endo- and meso- tissues, but sperm and egg are almost exclusively Yang and Yin, and occur exclusively in each gender.[110]

Why is one person a man (and thus inevitably challenged biologically by Yang experience, in addition to Yin experience which will also arise to varying degrees), and another a woman (and thus inevitably challenged biologically by Yin experience, in addition to Yang experience which will arise to varying degrees)? Is this accidental or random?

Stone explains human life as a quest for knowledge and experience. The fact of gender fits in with this quest idea. A student returning to college after vacation does not take the same courses, but rather goes to the next level in the progression of knowledge. Similarly, the soul seeks

---

[109] R. Stone, *Health Building*. CRCS, 1986. p. 23.

[110] Biological anomalies such as intersexism, rare in humans but common in other forms particularly invertebrates, defy clear classification. However many report having an inner feeling of one gender being correct more than the other even when the physical characteristics are mixed. See Elizabeth Reis, *Bodies in Doubt: An American History of Intersex*. Johns Hopkins University Press, 2012.

experiences that represent new challenges. In this view, the selection of a body gender for an incarnation is apparently a precise sequence.

In traditional Japanese folklore, as re-told in Macrobiotics, it is said that the gender of the child is a function of the challenge of the parents. A child will be born into a male body if the next progression of the soul's education requires Yang lessons (possibly having dealt previously and successfully with Yin challenges). Thus the child will be born to parents who, at that time, are creating a field of action in which the appropriate Yang challenges will manifest. If the parents are struggling with Yang issues, the child is more likely to be a boy. There is no way to test this folklore, but it does give food for thought, and supports the notion of purpose.

Substantial research describes significant gender variables, including behaviors, preferences and subtle differences.[111] Meanwhile other research has also emphasized the importance of individuality, indicating that gender is not so all-differentiating as often thought.[112] Obviously, gender does matter, but the context needs to be fully appreciated and the tendency to over-generalize or oversimplify needs to be firmly avoided. The goal of healthy living is to be able to manifest Yin and Yang and Neutral as appropriate, in all life's fields of action, in either gender. Stone gives us a big picture reminder by invoking the family unit:

> Male and female everywhere are the active factors with a neuter [neutral] field for gestation. Father, mother and child are the human family completed. In the Chinese system this was illustrated as the

---

[111] For example: Deborah Tannen, *You Just Don't Understand.* William Morris, 2001 and John Gray, *Men are from Mars, Women are from Venus.* Harper, 2003.

[112] For example: Cordelia Fine, *Delusions of Gender.* Norton, 2011.

yang (red, positive) and the yin (dark, negative) energy as its reflection entwined in endless motion.[113]

In this line of thinking, the fact of gender is a matter to be appreciated, not minimized. A significant amount of experience, from hormones to social roles, follows from the fundamental event of gender identity. As this book will show, the qualities of sperm and egg manifest throughout life, bringing particular lessons of life. We can observe Yin and Yang at every stage of the relationship process, from dating to raising children. The powerful magnetism and emotional force of sexual attraction and the miraculous dynamics of conception are perhaps the most remarkable demonstrations of the workings of Yin and Yang in human experience.

It is a measure of the grand illusion of life that so much controversy has arisen on issues of sexual identity and role. In a Yin and Yang approach, all options are open for inquiry, including all the possibilities of gender identity and relationship pairing. Equal rights constitute an essential property. Long before feminist advances of the 1960s, Stone emphasized that both sexes are on the same spiritual path, using his frequent all-capitalization style for emphasis:

> WOMEN, AS WELL AS MEN, have the same right and footing in both processes [involution and evolution].[114]

The body, male or female, is a meaningful temporary vehicle for the learning of certain lessons. The task is to

---

[113] R. Stone, *Polarity Therapy, Vol. 2*, Book 6, Chart 16. CRCS, 1986.

[114] R. Stone, *Polarity Therapy, Vol. 1*. CRCS, 1986. Book 1, p. 40. This passage includes a denunciation of his era's sexism (p. 39): "A great injustice was done to womanhood by the literal interpretation of the story of the Garden of Eden. WOMAN AS A PERSON WAS NOT THE CAUSE OF MAN'S FALL INTO MATTER." Stone's occasional use of all capitalization for emphasis is a peculiarity of his writing style.

embrace the situation and move forward in the search for understanding what are our individual lessons and how can we successfully learn them.

To again state the obvious, the Yin and Yang cosmology is at odds with materialistic medicine and science, including pure Darwinism.[115] It makes sense of some troublesome neuroscience anomalies, as well as being supported by venerable spiritual teachings that assert the reality of a non-physical dimension of existence. With the Yin and Yang cosmology, a theoretical bridge is offered to those who are open to exploring new territory. The proof is in the pudding because the methods that flow from the theories actually do work.

So, welcome to the School of Life! We come into being to gain experience, and we have bodies for that purpose. Through trial and error we learn to transcend the ego (the illusion of true self confused with senses, body and mind) and seek deeper meaning. Thus self-healing becomes the quest for self-realization. A health system merges seamlessly into a profound spiritual and philosophical understanding.

---

[115] While it has many virtues, Darwinism has two main problems:

1. Darwin fails to fully account for some obvious universal impulses, such as our longevity imperative in old age, altruism and the quest for meaning. In contrast, the wisdom traditions offer clear explanations for all of these. Darwinism implies "law of the jungle" materialism, whereas Yin and Yang theory uplifts us to "the journey of the soul."

2. Primate embryology contradicts Darwin's theory. The Victorian era phrase "ontogeny recapitulates phylogeny" ("Haeckel's Law") has been thoroughly disproven, beginning with the observations of Dutch biologist Louis Bolk in the 1920s. As late-term fetuses, chimpanzees show uniquely human anatomical features, which then disappear as the chimp matures. This is the exact reverse of what should occur under Darwin's Natural Selection. For a complete summary, see Jos Verhulst, *Developmental Dynamics in Humans and Other Primates: Discovering Evolutionary Principles through Comparative Morphology.* Adonis, 2003.

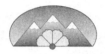

# Chapter 3

# Understanding Yin and Yang

*...Where to draw off excess energy and where to tonify or stimulate? Plus and minus, or "Yang" and "Yin" are the two main factors; why, where, when and how, the repeated questions and these no one fully answers, or the doctor could cure almost anything.*[116]

The study of Yin and Yang is so vast that exploration could take many pathways, from psychology to physical sciences, and using both ancient[117] and modern[118] sources.

The following four samplings from diverse sources show the true universality of the Yin and Yang idea:

***From Randolph Stone:***

Yang was the term used by the Ancient Chinese for this ever-expanding male principle. Yin was the female principle of contraction, concentration and resistance. These twin forces operate in all created forms, for without these two factors, neither function nor perpetuation of forms would be possible.

---

[116] R. Stone, *Polarity Therapy, Vol. 1.* CRCS, 1986. Book 1, p. 71.

[117] Alan Watts, *The Two Hands of God.* Collier Books, 1963.

[118] Fritjof Capra, *The Tao of Physics.* Shambala, 1975. There are many additional sources to add more detail; this was one of the first in the genre. Soon after came *The Dancing Wu Li Masters,* by Gary Zukav (Bantam, 1979).

There are three animating principles...They are the energies of the cosmos, by which man breathes and lives as a soul in human form.

1. [Yang] The fire energy of the sun is the warmth and expanding principle of motion in all living things.
2. [Neutral] Second is the hidden energy in the air as breath of life in the cosmic manifestation.
3. [Yin] The fluidic nature is a further step-down into the density of matter, it renews the finer energies for construction and maintenance of the body...[119]

## From Taoism:

Five thousand years ago, *The Yellow Emperor's Internal Classic*, the authoritative book of traditional Chinese medicine, released the Yin-Yang theory, which has guided the practice of traditional Chinese medicine ever since. To balance Yin and Yang is the major healing principle in Chinese medicine. Yin-Yang, the first Divine Universal Law, summarizes and describes everything in the universe, from the smallest to the largest, for both living and inanimate things. Everything can be divided into Yin and Yang...[120]

## From Western Science and Medicine:

At the very center of our being is rhythmic movement, a cyclic expansion and contraction that is both in our body and outside it, that is both in our mind and in our body, that is both in our consciousness and not in it. Breath is the essence of being, and in all aspects of the universe we can see the same rhythmic pattern of expansion and contraction, whether in the cycles of day and night,

---

[119] R. Stone, *Polarity Therapy, Vol. 1.* CRCS, 1986. Book 1, pp. 2, 16.

[120] Zhi Gang Sha, *Divine Soul Song of Yin Yang.* Institute of Soul Healing and Enlightenment, 2009.

waking and sleeping, high and low tides, or seasonal growth and decay. Oscillation between two phases exists at every level of reality, even up to the scale of the observable universe itself, which is presently in expansion but will surely at some point contract back to the original, unimaginable point that is everything and nothing, completing one cosmic breath.[121]

The wireless energies in the atom and in the solar system are the same as in the human body... The same energy which is in nature is also in us... The foundation for all therapies naturally rests upon the constitution of matter itself and its manifestation in organized forms as motion and function.[122]

## From Ayurveda and Traditional Chinese Medicine:

The principles of Yin and Yang are:
1) All things have two aspects, Yin and Yang;
2) A Yin or Yang aspect can be further divided into Yin and Yang;
3) Yin and Yang mutually create each other;
4) Yin and Yang control each other; and,
5) Yin and Yang transform into each other."[123]

## The Big Picture of Yin and Yang

Yin and Yang conveys an understanding of the grand design of the cosmology. Yang is the flow from spirit to matter and Yin is the return movement from matter back to spirit. Neither is "better" than the other; they both are essential for function and they are entirely interdependent. With diminished Yang, material security is reduced; with diminished Yin, spirituality is less accessible.

---

[121] Andrew Weil, *Spontaneous Healing*. Ballantine, 2000.

[122] R. Stone, *Polarity Therapy, Vol. 1*. CRCS, 1986. pp. 3, 11. Also, *Polarity Therapy, Vol. 1*, Book 3, p. 1.

[123] Ted Kaptchuk, *The Web That Has No Weaver*, McGraw-Hill, 2000. pp. 7-12.

The first inquiry about Yin and Yang is within ourselves. How is the balance internally? Are we able to flex and flow with events as a personal process? Are we able to take care of both material and spiritual levels of our lives?

A next level is interpersonal. How are we at both expressing our truth and also really hearing our partner's truth? The same questions extend to larger social situations. How does the group function in meeting the needs of the individual and also the larger needs of the whole? Even more widely, our whole society can be studied in terms of interplays between polarities such as structure and freedom, or opportunity and protection. The same patterns are there for us at every scale, if we pause to look for them.

To understand Yin and Yang, we begin with references to anatomy and morphology, guided by anatomist and embryologist Jaap van der Wal's teachings. "Anatomy" describes objective structure, whereas "morphology" describes activity and dynamic shaping under various conditions, a more subjective line of inquiry.

Morphology involves experiential performance more than flat facts, and its study derives from the larger topic of phenomenology, the study of consciousness. Using an experiential approach, we can see more than the anatomist, who tends to isolate the structure from the context. Yin and Yang are not pure structures; they are "process morphology." To comprehend Yin and Yang, we enter into the study of their most pure forms in the body, egg and sperm, and we study them as processes as well as tissues.

## Morphology of Yang

The most purely Yang anatomical parts in the body are those which are exclusively male, sperm cells. Sperm are active, numerous, dense, tiny and almost devoid of cytoplasm (the metabolically-active gel that gives cells their volume).

Lacking cytoplasm, they are relatively stable; with care they can be frozen, stored and manipulated without damage. Sperm are produced steadily in the male body and self-propel through rhythmic motion, guided by more subtle influences.

The whole sequence of the sexual process by which the purpose of sperm is fulfilled also reflects Yang attributes.[124] Safety as a prerequisite for arousal, passion as a gesture of involution, expansive density as a basis for delivery, forceful immersion as a gesture of contact and rhythmic movement as a pathway to fulfillment are all suggestive of the essential qualities of Yang.

The sperm cells' journey is fraught with obstacles such as problems with pH, temperature, distance and time. Even at the start, about 20 percent are not actually viable. As the self-propelled sperm approach the two entrances to the fallopian tubes, they must "choose" which fallopian tube to enter, possibly guided by subtle signaling from the female body and egg. In the end, the remaining sperm cells seem to exhibit a degree of mutual support, but eventually one will be admitted by a form of subtle agreement with the egg and the others will fall away having fulfilled their cooperative team mission.[125] The successful sperm cell will deliver its genetic

---

[124] G. van der Bie and M. Huber, Editors, *Foundations of Anthroposophical Medicine.* Floris, 2010. The fourth chapter, *Dynamic Morphology and Embryology* (p. 87), by Jaap van der Wal, MD, PhD, is a source for the sperm and egg information in this chapter.
Also see: Jaap van der Wal, *Human Conception: How to Overcome Reproduction?*, in *Biodynamic Craniosacral Therapy Vol. 1*, by Michael Shea. North Atlantic, 2007, Chapter 9, and *Human Conception: How to Overcome Reproduction: A Phenomenological Approach to Human Fertilization*, in *Energy & Character*, Vol. 33, Sept. 2004.

[125] Amusingly, the whole sequence bears resemblance to the action of American football, including the shape of the ball, the uniforms and helmets of the players, the swarming flow patterns of play, the layout of the field, design of the goal posts, cerebral head coaches and heroic scorers, cheerleaders on the sidelines, and many other attributes.

information and thereby "lives on" through its DNA contribution.

Like sperm cells, Yang is found in active, outgoing, goal-oriented, highly directional, risk-taking, materialistic kinds of activities. Sperm are produced steadily, not in cycles. Sperm cells are faced with making choices and then living with the consequences; therefore Yang has an inherent curiosity about its ability to respond to earlier actions ("response-ability"). Sperm are time-oriented; there is a limited window of time before the journey ends. The process of sperm has an urgency, and a competitive nature which manifests as individual effort but also as teamwork and playing a role in a group. Yang implies protection, as the chances of one sperm cell being successful depend on the support of the many. Yang is also inherently vulnerable, in that action has to be taken but the risks are high, and without a feeling of safety the whole process is jeopardized.

Yang is evident in all relationships. Yang is manifest in hierarchies and in the roles of speaker, leader, elder, teacher, father and husband. In public speaking, balanced Yang is easy to understand, attuned to the audience and not domineering. As a leader, balanced Yang is authoritative, decisive, focused and committed to the organizational goal, while also very skilled at receiving feedback and adapting its actions based on reflections. In elders, balanced Yang is protective and eager to guide. In teachers, balanced Yang is firm in providing structure and support. As fathers and mothers, balanced Yang creates steadiness and safety in the family, including modeling and creating mutual respect among family members. In husbands, balanced Yang is attentive, dependable, steady and responsible.

In a group, Yang will tend to be hierarchical and usually productive, but also vulnerable to making large-scale errors. For example a military organization (the epitome of Yang) can muster up enormous force and exert huge power, but if the leadership goes off track the negative results can be substantial because of the magnitude of the focused energy that is involved.

Of all adjectives, "responsible" is the first and foremost descriptor for balanced, healthy Yang. Just as the successful sperm must follow the subtle signals guiding its long journey, Yang is able to receive feedback and thereby channel its creative, impulsive surges of mental and emotional energy for beneficial purposes.

The understanding of Yang is complicated by the existence of two levels, a "Big Yang" and a "Little Yang." In human experience, Yang is the leader role, but in a larger sense, even the most powerful people are subservient to a higher power. As poet Bob Dylan put it, "You're gonna have to serve somebody."[126] "Big Yang" is "Father Sky," the power that created and sustains the universe and is the ultimate authority over all phenomena.

Meanwhile "Little Yang" refers to any person in a position of worldly authority. Ideally these leaders in society or the family are very respectful and clearly understand that their actions are secondary to the higher power. Major problems arise when "Little Yang" becomes delusional, imagining itself to be "Big Yang." The old adage, "absolute power corrupts absolutely," offered by British historian Lord Acton in 1861, can be interpreted in this light: "Little Yang" is susceptible to self-deception about its limitations. Napoleon's 1812 attack on Russia, ignoring the advice of his generals, is a prime example of how far off course unbalanced Yang can go; oblivious to a host of warnings and arrogantly believing he was invincible, he plunged ahead, with my teenage

---

[126] Bob Dylan, "Gotta Serve Somebody." *Slow Train Coming*. Columbia, 1979.

great-great-great grandfather in tow. Ninety percent of his army was lost and the whole region was devastated.

In the health care field, the direct action Yang players can go astray if they start believing they are omnipotent, and that the self-healing process is trivial compared to their pharmaceutical and surgical powers. The miracles of modern medicine might seduce some of its practitioners into believing that they are the true Source, a potentially disastrous error.

## *Morphology of Yin*

Yin is embodied in the female gender and its attributes can be studied by observation of the egg cell. The human egg is fundamentally hidden and mysterious, having only been "discovered" in 1835. Prior to that time, the process of conception was wrongly thought to be entirely the action of the sperm, with the female as a passive nutritive field. As a result, modern language has many biologically inaccurate terms. For example "reproduction" implies duplication, whereas new humans are unique. Similarly, "fertilization" implies the agricultural model of a complete seed placed in the passive ground, whereas in humans both sides are dynamic and the true "germ" appears only after fusion.

The egg is the largest cell in the human body, full of metabolic activity and cytoplasm. Its process is singular: usually only one egg at a time moves into a position that is receptive to the sperm. The egg is also cyclic, not steady-state: when its time comes, triggered by ovulation's complex hormonal changes, it is gently moved by cilia down the fallopian tube. It stimulates chemical changes to make the passages less hostile and more supportive of sperm, which seem to be guided by subtle gel-like filaments.

Jaap van der Wal emphasizes that conception involves mutual participation, not just "penetration" of the egg by the sperm, as conception is commonly described. The egg is fully participating, only in a more subtle way that involves reciprocal signaling by means of proteins, electro-chemical changes and some form of selectivity. Once the chosen sperm has entered, a powerful system-wide chemical signal creates dynamic changes throughout the body, which is now called a zygote. There is a quiet phase, the combining of DNA packages occurs, and the body for the new being begins to take shape with the first cell division.

Again using the biological story as a psychological metaphor, the attributes of the egg can be interpreted as attributes of Yin. Yin is fundamentally receptive, compellingly attractive and all-powerful as a basis for life. It is cyclical, hidden and mysterious. Its actions are metabolic and largely invisible to voluntary control, intertwined with the body's deep chemical interactions and not easily understood due to the enormous complexity of cellular and systemic processes.

Yin is paradoxical in many ways, exhibiting enormous power but through the indirect process of attraction and subtlety. Its magnetic energy is perhaps the strongest force in all biology. Yin is the base for the return pathway back to spirit, and therefore essential to the whole purpose of life. Yin can be interpreted as the "terra firma" foundation for an upward flow in the body from the mystery of the pelvis to the thoughtful observer perspective of the brain. Similarly, Yin shows the way for the pre-cognitive experience of the newborn on its journey to become the wisdom of the elder. Yin suggests evolution, pushing against the resistance of mother earth to find a path back to spirit. In this way Yin implies the progressive development of individual and collective consciousness. Yin's design is about creating a return to the source, so Yin tends to be more spiritually inclined and expressive while also often starting from a more emotional subterranean base.

In relationships, Yin manifests in nurturing, reflective activities, which may seem to be less powerful than Yang but are actually equally or more powerful. Ideally, balanced Yin will have a clear sense of values, an orientation to a higher power and an impulse to see life's big picture, in contrast to Yang's predisposition toward details and materialism. Yin's upward pointing flow in the body leads from the pelvis to the throat, which can express inner awareness as it talks about feelings and experiences. Thus Yin uses verbal expression to empty the system of metabolic and emotional debris accumulated from daily life. Females and young people are almost twice as likely to be diagnosed with mental-emotional disorders, possibly reflecting the pressure and complexity of the Yin role's challenges,[127] in addition to cultural misogyny problems. Yin processes feelings-level experience, in sympathy with the suffering of the world. Yin deals with paradoxes in search of meaning, while Yang is busy with worldly action.

Yin attributes are observed in the employee, the follower, the student, child, mother and wife. As employee, balanced Yin can give true, yet kindly feedback to keep impulsive Yang on track, like the passenger in a car who holds the map. As a follower, balanced Yin is the source of power in a democracy; a leader legitimately stays in office only with the consent of the voters. As a student, balanced Yin receives information but also is really the supreme power in the classroom, embodying the whole purpose of having an educational system. The student's (Yin) educational progress is the primary measure of the teacher's (Yang) success.

---

[127] USA Data from 2008:
http://www.nimh.nih.gov/statistics/pdf/NSDUH-SMI-Adults.pdf. These demographic groups are also more likely to be on the receiving end of exploitation and abuse, and therefore more likely to experience post-traumatic symptoms.

In children, balanced Yin learns how to be in the world by following the direction of the parents while also dealing with the resistance of childhood limitations. In a dysfunctional family the child is in a paradoxical bind, being too young to leave but too small to make changes. A common distortion happens when the insecure child becomes the dominant presence in the family.[128]

As mother or father, balanced Yin is nurturing and supportive, setting the subconscious emotional tone for the rest of the family. As wife, balanced Yin radiates safety, ease and wellness and renews her family's capability to go out and face worldly challenges. Because of the intimacy factor and the huge significance of relationships, Yin is especially challenged in a long-term intimate relationship, having to somehow reconcile "Little Yang" (limited capabilities of the partner) and "Big Yang" (unlimited potential of Spirit). The question is how to provide essential feedback without becoming a nagging "back-seat driver."

In a career context, Yin is about keeping your boss from making mistakes, not being a "Yes Man," while also advancing your own career: this makes quite a complex equation!

A normal conversation shows the paradoxical challenge of the Yin role. First one person speaks and the other listens. Ideally, they will then gracefully trade roles and the conversation will progress in a balanced and useful way. If one player has become fixated, he or she may continue talking obliviously, or only pretend to listen while the second person has a turn. Instead of listening, the dysfunctional person will be thinking of what to say next, instead of actually receiving what the second person is saying. Meanwhile the second person is put in a classic Yin bind,

---

[128] See Chapter 11 for more on Yin and Yang family dynamics.

whether to interrupt and point out the problem, or just go along with what is happening, to avoid conflict.

In terms of the challenge of Yin, the first option, interrupting to point out the problem, would be *True* and the second option, just indiscriminately accepting the imbalance, would be *Kind*. The first option has great value, correcting a problem before it increases, while the second option also has great value, keeping the peace. The optimum response would be to express the situation in such non-threatening language that the first person, the speaker, can receive the message and comprehend the problem. An insufficient Yin response would be to harshly criticize the offending speaker; an over-Yin response would be resentful acquiescence without saying anything. Unless Yin can find a balanced solution, or Yang can detect the problem, the conversation will probably not lead to new insights, deeper understanding or productive new action.

### *Yin and Yang Together*

All social interactions involve Yin and Yang action: giving and receiving, speaking and listening, leading and following. All the different roles played in life, including spouse, parent, employer and conversationalist, have identifiable Yin and Yang phases. Yin and Yang nourish and rely on each other: without the reflection of the moon, the sun may not know itself and may lose touch with reality; without the sun, the moon may be feel empty and cold. Even the sexual act and related biological processes exhibit rhythmic advance-retreat movements, another dance of Yang and Yin.

Dysfunctions of all kinds can be traced to fixations in this continual, polarized dance. From this perspective, there are only two imbalances, leading to four diseases: imbalances of Yin and imbalances of Yang, expressed as too much or too little of either.[129]

>"...when Yin or Yang are out of balance they affect each other, and too much of one can eventually weaken (consume) the other. Thus there are four possible states of imbalance: Preponderance (Excess) of Yin or Yang, and Weakness (Deficiency) of Yin or Yang.[130]

The thousands of physical, emotional and mental symptoms are just subsets of these, varying by location and degree of development, from acute to chronic. If Yin and Yang are in functional reciprocal tension, we will be able to smoothly and gracefully adapt appropriately to different life circumstances, moment by moment as they occur. In the great dance of life, we can lead or follow, according to the music and the context. More mental/emotional ease and coherence will result, with greater wellness as a natural by-product. As van der Wal puts it, "The stability is in lability," meaning that stability derives from flexibility.

This explanatory model provides a frame of reference to make sense of the seemingly random events in our lives. Health problems can seem to be entirely accidental, as if they fell from the sky for no apparent reason. Understanding Yin and Yang can be a revelation. Suddenly many baffling experiences become comprehensible. Yin and Yang offers an expansive understanding for effectively resolving physical, emotional, and mental problems. If Yin and Yang imbalances can be corrected, better health is likely to follow.

In addition, the functioning of the mind itself is also a polarized dance. Yang may initially have a more cerebral

---

[129] Michio Kushi and Phillip Jannetta, *Macrobiotics and Oriental Medicine: An Introduction to Holistic Health.* Japan Publications, 1991.

[130] Thomas Dehli, L.Ac., www.sacredlotus.com.

approach to life but be susceptible to materialism; this is observed in Yang's tendency to focus its attention on wealth, power, prestige and goal-oriented projects. Conversely, Yin may tend to operate on a more emotional level while also being more called to family connections, spirituality and understanding the big picture; this tendency can be observed in predominantly Yin interest in personal and spiritual growth seminars. Similar clues are everywhere in the popular media, including the content of advertising for Mother's Day and Father's Day, or the choice of Yin-attraction physical beauty for magazine covers; these are reminders about the universal subliminal presence of Yin and Yang in everyday life.

Yin and Yang together will have to overcome the problem of their differences. In an intimate relationship, both can wish the other could be more like themselves. One may want more physicality and the other more connection and communication; one may want more productivity while the other wants more vacations. One may want more autonomy while the other thrives on participation. In a Yang role we want to analyze and take action (antipathy), while in a Yin role we wish Yang could "really feel how we are feeling" (sympathy).

The dance is to adapt, compromise and embrace the differences. We are much less likely to be disappointed if our expectations are realistic. Wanting our partners to be like us is like "trying to find gold in a silver mine,"[131] as songwriter Elton John put it. Hopefully we can find some fulfillment of the impulse for like-minded sympathy with friends of similar positioning, such as a man with his sports buddies and a woman with her social circle, to reduce some of the pressure.

---

[131] Elton John, "Honkey Cat" on *Honkey Chateau*. Uni, 1972.

### *Plato's Cave: the Yin and Yang Version*

In the famous allegory in *The Republic*, the Greek philosopher pondered the concepts of perception, perspective and reality. In the dialogue, our normal perception is actually just our interpretations of shadows on a wall in the back of a cave, rather than arising from our direct experience. Plato described the enlightened philosophers as those who were freed from being chained to the cave wall, and who could go outside the cave, experience reality directly and form their own insights.

The Yin and Yang version of this story is that of two people in a room with a big south-facing window. Yin and Yang each have perspectives that affect their perception, experience and reality. The Yang perspective is that of a person standing at the window and looking into the room; the Yin perspective is a person seated in the center of room looking at the Yang and also simultaneously looking out the window. Over a long period of time, and unable to turn

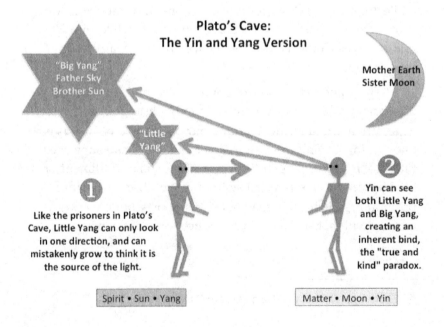

Plato's Cave:
The Yin and Yang Version

"Big Yang"
Father Sky
Brother Sun

Mother Earth
Sister Moon

"Little Yang"

① Like the prisoners in Plato's Cave, Little Yang can only look in one direction, and can mistakenly grow to think it is the source of the light.

② Yin can see both Little Yang and Big Yang, creating an inherent bind, the "true and kind" paradox.

Spirit • Sun • Yang

Matter • Moon • Yin

around to look through the window to see the real sun ("Big Yang"), the "Little Yang" position can mistakenly think that the light streaming into the room from the real sun is the result of its own power. For example, a delusional Louis XIV in France declared himself to be the Sun King. Healthy Yang can generate energy flowing to enliven the room but will never forget that there is a real sun and that larger forces are at work; dysfunctional Yang can become arrogant about its role and significance.

Meanwhile the Yin perspective is sitting in the room. Yin simultaneously observes the Yang entity performing the gestures of creativity and action, while also being aware of the "Big Yang," the plainly-visible real sun behind the Yang, outside the window. Thus Yin is in the fundamental bind described earlier: how to stay in relationship with human-level "Little Yang" while also continually being called and oriented to universal-level "Big Yang" by its inherent spiritual tendencies.

Again, the positioning for Yin is paradoxical and complex. Yin could discount the human-level (but thereby lose relationship), finding fault constantly, especially in comparison to the universal-level Yang. Conversely, Yin could become entranced by the human-level entity and lose its relationship with the higher forces. The solution is in the paradox, a both/and approach that honors both aspects of Yang. Quoting a student, van der Wal comments: "It is not either/or, it is not neither/nor, it is both, and that is more!"[132] The complexity of embracing such a paradox in real life situations makes functional Yin a high art, all the more difficult in a long-term relationship.

---

[132] Jaap van der Wal, lecture at Colorado School of Energy Studies. June 2012.

Yin has enormous power. From its position in the room, Yin holds a mirror that enables Yang to see what is happening behind, outside the window. Yin thus serves as a medium for Little Yang to see and know Big Yang. Additionally, having a mirror makes it possible for Yin to manipulate Yang. Yin can easily bend the mirror to create distortions in the reflection, similar to a carnival funhouse mirror that can make a short person seem tall. Because its perspective is limited to one-directional looking into the room, Yang is at the mercy of this powerful reflective function; great stress can arise when Yin reflects inaccurately or vindictively.

In a theater performance, who is more important? The writer, director or actor on the stage would seem to be obvious choices, but the critic in the audience, who will write a review for the next day's newspaper, actually wields decisive power to make the event, and even the creative team's whole career, a success or failure.

## The Dance of Yin and Yang

Throughout life, we all constantly experience both Yin and Yang roles, and it is crucial to wellbeing that we learn how to navigate the strengths and weaknesses of each role. Much suffering arises from being out of sync, or unable to respond appropriately, with the requirements of a specific situation. The challenge arises both internally, just within ourselves, and externally, with others.

If an event calls for Yang attributes, such as responsibility and action, and if we are unable to find a way to manifest these in a balanced way, stress and chaos will probably follow. Similarly, if an event calls for Yin action, trusting and yielding with discrimination and wise reflection, equilibrium may be threatened if Yin sensitivity is lacking. The more Yin and Yang dance gracefully together, the more coherence and prosperity will emerge in a system.

For example, successful driving depends on being adept in using both the accelerator (Yang) and the brakes (Yin), and being able to deploy the right method at the right time. In addition, successful travel depends on having a skilled driver (Yang) but also a skilled navigator (Yin). One without the other is likely to be problematic. This holds true both internally within the conduct of our own lives, and externally, in the context of a relationship, or more widely, within an organization.

At all scales from personal to social, the key is the dance, the ability to flex and flow as circumstances require. Yin and Yang are highly interactive in all cases. When one player shifts, the linked partner must follow at least to some degree, or the relationship will start to break down. Too much Yang tends to engender too much Yin, and too little Yin tends to engender too little Yang.

In many dysfunctional relationships, it may seem at first glance that one person is the primary problem. In actuality, the other partner is usually an equal player. The Macrobiotic aphorism, "The bigger the front, the bigger the back," [133] profoundly describes this fact. When interdependence is really understood, both partners are pushed to accept responsibility for the dysfunctions in the mutual system. When both people really see and accept their roles in the situation, they can stop blaming each other and begin the real work of consciously creating harmony.

The interdependent spirals of the Tao symbol each contain a smaller circle of the opposite color, a reminder that when maximum density or spaciousness is achieved, the reversal process will

---

[133] Verne Varona, *A Guide to the Macrobiotic Principles.* www.macrobiotics.co.uk/articles/principles.htm. The statement is attributed to George Ohsawa and earlier teachings of Judo.

inevitably begin. This insight can be observed in several scenarios, including birthing (the Yin fullness of full-term pregnancy contains the enormous muscular Yang forces of delivery) and development (the baby is super-Yang in vitality but super-Yin in dependence).

The lens of Yin and Yang provides ever-increasing insight as it is used to understand any field of inquiry. All systems have "interactive complementarity" in always having polarized factors that are constantly self-adapting to the other and thereby maintaining equilibrium, like a balance scale with small weights being added and subtracted on each side in order to keep an overall balance.

All fields of action, not just interpersonal dynamics, can be studied in this light: political, economic and historical studies lend themselves to Yin and Yang interpretations. Authors such as Leonard Schlain and Riane Eisler have explored the long-term reality of Western history struggling to manage the dysfunctional dance between Yang tyranny and suppression of Yin.[134] They note how balanced Yin is particularly difficult in the modern era, when Yang has been quite dysfunctional. After centuries of war and exploitation, we are rightfully skeptical about Yang. Observing the carnage of modern history, sensitive and idealistic Yang players might be tempted to shrink from any action at all, for fear of offending. This is a recipe for problems because society is then deprived of some of its potential best leaders.

### Neutral Is the Key to Functionality

The Neutral Principle is like the tipping point of a balance scale, and it has great leverage: the touch of a feather can shift the flow pattern. Poet T. S. Eliot eloquently approached the concept:

---

[134] Leonard Schlain, *The Alphabet Versus the Goddess*. Penguin, 1999. Also: Riane Eisler, *The Chalice and the Blade*. HarperOne, 1988.

*At the still point of the turning world.*
*Neither flesh nor fleshless;*
*Neither from nor towards; at the still point, there the dance is,*
*But neither arrest nor movement.*
*And do not call it fixity,*
*Where past and future are gathered.*
*Neither movement from nor towards,*
*Neither ascent nor decline.*
*Except for the point, the still point,*
*There would be no dance, and there is only the dance.*[135]

Neutral is the solstice and equinox in the seasons, or noon and midnight during a day. Neutral is seen in all life processes, just as Yin and Yang are also always present. In embryology, it is the gentle balanced dance between sperm cells and egg,[136] the "pre-conception attraction complex," that can go on for hours. Just after union, Neutral is found in the twenty-four hours of dynamic stillness before cell division. In breathing, the Neutral Principle is the moment of reversal at the fullness of inhalation and emptiness of exhalation. In the circulatory system, Neutral is the heart's resting moment between diastole and systole, and the micro-transfer point in the capillaries where the blood flow shifts from arteries to veins.

Neutrality is about balance, freedom, choice and the capacity to move in any direction. It is a powerful, ever-present aspect of all experience, although it is sometimes missed because of its subtlety and temporary nature. Neutral is the essential ability to shift as needed in the dance of Yin and Yang, according to conditions. Without a functional Neutral, we are likely to stay in the role of the moment out of habit or inertia, and miss our cues for change and growth.

---

[135] T.S. Eliot, *Burnt Norton*, in *Four Quartets, The Complete Poems and Plays: 1909-1950.* Harcourt Brace, 1971.

[136] See http://www.youtube.com/watch?v=ISoHUIGY1EM

All systems have all these three "poles," embedded within each other. In science class we learned that dividing a bar magnet creates new complete magnets, with new positive and negative poles, and a new neutral in the middle.[137]

In a relationship, neutral is represented by the ability to gracefully make the transition between giving and taking, speaking and listening, observing and participating, attending to self and attending to other.

Neutral is also found in ideals and intentions. These form a "third presence" that gives us a point of reference for decision-making and action. Having a common agreement in a relationship allows the partners to ebb and flow within a safe container, whereas without a clear agreement, a relationship is more vulnerable to drama and cycles of attraction-repulsion intensity.

Neutral happens in the "aha!" moment of new insight and the settling from busy active daytime awareness into quiet, reflective, regenerative rest. Neutral is also present at a time of transition, such as before the start, during the middle or after the end of an event.

In a business, neutral exists as an overall goal for all participants, such as the mission statement of an organization. Neutral in a business is also indicated by the ambience of the workplace, including the corporate culture that permeates the experience of work for the employees.

The heart has a special significance in the Neutral Principle. Embryologically, anatomically, morphologically and functionally, the heart is the primary organ of Neutral. The heart manages the body's polarized cycle of expansion and contraction and has justifiably been called the

---

[137] "Any Yin or Yang aspect can be further divided into Yin and Yang." Ted Kaptchuk, *The Web That Has No Weaver*, pp.7-12.

fundamental engine of life,[138] a status reflecting the power of Neutral. Stone considered the heart to be the subtle basis for all health.[139] He observed:

> The outward and inward currents must move in all fields if there is to be health and happiness... The heart center is the pivot for the circulation of these energies through the blood... and becomes the control center for these energies. [140]

The absence of a functional Neutral leads to fixation in either Yin or Yang. Lacking a Neutral, we feel that we have "no choice" in difficult situations, and we are highly susceptible to all the dangers of disturbed Yin and Yang. Stone considered "no choice" to be a primary warning sign of mental-emotional problems. He taught that working with the Neutral Principle is a top priority in the therapeutic process, and used both talk and touch to support the restoration of Neutral in all disease conditions.

In this context, Neutral marks the path to wellness. Neutral facilitates being adept at both Yin and Yang, and transitioning between the two as needed. If one can be skilled at recognizing which mode is relevant for each life situation, and graceful in switching into the appropriate part of any polarized field, life will become more coherent. Time spent cultivating sensitivity and awareness of Neutral will pay off in less fixation throughout life, and reduced risk of behaviors becoming habitual and unconscious. Practicing some stillness every day, such as taking time for meditation or relaxation, can refresh our flexibility and range of motion for coping with the next cycle of Yin and Yang challenges.

---

[138] Gary Zukav, *The Dancing Wu-Li Masters,* p. 206.

[139] Irving Dardik, *The Origin of Health and Disease, Heart Waves.* The Center for Frontier Sciences Vol. 6 No. 2, 1997.

[140] R. Stone, *Polarity Therapy, Vol. 1,* Bk 3, CRCS, 1986. p. 36.

The Yin and Yang approach is different from non-dual or transcendent approaches, and Neutral is also different. Yin and Yang is about having a full range of motion from full Yin to full Yang, not about trying to suspend that flow or float above it. Neutral is dynamic, providing a pivot effect that manages the swings of the pendulum between the polarities. "The outward and inward current must move in all fields if there is to be health and happiness" is Stone's call to embracing the differences, not trying to mute them. The sweet, temporary calm of Neutral may resemble transcendent or non-dual states, but it is really very different. We may walk on the north or south sidewalk back and forth to work, and we may cross the street occasionally as needed, but walking in the middle of the street is unlikely to be sustainable.

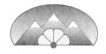

## Chapter 4

# Yin and Yang Archetypes

Now that we have a general sense of Yin and Yang, we can turn our attention to practical applications. A first step for this relates to recognition. We need an easy, common-sense way to identify Yin and Yang in everyday life, particularly in areas affecting mental and emotional health. For this purpose, archetypes and their related symbolism are immediately helpful, giving us a practical frame of reference for Yin and Yang in real life.

In the language of psychology, "archetype" refers to a model that has become widely popular and embedded in collective consciousness. An archetype takes on symbolic meaning. Psychologist and philosopher Carl Jung identified numerous states of being that he considered to be so universal that they existed in a "collective unconscious" or a primordial truth that is shared by everyone in their myths and dreams. These dreams inform and help us process our experiences. He identified archetypal personality types, such as the hero, the wise man, the great mother and the trickster. Jung also spoke of archetypal crucial events such as "initiation" and "rites of passage."

Archetypal figures populate the myths and fables of many cultures and eras. Even today, Zeus, Aphrodite, Apollo, Dionysius, Snow White, Pinocchio, Cinderella and countless other fictional characters can help modern people in the process of understanding their life experiences, serving as a quick reference to convey meaning with evocative abbreviations.

Historical characters also serve as archetypes, in both positive and negative lights, as either super heroes or super villains, and sometimes both. Attila the Hun, Genghis Khan, Joan of Arc and Queen Elizabeth I have "identities" in the popular imagination that convey more meaning than just their actual biographies.

Early pioneers in psychology, like Freud, used archetypal characters such as Oedipus and Narcissus to explain instinctual behaviors. Several systems of psychological thought have also embraced archetypes as a way to describe common states. For example, among siblings, therapist Virginia Satir described how there might be a family hero, a rebel, a scapegoat, a mascot or a lost child.[141]

In popular culture, Tarot and Enneagram systems use archetypes to help describe character styles and events in life.

Even contemporary characters can become archetypes in popular culture. Athletes, movie stars and politicians become iconic examples of particular traits, with meanings that are well known and easily recognized. For example, "Marilyn Monroe" readily conjures up a whole cascade of psycho-emotional impressions.

Yin and Yang counseling has its own set of archetypes that serve to guide understanding of life's experiences. For the Three Principles, the archetypes begin with the Sun and Moon. The Sun is the primary archetype for Yang in a balanced state, and the Moon is the primary archetype for Yin in a balanced state. The Sun is an outgoing, heating, constant,

---

[141] Virginia Satir coined these terms; for a modern example, see Lynne Forrest, *Which Child Were You? Roles by Birth.*
http://www.lynneforrest.com/articles/2011/06/which-child-were-you-roles-by-birth/

active force, while the Moon suggests a reflective, cooling, cyclic, quiet process. Versions of these archetypes are found in virtually all ancient cultures, and on every continent. In India, *Ha* and *Tha* mean Sun and Moon, hence *Hatha Yoga* can be translated as the "Union of Yang and Yin."

Archetypal names are also available for Yin and Yang imbalances, and these have a long history of usage in psychology. For Yang, the *Tyrant* and the *Wimp* archetypes suggest the experience of too much and too little Yang (also known as Yang Full and Yang Empty) functioning. For Yin, the *Critic* and the *Doormat* can describe the experience of too little and too much Yin, respectively.[142] These terms give quick, emotionally engaging, meaningful words to use when trying to identify Yin and Yang in action, especially in relationships. Since relationships are a primary source of psychological distress (to be discussed in the next chapter), these easy archetypes are a shorthand language to guide repair.

## How to use archetypes

This understanding can be quite enlightening. When relationships are not going well, common psychological terms such as Oedipus complex and Avoidant attachment style may add to the confusion. In contrast, Sun/Tyrant/Wimp and Moon/Doormat/Critic cut to the central issues, in plain colloquial language that everyone understands. Clients do not need a complicated theoretical model to understand the meaning. The most frequent application for the archetypes is in the two-chair process,[143] in which the client has a tangible, embodied experience of an archetype and its complementary

---

[142] Users of these particular terms include Family Systems Therapy, Recovery Therapy and Christian pastoral counselors. From Polarity Therapy, the same terms are found in Morag Campbell's *Sink the Relation Ship: Transform the Way You Relate* (Masterworks, 2010).

[143] Described in Chapter 10.

unbalanced correlate, in a memorable summary. The words are intentionally extreme in terms of impact; their "psycho-semantic" force can help push through inertia and habitual resistance in order to elevate self-awareness.

Once the archetypal state is experienced consciously, as a psychological and embodied experience, and the process is named, the chances of more conscious self-regulation go up significantly. When the same dynamics begin to be expressed in a future situation, there will be an additional capacity to self-correct and ward off the negative consequences of the unbalanced state.

Many relationship problems arise from not knowing what to expect. The Sun/Tyrant/Wimp and Moon/Doormat/Critic archetype system makes it simple. If, for example, I am an employee, my job is to manifest Moon and avoid Critic or Doormat. As a father, I need to manifest Sun and avoid Tyrant or Wimp. In a relationship, I refer to the appropriate set of archetypes to form expectations of my partner's behaviors. These are likely to be the reverse, not the same, as my own set of tasks. Thus I am helped to bypass the common problem described above, expecting my partner to be like me, a situation known as "de-polarization."[144] Yin and Yang implies attuning to complementarity more than similarity.

Similar exaggerated language occurs when the Edgar Rice Burroughs character declares, "Me Tarzan, you Jane!" Setting aside its chauvinistic modern interpretations, Tarzan was an effective archetype for conveying the meaning of the lost primitive purity of masculinity in an alienated and repressed Victorian society, including the sense of highly charged sexual potency that accompanies strongly polarized interpersonal dynamics. In just four words, Tarzan's short

---

[144] David Deida, *Intimate Communion: Awakening Your Sexual Essence*. HCI, 1995.

phrase re-established the simple reality of *"Vive la différence"* and evoked a contrast between modern and primitive states. Tarzan's abiding popularity, spanning decades, confirms that the character is subliminally on target for his audience.

A more modern expression of strongly polarized dynamics in corporate and political culture is represented by the aphorism, "Lead, follow or get out of the way," attributed to Thomas Paine, a leader of the American Revolution. The phrase also illustrates the delicate challenge of Yang, in that it

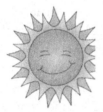

**Archetypes of Yin and Yang**

| Key Topics | YANG : SUN | YIN: MOON |
| --- | --- | --- |
| **Too much** | Tyrant: domineering | Doormat: self-denying |
| **Too little** | Wimp: paralyzed | Critic: nagging |
| **Essence** | Action: motor | Reflection: sensory |
| **Purpose** | Manifestation: "involution" | Spiritualization: "evolution" |
| **Process** | Action, steady output | Attraction, fill & empty cycles |
| **Main Task** | Responsibility | Contentment |
| **Roles** | Elder, boss, teacher | Younger, employee, student |
| **Danger** | Illusion of materialism | Fixation in empty or full |
| **In Weakness** | Becomes ...aholic, oblivious | Can't be both true and kind |
| **Physical areas** | Heart, back, eyesight | Digestion, lymphatics, cancer |
| **Challenge** | Act and learn from mistakes | Reconcile Little & Big Yang |
| **Expression through** | Physicality, doing | Emotionality, being |
| **Perceptual process** | Antipathy, witness | Sympathy, participant |

has been publicly quoted by such modern Yang-full personalities as George Patton, Ted Turner and Mitt Romney.

How archetypes are used in Yin and Yang counseling is fairly simple, especially using the two-chair method described in Chapter 10. I had a male client in his mid-30s who sought marriage counseling. Sitting in the first chair, he felt depleted and disoriented, but when he imagined his wife in the second chair, he immediately felt himself cringing and "walking on eggshells." When he switched chairs to be in her position he could feel her frustration and bitterness. Subsequently we talked about what he had felt; he could readily identify the exchange as a wimp/critic scenario. Just a few words conveyed a wealth of meaning. I was careful to keep the conversation free of judgment, blaming or shaming, following with the guiding Yin and Yang theme that all behaviors are intelligent attempts to maintain equilibrium. The situation was de-pathologized, and he could see that he and his wife had slipped into some old habits, familiar because their parents had done something similar, and their relationship was being subtly undermined.

When he went home he had a great conversation with his wife and they mutually saw what was happening: the "light went on" for them and they resolved to apply themselves to be aware and re-align more with sun and moon. Armed with identifiable categories, they had a clearer idea of what to do and what not to do with each other, and what to expect from the other. Neither one wanted to be in the dysfunctional category, for themselves or for each other. By the time of the next session, the situation had improved and he was ready to take additional steps to correct other imbalances in the relationship. Within four more meetings the domestic problems had been resolved enough for the sessions to be discontinued. The simplicity and effectiveness of this approach thus helped a young family with limited resources improve their situation without long-term counseling.

As stated in Chapter 1, naming a condition increases self-awareness. Of course, just naming something does not change it. There is a gap between an unconscious autonomic state and the conscious intention to change that state; one cannot simply tell the unconscious to stop being anxious. The conscious function does not reach deeply enough into the subconscious function to be able to change an autonomic state directly. However, if there is a script, we can read the lines, and reading lines appropriate for a balanced state tends to engender a more harmonious response in the other person. This is a "top-down" approach to therapy, using strategies that gently shift the more subconscious experience. Through repetition the brain can re-wire itself into a less troubled configuration. The same sequence has been studied in meditation, in which a particular discipline, such as watching the breath or the repetition of a mantra, is practiced repeatedly and the underlying landscape starts to change.[145]

With recognition, long-term relationships can be a practice to gently re-mold underlying states. Mutual intention and gentle repetition gradually cause real change. The process can feel artificial at first, as if a Yang-role player is just acting the role of the Sun, and artificially reducing the incidence of tyrant or wimp. To some degree, however, we can "fake it until we make it." If we can stay with the practice, our involuntary system gradually re-configures its processing, and we become what we envisioned, instead of continually playing out the behaviors that we inherited from our parents. By building up consistency in functional behaviors, our subconscious naturally begins to trust in their presence. If children are present, they will imprint the new

---

[145] The Dalai Lama, *Destructive Emotions: How Can We Overcome Them?*. Bantam, 2003. Narrated by Daniel Goleman.

programming and be released from ancestral dysfunctional patterns, at least to some extent. This topic will be expanded later in Chapter 10.

## Yang Imbalance Archetypes

"Too much Yang" (also known as "Yang full") dominates Yin and becomes oblivious to feedback. People with too much Yang tend to be forceful and insensitive, expressing themselves in domineering, willful, loud, intimidating styles, such as "Type A" behaviors. The behavior may be disguised or even intentionally hidden, but a tyrant is readily recognizable by an astute observer. The tyrant may show symptoms such as being compulsive, agitated and hyperactive. In a relationship or family, the tyrant will tend to bully and dominate the other members of the household, especially the partner. Tyrants are not able to receive feedback; instead they plow ahead regardless of the effects on others.

The inverse state, too little Yang (also known as "Yang empty"), appears as shy, withdrawn and suffering from low energy. They lack a capacity for risk-taking and bold decisive action. Their facial expressions may also seem dissociated or avoidant; they may not be able to look others in the eye. In a wimp archetype, we may avoid taking chances or distract ourselves to avoid responsibility. In a relationship, the wimp will be low-energy and acquiescent, trying to avoid conflict but also generally not stepping up to take an active role in the family's needs. The wimp may also "disappear" from responsibility through distractions, intoxication, absorption in work or similar activities. Generally, the presence of an addiction or low willpower suggests a Yang-deficient condition.

When a person is in a Yang role (such as being a teacher, parent, or boss), the healthy intention is to avoid the extremes of too much or too little. Action and decisiveness are strengthened by the capacity to receive feedback and adapt to changing circumstances. Balanced Yang follows through with dependability and steadiness. Part of the therapeutic process is to intentionally practice actions that are closer to the optimum, even if doing this feels awkward at first.

## Yin Imbalance Archetypes

Again, the Yin position is complex and involves some paradox. The challenge is how to be both true and kind in relationship with Yang, and how to maintain contact with equanimity in the presence of Yang's behaviors and activities. Yin faces a difficult task of balancing these potentially contradictory actions.

"Doormat" is the condition of too much Yin ("Yin full"), when we yield excessively and comply without discrimination, thereby being "kind" in a relationship but not "true." The doormat puts up with abuse particularly from a tyrant-type partner. Having a tendency toward submissive positioning can lead to feeling like a victim in a difficult situation. Doormat types may feel that they are magnets for predators and abusers, and they may need to get to the sidelines and regroup before continuing activities. Operating under a self-aware, balanced Moon script can do wonders for relational coherence without necessarily having to totally excavate all the ancestral garbage that preceded the imbalanced condition.

This archetypal character can be found in a family, obviously, but also in a corporation, team, social group or club. Doormats may keep a low profile, but underneath the surface, they struggle with anger at authority figures, especially their partners and close associates.

Being overly submissive for a long time is actually dangerous, because at a critical tipping point, the condition may swing to the other extreme and all the pent-up anger may erupt. "Revenge of the Yin" is a phrase for when pent-up resentment boils over. The indiscriminate rage of the French Revolution's Reign of Terror is an example of a large-scale Revenge of the Yin sequence. Innocent bystanders were badly hurt. Pent-up long-term doormat types need special attention to avoid being swept up in "mob psychology," backing away from explosive situations until they have time to regroup. For example, a long-suffering employee may snap and commit workplace violence; with recognition of the condition, we may be able to persuade our clients to back away from the situation. In another example, a long-suffering family member may suddenly lash out, not only at the tyrant, but also at the whole family even though some of the others were not directly part of the problem.

Too little Yin manifests as the critic archetype, a person who is hyper-complaining and cannot be satisfied. The critic could be said to be true but not kind in interacting with others, quick to express discontent and say what is wrong (and the criticisms may actually be correct, but not delivered gracefully or effectively), but slow to offer encouragement and nurturing. Critics (too little Yin) are often linked with wimps (too little Yang) in cycles of mutual dysfunction that eventually may lead to illness. The critic can be nagging, manipulative, emotionally cold and constantly complaining, to the detriment of everyone nearby.

### Dysfunctions in Pairs

The four dysfunctions all put pressure on nearby players. Tyrants attract and encourage doormats, critics create wimps, and the reverse sequences are equally possible. An analogy is the action of walking: when one foot steps forward, the pressure is naturally on the other foot to make the next move. The effect is like a vortex, drawing two partners from an initial subtle hint of the imbalance into ever-deepening stress.

In dysfunctions, the main attributes of Yin and Yang become liabilities. We lose the capacity to recognize and address the other person's needs; unmet needs of Yin and Yang become weapons, with Yin often using words and Yang using physical action or avoidance and withdrawal.

In dysfunctional dynamics, something eventually has to give; the relationship ends or some major interruption arises, such as an illness or accident. Healing begins when one of the individuals initiates a shift toward a functional state and encourages the other to move as well. One has a fresh insight and initiates change, and the other cares enough and has enough emotional resources to overcome inertial resistance and respond, maintaining overall balance in the system.

In the dynamic of couples in relationship, the effect is direct. Often, the one who sought help takes the first step with the other sometimes reluctantly following. In groups, such as a workplace, a correction arises when a player on either Yin or Yang side finds a way to communicate the dysfunction to the other side, such as when an employee has particular access to a boss to bring awareness to the problem without a destructive reaction, finding a way to be both true and kind in the process. Once the state has been named, the healing process can begin.

## *The Importance of Relationships*

Completing the Yin and Yang discussion, the importance of relationships is clear. Aside from our own inner self-respect and integrity, there is no higher impact on health than the experience of our significant relationships. If a client has a health problem, including mental, emotional or physical, a few open-ended questions about what is happening in intimacy often reveals a bind of some kind; a Yin and Yang dysfunctional archetype is likely to be present.

In any relationship, the basic dualistic arrangement is partially externalized. Instead of a purely internal duality, in a relationship we exist in an externally polarized field with another person. We will have Yin and Yang positioning depending on numerous factors. Generally the masculine, older, bigger, more directive position is pulled to be more Yang, and the reverse applies for Yin.

A system with two people making up one field together is complicated. It is no wonder that real intimacy (being vulnerable and receiving direct feedback) can be so challenging. A disturbance in the other person, who cannot really be controlled, is directly affecting the first person's energetic stability and coherence. As stated above, people in intimate relationships can abruptly act in ways that are inconceivable to those who know them. The news headlines often show this effect, in reports of severe domestic violence. Being in close proximity to a dysfunctional person can make the other physically or emotionally ill. A family can seem to explode in chaos without knowing why. The answer is in the subtle interpersonal dynamics of the central pair. Correct the main polarized field and a healing process is likely to follow.

In the first part of his poem, *The Second Coming*, William Butler Yeats provided an eloquent summary of the interplay between Yin and Yang, including a vivid depiction of what happens when the polarity relationship breaks down:

> *Turning and turning in the widening gyre*
> *The falcon* [Yin] *cannot hear the falconer* [Yang];
> *Things fall apart; the centre cannot hold;*
> *Mere anarchy is loosed upon the world,*
> *The blood-dimmed tide is loosed, and everywhere*
> *The ceremony of innocence is drowned;*
> *The best lack all conviction, while the worst*
> *Are full of passionate intensity.* [146]

---

[146] W. B. Yeats, "The Second Coming." *The Collected Poems of W. B. Yeats*. MacMillan, 1956.

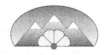

# Chapter 5

# Hierarchy of Action Fields

One more theoretical piece is needed to fill in the basic foundation for Yin and Yang psychotherapy, the "Hierarchy of Action Fields."

The most well known version of a psychological hierarchy model is Abraham Maslow's Hierarchy of Needs.[147] Maslow taught that people's essential requirements for wellbeing existed in a progressive continuum including five needs, with later stages being dependent on successful attainment of the preceding stages:

- Basic physiology (hunger and thirst)
- Safety (freedom from threat)
- Belonging (familial and social connection),
- Esteem (self-worth)
- Self-actualization (self-purpose)

This model correlates well with a Polarity version derived from the Five Elements. In Stone's version, the stages are similar but not exactly identical:

- Safety and material survival (Earth)
- Connection and belonging (Water)
- Action (Fire)
- Idealism and inspiration (Air)
- Self-expression and self-realization (Ether)

---

[147] Abraham Maslow, *A Theory of Human Motivation*. CreateSpace, 2013. Originally published in 1943.

One more example reinforces the notion of a hierarchy of needs. In Developmental Bodynamics, Lisbeth Marcher identifies a similar set of stages for babies to move through in order to attain healthy maturity:[148]

- Existence
- Needs
- Autonomy
- Will
- Love

The hierarchy of needs idea points to an interesting side discussion, specifically relating to what psychotherapy is aiming to accomplish with different populations. Counseling for an individual in desperate circumstances, such as constant physical threat or severe poverty, will be different from the therapy methods for a person who is physically secure.

At each stage in the hierarchy, the immediate focus is just the next step up the stairs, not necessarily trying to get all the way to the top in one leap. At the bottom of the staircase, to stay with the imagery, basic needs are the agenda; at the top, the deepest mysteries of life's meaning can be contemplated, to the degree that there is a steady foundation in place. The Yin and Yang model guides the building of a foundation so that the evolutionary progress has stability and longevity for enduring development.

In a Yin and Yang version of the hierarchy of needs, a different approach is used. Here, the "fields of action" are the primary focus. In this approach, "hierarchy of needs" is reinterpreted to mean "needs of orderly living." They are studied in *descending* order, with the most significant and higher-impact issues at the top, while the less significant follow at the bottom of the model. The hierarchy of action

---

[148] Lisbeth Marcher, *Body Encyclopedia: A Guide to the Psychological Functions of the Muscular System*. North Atlantic, 2010.

fields enables us to efficiently prioritize the psychotherapy inquiry, removing the biggest pebbles from the client's shoe first.

### Hierarchy of Fields of Action
- **Self** (sense of self-worth, value and integrity)
- **Intimate Relationship** (relationship with a spouse, partner, significant other)
- **Family** (children, parents, siblings, extended family)
- **Work** (career and vocational relationships)
- **Play** (recreational and entertainment activities)

We all have various fields of action in which we experience life's challenges. The different fields have different impact levels and need to be addressed in sequence. People mishandling a high-impact field with dysfunctional Sun and Moon behaviors are much more likely to experience disturbances and health problems, while those having problems in a low-impact field of action may be able to persist for years without a breakdown. When there is a disturbance in a low-impact field of action, I gently ask questions about current events in the client's life, particularly in the inner three rings. Doing a "hierarchy inventory" can greatly expedite the therapeutic process.

Typically, I ask a client who has a particular health problem, "When did this condition first appear and what was going on in your life in the months prior to the first symptoms?" A theory for the condition's context may be revealed by this kind of inquiry. Often, when a condition is more fully understood, the symptoms begin to recede, as if they were serving as a "wake-up call" to address some imbalance in life experience.

Yin and Yang therapy is not alone in such modes of inquiry, but the addition of this hierarchy model provides great efficiency. Clients often say that they are amazed at how quickly core issues are identified, often in the first half of the first session. The efficiency arises from the model and the method, another confirmation of the validity of the system.

Similarly, the hierarchy of action fields model gives a sequence for therapeutic support, as we guide clients to explore the highest-impact levels first. Lower-level issues and conflicts may naturally resolve when upper-level changes are made.

A coherent life arises naturally from attending to each field of action, in this sequence of priorities, from core to periphery. One must not elevate one field of action above the more central others, for example children/parents before spouse, work before family, or play before work. We watch for clients who put the fields of action steps out of order, such as when work activities are given more time, attention and resources than intimate relationship challenges, a so-called "workaholic" behavior. The therapeutic sequence ideally builds coherence from the center out, by conscious allocation of attention, time and resources to the fields in their proper order.

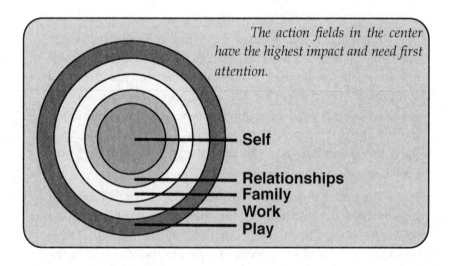

*The action fields in the center have the highest impact and need first attention.*

Self

Relationships
Family
Work
Play

## *The Self Field of Action*

In this context, "self" refers to our own inner values and attitudes; actions counter to our deepest beliefs can create tremendous turmoil. Lack of integrity or coherence at this level undermines everything else; for example, living a lie that violates fundamental values is corrosive to intimate relationships and life in general. For the inner circle of self, the relationship is between one's normal waking consciousness and a "higher power." This higher power may be our experience of our true nature, or a set of values that guides our daily actions.

Disturbances at the level of self can originate from within, such as in lying or cheating, or from outside, such as when we feel victimized and cannot find completion or re-establish balance. For example, if we experience some terrible betrayal, tragedy or loss and cannot resolve the feelings of anger at the injustice of extreme events, we may develop a "broken relationship with God," whatever that means to us. These disturbances may show up a few months later in destructive behaviors or physical health problems.

For the core level of self, it is useful to ponder our values. We can ask ourselves questions such as, "What is actually most important?" and, "What is the real purpose of life?" The answer to these questions will vary for each person, but often the question has never fully been contemplated consciously. When core values are actively protected, we feel stronger and more able to meet life's challenges. In contrast, feeling guilty, angry, fearful, remorseful or deficient in key areas can reduce our capacity to be in an intimate relationship, particularly if secrecy is part of the process. A self-inventory of this most central field of action can be very revealing and supportive of putting our lives in order.

The layer of self also includes issues relating to self-esteem. In Pia Mellody's system (Chapter 13), self-esteem issues arise when the child is denied experiences of being valued, leading to Pia Mellody's phrase "permission to be precious."[149] Many psychology systems have confirmed the primary importance of self-esteem as a cornerstone of all other layers of mental-emotional function. As visionary counselor Edgar Cayce stated, "There must be first the quiet or harmony in one's own self if one would find harmony with the association with others."[150]

As discussed before, having a sense of purpose in life is directly connected to longevity, heart health, immune system function and other important indicators. Stone thought that a clear sense of purpose should be elevated in the healing process and made a factor in treatment.

The Self layer also implies the "Journey of the Soul." As Tao Master Zhi Gang Sha says, "The Soul is the Boss,"[151] meaning that if the expression of the soul's purpose is blocked, the rest of life will become problematic.

## The Relationships Field of Action

"Intimate relationship" refers to the "significant other," or spouse, particularly a person with whom intimacy is happening. A Yin or Yang dysfunction at this level has major effects. Therefore the circumstances pertaining to the client's intimate relationships are given high priority, including specific recommendations for common intimacy experiences. Stress at home is a subtle factor in many health conditions. Asking the right questions using this model often cuts right to the chase. Perhaps the day will come when people in any kind of health crisis will routinely be asked, "What is happening in your life, and especially in your relationships?"

---

[149] Pia Mellody, *Permission to be Precious*, Audio CD set. Encore, 1987.

[150] Edgar Cayce Reading 1540-7. See www.edgarcayce.org.

[151] See www.drsha.com

Family is a secondary layer in the Relationships area; it is less impactful than the main partner experience. Family includes our children and parents, in that order. If children are having problems, the impact will be significant, and the same can be true when our relationship with parents is stressed, but these impacts are smaller compared to those from turbulence with one's intimate partner. We need a high focus on how to manage the birth process and early childhood responsibilities, and also a strong focus on how to care for the aging and dying. The often severe toll of divorce on children also deserves our attention; the distress of children subsequent to a client's divorce can cause problems that last for decades. There are many variations on this theme, to be discussed in more detail in Chapters 10 and 11.

The sequence of first caring for the children, then caring for the parents is significant. The primary attention needs to be "downstream," to the next generation. Reversing this order, such as when adults neglect children due to the strain of caring for needy parents, leads to more long-term problems as the children try to mature with only part of the necessary resources.

### *The Career Field of Action*

Career problems have a relatively smaller impact. Financial problems are highly stressful; however, some of the impact relates to the effects on a person's sense of self-worth (highest impact) or relationships with key people (such as spouses and children). Self and Spouse are much higher-impact fields of action compared to stress at the workplace. For example, poverty is extremely debilitating on all levels but the impact on self-esteem and relationships may cut more deeply than the experience of low income.

In general, vocational experiences fall within the territory of Yang. Supportive inquiry about the Sun archetype is likely to be helpful when there is disturbance in the career field of action. The basic nature of Yang is about manifestation, including being able to acquire adequate financial security and a sense of personal fulfillment in working life. Some people who place a high value on spirituality may find themselves becoming Yang-deficient over time, enjoying meditative states and retreats but unable to consistently pay the bills; this condition responds well to Yin and Yang counseling once the client understands the underlying problem.

The career theme is in play when we are unemployed or have an unfulfilling career, when there are arguments and frustrations with supervisors, co-workers or employees, or when our career is not moving forward as desired. Ideally, we can leave these stresses at work and return to a coherent and integrated home life that acts as a buffer against the excessive impact of disagreeable workplace experiences. However, we may need help to do this.

### The Recreation Field of Action

The most distant field of action, in terms of impact, is recreational activity. Therapeutically it is almost an afterthought and rarely a factor in health problems. Recreational activities include those that are for amusement and play, such as sports (participatory or spectator) and hobbies. Issues arising at this level are often a nuisance but usually not threatening to one's health. Problems arise when these activities absorb an inordinate amount of time, compared to the time and attention devoted to the inner fields of action, or if the pursuit of perfection in them becomes compulsive. In these cases the issue is probably not with the recreational activity itself; it is with the other field of action that is being avoided. Allocation of time and attention needs to match the hierarchy, or problems are likely to follow.

Problems also arise when there is no time for play at all. The word "recreational" can be interpreted quite literally, and there are many health benefits in having fun and trying new activities just for inspiration, learning, enjoyment and refreshment. Playful novelty nourishes and enhances our brains for optimum functioning and wards off degenerative cognitive problems.[152]

The notion of work and play has attracted interesting comments, such as metaphysician Rudolf Steiner's advice that the difference between the two should be dissolved. In an ideal world, work and play are actually the same feeling of inquisitive engagement and meaningful service to society. In our early working life, we are inclined to take whatever is available, just for the compensation; later in life we may feel more flexibility and seek an occupation that feels compatible with our personality and purpose. Poet Robert Frost wrote:

> *My object in living is to unite*
> *My avocation and my vocation*
> *As my two eyes make one in sight.*
> *Only where love and need are one,*
> *And the work is play for mortal stakes,*
> *Is the deed ever really done*
> *For Heaven and the future's sakes.*[153]

## Summary

The theme here is about priorities and taking care of business in hierarchical order. To avoid dealing with difficulties at home, I might stay late at the office. I might justify and rationalize this behavior as a financial necessity, but the hidden agenda is avoiding essential challenges. In the Yin and Yang approach, putting life's actions back in order is a top priority. If we take care of self and other, the rest will probably begin to sort itself out.

---

[152] Science News, *Pure Novelty Spurs The Brain.* Aug. 27, 2006.

[153] Robert Frost, "Two Tramps in Mud Time." *The Poems of Robert Frost.* Coyote Canyon, 2009.

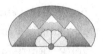

# Chapter 6

# The Autonomic Nervous System

A true revolution is unfolding in health care with the rise of a more accurate understanding of the autonomic nervous system (ANS) and comprehension of its significance. The ANS was under-appreciated in psychology's early history.[154] Now we can say with certainty that most health problems, including psychological conditions, arise from ANS functions. Understanding the ANS is crucial to clinical effectiveness because the ANS and its "survival imperative" form the substrate for most behaviors and responses, including the immune system. According to Franklyn Sills,

> The autonomic nervous system is pivotal in the regulation of survival functions. Its importance cannot be overstated. The entire field of post-traumatic stress disorder certainly falls in its scope, along with most degenerative diseases, all stress-related situations, autoimmune diseases, and many others.[155]

Randolph Stone anticipated the revolution, describing the difference between voluntary and involuntary function and giving specific, effective methods for ANS support.

---

[154] Roy Porter, ed., *Medicine: A History of Healing.* Ivy Press, 1997. Chapter 6, "Healing and the Mind," gives a concise history of psychology, and the autonomic nervous system is never mentioned.

[155] Franklyn Sills, *Foundations of Craniosacral Biodynamics, Vol. 2.* North Atlantic, 2012. p. 527.

No relaxation of the voluntary nervous system and muscles can take place as long as the involuntary ones are locked and tense... Merely telling the patient to relax is useless. Tension usually goes much deeper than the voluntary muscular control.[156]

The ANS controls most of the body's involuntary activity, including the essential survival functions including circulation, respiration, digestion, metabolism, daytime alertness and mobilization, nighttime sleep and regeneration, and more. In addition, the ANS operates our stress responses, such as "fight-or-flight" as well as "freeze." The ANS has the goal of assuring survival, achieved through constant adaptation to changing conditions. This biological imperative is too important to be left to chance or voluntary control; the ANS is the hard-wired, fail-safe mechanism to avoid disaster.

Most health care professionals will answer the question, "What is the ANS?" by saying it is the reciprocal action of

## Summary: Old & New Views of the ANS

| Aspect | Old View | New View |
|---|---|---|
| Importance | Under-appreciated | Supreme Importance |
| How many parts? | **Two** (Sym-, Parasym-) | **Three** (Social, Sym-, Parasym-) |
| Action | **Reciprocal** (Sym- and Parasym- are seesaw, on/off) | **Sequential** based on phylogeny (evolutionarily newer vs. older) |
| ANS Categorization of Vagus Nerve | **All Parasympathetic** | **Mixed** (Ventral branch of Vagus is not Parasympathetic) |
| Therapy goal | Parasympathetic relaxation | Re-establish newer branches |
| Babies | Feel no pain and have no memory | ANS is hyper-sensitive & records experiences, particularly betrayals |
| Popular characterization | Parasympathetic "**Rest & Rebuild**" Sympathetic "**Fight-or-Flight**" | Differentiate "normal functions" from "stress responses" |

[156] R. Stone, *Polarity Therapy, Vol. 1.* CRCS, 1986. p. 85.

sympathetic and parasympathetic branches, particularly fight/flight for the sympathetic nervous system and rest/rebuild for the parasympathetic nervous system. They may also add that a goal of therapy is to reestablish a parasympathetic state and reduce the over-expression of a sympathetic state, which is corrosive for the body if sustained for too long. This description has been around so long that it is accepted without question and recycled in textbooks and classrooms. However new information shows that the familiar explanation is only partly true.

### Stephen Porges and his Polyvagal Theory

The "Polyvagal Theory" is a new understanding of the ANS, arising from the research and writings of psychiatry professor Stephen Porges. He conducted research that changes the standard view, with huge implications for psychotherapies and health care in general. Based on Porges' findings, the ANS has three branches, not two, and they are sequential, not purely reciprocal.

"Polyvagal" derives from Porges' observation that one branch of the vagus nerve (Cranial Nerve X) does not fully conform to the expected standard classification as parasympathetic like the rest of the vagus. Porges sought an understanding of the true function of this branch, known as the "ventral vagus." He found that it is still autonomic in that

**"POLYVAGAL"– FOUR NUCLEI OF THE VAGUS NERVE IN THE BRAIN STEM**

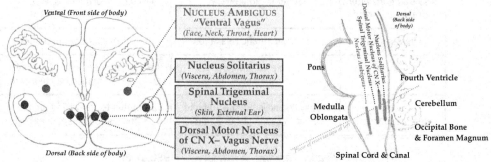

Note: All ANS diagrams in this chapter have been consolidated into one 18x24 full-color wall poster, available from www.energyschool.com.

it regulates involuntary survival functions, including a previously under-appreciated role in heart regulation, but that it has other functions as well.

Exploring further, he found that the ventral vagus branch was interconnected with involuntary facial gestures, listening, vocalizing and other faculties. Considered in combination with other involuntary nerves in the face, throat and neck (Cranial Nerves V, VII, IX, X and XI), the ventral vagus participates in a unified complex that has a critical but previously unrecognized survival function in mammals and especially in primates. Together these nerves provide mission-critical functions for infants (securing maternal bonding), and later for adults (enabling speech and social communication).

Primates need maternal bonding more than other animals because their much more complex cortex needs time to mature. A bird or fish newborn is relatively functional soon after birth, but mammals need more time and humans need literally years before their survival capabilities are fully available. The ventral vagus nerve group secures the mother's loyalty and nurturance to make sure that the vulnerable new baby is able to survive, and then throughout later life it enables communication functions that are key to our astounding biological success. New infants need no coaching to orient toward their mothers and engage in loving interchanges through voice, listening and facial gestures. Their mothers are just as involuntarily captivated and expressive.

A great chain of benefits ensues from our unique polyvagal anatomical design: maternal bonding enables the maturation of our large cortex and development of language. These facilitate the transfer of knowledge, which, in turn, enables the efficient development of social structures and technology, leading to ever-increasing security ascending the ladder of needs to richer access to the purpose in life.

Embryological and anatomical evidence strongly supports the theory that the Social Nervous System is the ultimate development in regulatory design. A Social ANS function, communications (especially speech), has been convincingly discussed as being the supreme functional purpose of the numerous anatomical specializations that are uniquely human, bestowing major survival advantages such as transfer of knowledge.[157] The design works: humans are the ultimate biological success story, even to the point of threatening ourselves through overpopulation.[158] Our success is due to our brainpower, thanks significantly to this third branch of the ANS.

### Phylogeny and the ANS

Porges' inquiry led to an examination of *phylogeny*. Phylogeny refers to the study of the development of functions across different life forms. For example, all animals have some form of digestion and circulation; even a single-celled organism floating in a liquid medium has some way to take in nourishment and discharge waste. As creatures progressed through evolutionary stages, these systems became more sophisticated, all in the service of enhanced survival. What is true for the digestion is also true for the nervous system; greatly increased complexity has led to enormous improvements in adaptability and biological success.

---

[157] Jos Verhulst, *Developmental Dynamics in Humans and Other Primates: Discovering Evolutionary Principles through Comparative Morphology.* Adonis, 2003. Page 348 contains an intriguing diagram showing that human morphology seems to have speech as its ultimate functional goal.

[158] The situation poses an unanswered question in the evolutionary story: can our expanded cortex capabilities, which brought us such success, solve the overpopulation problem?

## Phylogeny of Heart Regulation in Vertebrates

Stephen Porges, "The Polyvagal Theory: Phylogenic Substrates of a Social Nervous System," *Int'l Journal of Psychophysiology.* 42 (2001) 123-146, 2000.

**Key:**
**Arrows** indicate the presence of heart regulating functions. Up-arrow means faster heart rate, down-arrow means slower heart rate.
**Asterisks** indicate which autonomic branch is deployed: ***Social, **Sympathetic, *Parasympathetic.

| Definition of Phylogeny (American Heritage Dictionary) 1. The evolutionary development and history of a species or higher taxonomic grouping of organisms. | Mechanisms of Heart Regulation | | | | |
|---|---|---|---|---|---|
| | Chromatin Tissue (CHR) | * DMX Dorsal Motor Nucleus of CN X (Vagus) | ** Sympathetic Nervous System | ** Adrenal Medulla (Produces Catecholimines) | *** Nucleus Ambiguus Ventral Motor Nucleus of CN X (Vagus) |
| Cyclostomes- Jawless Fish (Lampreys) | ↑ | | | | |
| Elasmobranchs- Cartilagenous Fish (Sharks) | ↑ | ↓ | | | |
| Teleosts- Bony Fish | ↑↑ | ↓ | ↑ | | |
| Amphibians | ↑ | ↓ | ↑ | | |
| Reptiles | ↑ | ↓ | ↑ | ↑ | |
| Mammals | ↑↑ | ↓ | ↑ | ↑ | ↓ |

*More Modern*

*CHR– Chromatin is non-neural tissue that stimulates the heart by releasing noradrenic amines directly into blood in the heart.*

Porges found that the phylogeny of heart regulation in vertebrates showed this kind of increasingly sophisticated progression, and that the ventral vagus appeared only in the most recent creatures in the evolutionary chain: mammals, primates and especially humans. The resulting picture of heart regulation, shown above, shows alternating mechanisms for increasing and decreasing heart rate, each new layer adding greater resiliency and range of motion.

### Three Branches of the ANS

The **parasympathetic** system is the oldest part of the ANS, reflecting the survival needs of a primitive passive feeder. It innervates essential baseline metabolic functions, delivering nutrient-rich, oxygenated blood to the system, particularly the brain, and its components regulate heart, lungs and viscera. Normal parasympathetic functions are relatively limited, such as waiting for food and opportunities to mate. Parasympathetic stress responses are limited to adjusting the metabolic rate within a fairly narrow range, such as in "death feigning" survival tactics. In mammals the parasympathetic stress response appears as "playing possum" behaviors; in extreme cases it is known as parasympathetic shock.

The **sympathetic** nervous system is a later development of the ANS, adding mobilization and a wider range of possible responses. More sophisticated animals gained more survival options in essential feeding, protective and mating behaviors. With a sympathetic ANS branch, creatures can pursue food and mates, evade predators and adjust to environmental conditions with greater adaptation and success. The capacity for movement and increased sensory awareness developed, and muscular/structural tissues became more sophisticated. The sympathetic system acts as a controller on the primitive parasympathetic to give a wider range of metabolic responses, a faster heart rate for higher exertion, and the ability to shift resources to muscular, visceral or other systems as needed in response to survival challenges.

"**Social** nervous system" is a prospective term for the third branch of the ANS. This most modern branch confers supreme survival advantages. The social nervous system is a controller over the sympathetic to greatly expand the functions of the more crude "fight/flight" responses and fulfill the purposes described above.

### Hierarchical Interactions of the Social Nervous System

The anatomy of the social nervous system consists of mechanisms that create the all-important protective bond between newborns and their mothers. These include vocalization, hearing, visual contact and facial expression, which are each capable of triggering hormones inducing pleasurable sensations in both infant and caregiver. These are hardwired, involuntary, precognitive functions that exist in

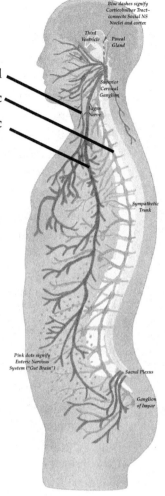

**The New ANS Anatomy**

Social

Sympathetic

Parasympathetic

*"Three neural circuits form a phylogenically ordered response hierarchy that regulates behavioral and physiological adaptation to safe, dangerous and life-threatening environments."*

–Stephen Porges, <u>Polyvagal Theory</u> (Norton, 2011)

**Parasympathetic** (most ancient)
"A primitive passive feeding and reproduction system creating a metabolic baseline of operation to manage oxygen and nourishment via the blood."

**Sympathetic** (newer)
"A more sophisticated set of responses enabling mobility for feeding, defense and reproduction via limbs & muscles."

**Social Engagement** (most modern)
"A sophisticated set of responses supporting massive cortical development, enabling maternal bonding (extended protection of vulnerable immature cortex processors) and social cooperation (language and social structures) via facial functions."

newborns and have a compelling power to engender biochemical changes that create emotional bonding during the vulnerable period. Healthy babies exhibit these capabilities instantly at the time of birth. Infants experience compromise or failure of these strategies (such as betrayal by or alienation from the caregiver) as life threatening, and justifiably so.

Drawing on the "Theory of Dissolution" (developed by British neurology pioneer John Hughlings Jackson, ca. 1910), Porges also explains a sequence of operation. Under stress, we involuntarily try our newest, most sophisticated and efficient equipment first. If that doesn't work, older strategies are attempted, and if they don't work, the oldest resources are employed. Therefore, under stress, humans first use our social/relational tactics, then fight/flight, then immobility, as survival strategies. Each of these stages has characteristic indicators for accurate identification.

The sequence bears repeating and elaboration because it is so important in therapy. The hierarchical scheme is undermined by traumatic experiences. If social engagement did not work in the past, we are less likely to try it again in the present. Instead, we go to the next, older strategy, sympathetic's fight/flight neurochemistry and anatomy. Furthermore, if these did not work earlier in life, we may skip the sympathetic stage and simply go to the last ANS level, parasympathetic. Parasympathetic stress responses (freeze, immobilize, dissociate) are the final functioning points in the model. If these kinds of responses are also overwhelmed, the situation can be fatal, as in parasympathetic shock. Averting parasympathetic shock is justifiably well known as a top priority for emergency response personnel, because shock can be fatal.

Robert Scaer, neurologist and trauma expert, has identified dissociative, depressed states as the fullest expression of post-traumatic stress disorder and the proper primary target of PTSD therapies.[159] Among many studies described by Scaer , two stand out:

---

[159] Robert Scaer, *8 Keys to Brain-Body Balance*. Norton, 2012. Scaer's books describe all these parasympathetic research items.

• The phenomenon of "voodoo death," in which a tribe member would receive a curse from a shaman and just lie down and die, was investigated by physiologist Walter Cannon in the 1930s. Cannon, who coined the phrase "fight or flight," wondered what could be the mechanism of such a sequence; the hierarchical arrangement of the ANS explains the mystery. At the low end of the sequence, there is no further ANS option and the system shuts down.

• In autonomic experiments, lab rats put in a deep basin of water swam indefinitely because they knew the routine of being subjected to experimentation during the day and cared for at night; in contrast, wild rats swam once around the edge to determine that there was no escape, and simply gave up and sank to the bottom. They had no expectation of a survival alternative.

The whole sequence is played out in a sub-optimum hospital birth. Newborn babies come out pre-programmed for maternal bonding including skin-to-skin contact and nursing. Instead they are often separated from their mothers ("infant quarantine") and subjected to painful unnatural procedures, facilitated by medicine's obsolete belief that babies are insentient. Since the social engagement system impulses are thwarted, babies then try the older strategy, the sympathetic ANS in the form of angry-sounding crying. When that doesn't work, and it cannot work unless the adults are sensitive and discerning about such sounds, all they have left is the parasympathetic freeze/immobilization response. The misunderstanding caregivers may interpret this seemingly quiet state as being "good babies," when actually they are seriously compromised. Potential long-term implications include reduced immune system, limited heart rate variability and loss of other ANS functions. Many research studies have confirmed the reality and value of a functional social engagement system: patients with strong and active social connections recover faster and live longer.[160]

A beautiful case study was accidentally created by "The Rescuing Hug."[161] Twin newborn girls were in their hospital bassinets after a difficult birth, and one was not flourishing. A nurse intuitively had the insight to put them together in one bassinet instead of being separated. The stronger one flopped an arm over the weaker one in a heart-touching embrace. With the social engagement system stimulation stimulated by her sister's touch, the weaker sister's heart rate stabilized and her temperature returned to normal. These are remedial effects beyond the capability of modern medicine, a perfect example of a Yin approach being able to solve a situation that a Yang approach cannot. Seventeen years later, journalists tracked down the sisters and reported the story again with a fascinating video interview. Porges, with an expert eye for micro-cues given during the interview, readily identified which girl had been the weaker one at birth.

In another compelling example, the famous baby doctor Benjamin Spock (1903-1998) actually filmed a close-up view of the three-step sequence of ANS progressive degradation during a circumcision surgery.[162] The steps are clearly visible exactly as described by Porges. In his late eighties at the time, Spock commented poignantly about its effects, expressing extreme remorse for some of his earlier beliefs about babies. At the time of the movie filming he did not have a context to really explain what was happening, but it is excruciatingly obvious after learning about Porges' work. I am unable to show this video clip in class because the students become too

---

[160] Dean Ornish, *Love & Survival.* William Morrow, 1999. pp. 34-51.

[161] To follow up, use *The Rescuing Hug* as internet search terms.

[162] Benjamin Spock, *The Circumcision Question* (VHS). Wilbert Productions, 1994.

distressed for any further learning and we have to spend the rest of the day restoring their ANS range of motion.

## *Implications of the New ANS Understanding*

The new ANS understanding firms up a field that was previously considered to be "soft science." Science seeks precision, in the form of measurable results, isolated variables and double-blind methodology. Human behavior does not readily fit in with such constraints, due to having too many variables. As a result, the fields of psychology, sociology and related topics have suffered from second-class status in the science community. With a fuller understanding of the ANS, a door is opened for more measurement and credibility and perhaps real progress in changing destructive practices. The ANS is not hard to measure: even a saliva sample shows instant changes, and biofeedback methods for measuring ANS activity are being constantly improved.[163]

Counselors have known for years that creating rapport and supporting safety were important for clients; now they gain credibility with a physiological explanation and a precise way to identify and measure the effects.

As new ANS theories are confirmed and applied, major changes can be expected. The first applications would be in health care, particularly with young children and post-trauma treatment, but further applications are also easily envisioned. Basically, there is now a compelling reason to treat babies with much more attention to maternal bonding and avoiding painful interactions, so that the "trump card" of the all-important ANS will thereby be preserved. This is a revelation in health care: it was not until 1998 that the

---

[163] Minimally invasive ANS measurement methods include heart rate variability (HRV), galvanic skin response (GSR), muscle activation (sEMG), body temperature, brain wave (EEG), cortisol levels in saliva and carbon dioxide measurement. Dark field microscopy of fresh blood samples is a more high-tech method.

American Medical Association even agreed that babies could feel pain, and the medical profession is still not unified about such ANS-damaging practices as infant quarantine, umbilical cord cutting and circumcision.

In the future, a newborn baby could be tested for autonomic markers from the first moment (using a non-invasive saliva swab test), and biofeedback could give caregivers instant ANS status reports to guide optimum handling. Procedures would be applied more gently, and some procedures would be stopped altogether if the actual autonomic effects were made visible.

Similarly, environments of the future for young children and emergency medicine are likely to be re-designed to optimize for the social nervous system, in the knowledge that if this part is highly functional, the older sympathetic and parasympathetic systems will work better. The effect has been demonstrated very effectively by the "Roots of Empathy" program in which new mothers bring their young babies into

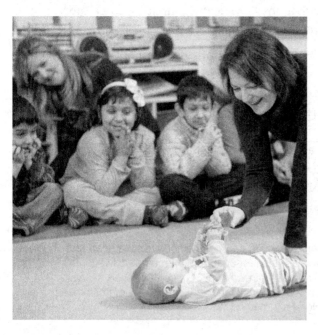

**Research on the Roots of Empathy program found increases in these qualities:**

Emotional literacy
Neuroscience interest
Temperament
Curriculum connection
Participatory democracy
Infant development interest
Violence prevention
Perspective taking
Prevention of teen pregnancy
Attachment
Male nurturance
Inclusion
Infant safety

K-12 classrooms.[164] The mere presence of a baby triggers involuntary neurochemical changes throughout the whole classroom, with enormous benefits in learning and behavior that have been repeatedly confirmed in scientific studies. This program is another example of conscious actions (bringing a baby into the room) being able to reach into subconscious processes and definitely change ANS states and behaviors.

Uplifting the social engagement system is the new "holy grail" of therapy, health care and child care. When the highest resource of the whole ANS is fully operative, the immune system, neurological function, self-empowerment and related indicators all improve. These new methods have even worked with autism, using specific sounds to induce nerve signaling along the social group anatomy.[165]

To illustrate the significance of this new understanding, a male client in his mid-60s came for sessions complaining of heart problems, particularly irregular heartbeat and episodes of not feeling well, including fatigue and mild depression. His family history featured an abusive, alcoholic father, so there was plenty of material for traditional psychotherapy and the trauma history was acknowledged but it was not the first emphasis of inquiry.

Instead of trying to resolve the past, we inquired into the surrounding context of his current life, focusing on the hierarchy of action fields and the ANS. He told a story of multiple disappointments in intimate relationships, including a marriage that "lost its spark" and ended in a disappointing divorce, followed by a more recent breakup of a subsequent relationship. Through a two-chair Yin and Yang counseling process, he gained insights into why these relationship patterns had developed in the past, and how to recognize

---

[164] http://www.rootsofempathy.org

[165] http://www.education.umd.edu/EDHD/faculty2/Porges/tlp/tlp.html

them in the present. He became more self-aware about the complexity of relationships and observed that his own social engagement system was under-nourished and under-utilized, especially since he was retired and living alone.

The deficiency of social stimulation was understandable in light of his history of disappointments, but once he became aware of the situation he resolved to consciously undertake remedial actions, such as going out into social situations more frequently. Over time he was able to make major changes, including creating a new relationship with a much stronger sense of purpose and an intentional basis informed by understanding Yin and Yang archetypes. Within a year his heart symptoms faded and then disappeared altogether.

In another example, a female client in her 30s sought help with severe depression. The initial sessions went fairly well, leading to resolving binds with her highly-inappropriate boyfriend as well as her parents who had been through a divorce a few years earlier. She was beginning to exercise more and get out in nature; these are signs of re-establishing sympathetic autonomic fulfillment, one step up the ladder from parasympathetic's bottom rung. She was improving but progress was slow. Then one week she arrived for her session and was visibly much better. When I asked what had happened, she reported that her sister and her best friend had both given birth that weekend, and she had spent the entire week holding newborn babies. In holding the babies, she was inadvertently stimulating her own ANS via the neurochemistry of the social nervous system, and her depression lifted. She did not have a relapse and discontinued the sessions to focus on her career.

## *Differentiating Normal Function from Stress Responses*

The new ANS understanding also remedies a common error, confusing "normal functions" with "stress responses." This is an example of familiarity and habit obscuring critical thinking. For decades the characterization of the ANS has been mixing apples (sympathetic's fight/flight, a stress response) with oranges (parasympathetic's rest/rebuild, a normal function).

Another effect of the new ANS understanding is to put the sympathetic branch in a new light. Previously, sympathetic was primarily known for its stress response, and its normal function was under-appreciated. Meanwhile parasympathetic's stress response, the freeze/dissociation response, was under-recognized as a more serious survival problem, the last resort for the ANS survival sequence.

Resolving this error overturns a popular therapy model misconception about the ANS, that the sympathetic, fight/flight autonomic response is worse for health than the parasympathetic. In fact, therapists of the future will try to re-establish the sympathetic through enabling thwarted defensive responses. The whole ANS can be seen as a three-step ladder, with parasympathetic being the lowest and last rung. The parasympathetic can appear to be calm and placid and thereby possibly "better" but in fact if the state is involuntary, such as in depression, it is far worse biologically and more challenging therapeutically.

The diagrams below summarize ANS functioning. For efficient ANS therapeutic support, I suggest that the information in these charts be memorized in its entirety, so that ANS clients are correctly identified and appropriate therapeutic strategies can be deployed. I have made these into a poster (see the back of this book) so that they can be viewed repeatedly until they become second nature.

### Reviewing the Stress Response Sequence

Because of its importance in health care, the sequential operation of the ANS deserves repetition and embellishment. Again, the ANS stress responses are organized in involuntary sequences. At the first moment of perception of novelty or threat in the environment, a precise set of step-by-step actions will ensue.

This can be readily experienced in everyday life by making a loud noise in a room of people, whether or not they are primed to study the topic. The fact that the responses are the same with or without prior warning shows that the sequence is involuntary and therefore autonomic; the same sequence appears because cognitive control does not reach deeply enough to manage the reactions. I first instruct the

## Differentiating Normal Functions from Stress Responses

Although the terms are commonly used, "Fight-or-Flight vs. Rest & Rebuild" is a confusing and outdated characterization of Sympathetic and Parasympathetic ANS branches. Fight/Flight is a **Stress Response** whereas Rest/Rebuild is a **Normal Function.**

|  | **SOCIAL** | **SYMPATHETIC** | **PARASYMPATHETIC** |
|---|---|---|---|
| **Normal Functions** | "Love" <br> Communication & Language <br> Social Organization <br> Sex- Flirting, Afterglow <br> Prosody, Vocalization <br> Reciprocal Play <br> Contact & Interaction | Mobilization <br> Daytime Alertness <br> Recreational Excitement <br> Vocational Initiative <br> Muscular activity <br> Sex- Climax | Baseline metabolism <br> 'Rest & Rebuild <br> Meditative States <br> Sex- Arousal <br> Sleep (4 stages) |
| **Stress Responses** | In-crisis contact & <br>   Communication <br> First Aid "Tend & Befriend" <br> Empathy, Comfort, Touch <br> Emergency Teamwork <br> Group Psychology | Alarm, Anxiety <br> Orient <br> Fight/Flight <br> Discharge (shaking) <br> Rest | Immobility (Freeze) <br> Dissociation, Depression <br> Catatonia <br> Sleep Disorders <br> Parasympathetic Shock |
| **Fast Involuntary Transfers** | Mob Behavior ⟶ | ⟵ Eye & Verbal Contact <br> Freeze ⟶ | ⟵ "Startle Awake" |

### Notes:

- A high percentage of health conditions are Autonomic Nervous System events, including immune system disorders, attention deficit conditions, psychosomatic issues, post-traumatic stress effects and others.

- Normally, ANS stages flow and interchange rhythmically based on routine stimuli and biological sequences such as circadian rhythm, digestion and sexual processes. ANS fixation or loss of flow is a sign of PTSD.

- Voluntary and involuntary functions overlap significantly, and most of the functions listed here could be either. But voluntary and involuntary can be distinguished by close observation. Involuntary (autonomic) responses are immediate and universal across differences of age, gender, education and culture. The conscious mind cannot fully control face and body expressions. The ANS seems to be mainly incapable of inauthenticity or deception (Paul Ekman (2009).

- In the presence of novelty or threat, we try our phylogenically newest, best strategy (Social) first. If that does not work, or has not worked in the past, we try our older, second strategy (Sympathetic). If that does not work, we try our most primitive, last strategy (Parasympathetic). If that does not work, we are in great danger and we experience Immobilization, deep depression or parasympathetic shock.

- "The higher nervous system arrangements inhibit (or control) the lower, and thus, when the higher are rendered functionless, the lower rise in activity." –John Hughlings Jackson (1835-1911), Neurology Pioneer.

## Recognizing ANS stress responses

| Parasympathetic | Flat affect, depression, pale, quiet; degenerative conditions |
|---|---|
| Sympathetic | Agitation, anxiety, speediness, eyes hyper-active; inflammation conditions |
| Social | Lack of eye contact, unclarity of speech, incapacity for rapport and feeling at ease in the relationship |

group to take an internal inventory of sensations and self-awareness, to get a baseline state. Then I make a loud noise, and each person closely observes what happens next. Regardless of education, age, gender, religion, culture, belief system or any other demographic variable, everyone will have similar physiological involuntary responses.

First is an instantaneous elevation of the head, neck and shoulders (the "alarm" phase), quickly followed by a sharpening of the senses, especially eyes and ears, with a turning of the head to locate the sound (the "orient" phase). Less frequently, the head and neck may quickly contract downward, in a "duck and cover" gesture; the simultaneous up and down impulses may be a key to neck tension, because realistically the muscles can only do one at a time. Next appears one of two possibilities: a turning toward relationship, such as eye contact with other people and some form of the question, "What was that?" or a turning toward the disturbance, beginning a mobilization for action. The sequence continues with a sense of muscular engagement for fight or flight, whichever the ANS determines has the best chance of survival based on each individual's prior history. In a real emergency there may be a quick deployment of teamwork strategies at this time, an expression of the social engagement system: one person is designated to telephone for help while another runs for the fire extinguisher.

If neither fight nor flight is effective, next there will be a "playing possum" state, in which the system suddenly "puts the brakes on" all the mobilization that was present an instant before. This is the moment of stepping down to a lower, less functional, more dangerous state, the parasympathetic stress response. It can be effective in dealing with a threat, because a frozen, dissociative "duck and cover" strategy can constitute a form of "death feigning," making some predators lose interest. Unfortunately the dissociative state can become habitual, with severe health consequences. The analogy is a car with both accelerator and brakes both pressed to the floor: something has to give.

After the crisis has passed, the threat has been identified and removed, and the ANS perceives a return to safe conditions, shaking or micro-fibrillations in the tissues will begin. This movement discharges the intense ANS energy that was mobilized. Ideally the system will later experience a deep restorative sleep.

If every step is deployed, including subtle or obvious shaking and discharge moving to rest, the system is likely to re-set back to normal, ready for the next challenge. Problems arise when there is not enough time or capability to go through the whole sequence. Then the system will seem to get stuck at one point. For example, in a car accident, the person may have just noticed the impending problem and not have had time to swerve with the steering wheel or stab at the brakes; the ANS system tries to fulfill its program with defensive responses by the hands, shoulders and legs, but it cannot. Months or years later these parts of the body may be still trying to do what was intended before the response was interrupted. Physical problems may appear in the exact places, such as arthritis in the hands that gripped the wheel and circulatory or structural problems in the leg that stabbed for the brakes.

Peter Levine has discussed the effects of "thwarted defensive responses." The phrase refers to how there is a great value in helping clients experience fulfillment of defensive responses so that those impulses can be "retired" from continual effort. This can be done any number of ways; authors such as Levine and Diane Heller have given excellent descriptions, which will be explored later.

## ANS portals

Another new concept for therapy arising from Porges' work is the concept of "portals" for affecting the ANS branches. "Portals" refers to anatomical components of the ANS that can be physically stimulated to support a particular layer. By stimulating specific locations in specific ways, ANS changes can be created. Creating signaling along a portal pathway is very useful therapeutically because it is effective without cost or risk; methods for this are discussed in the following chapter.

For example, in The Listening Project research at the University of Maryland, Porges found that stimulating nerves of the social nervous system through specific muscular activation created profound improvement in the relational behaviors of autistic patients.[166] The effect is also seen in the use of vagus nerve stimulation, in which a pacemaker-like device is implanted adjoining the vagus nerve in the neck to relieve neurological and behavioral symptoms.[167]

The portals for the parasympathetic system, based on anatomy, are the vagus nerve, accessible on both sides of the neck, and the sacral plexus. For the sympathetic ANS branch,

---

[166] https://clinicaltrials.gov/ct2/show/NCT02398422

[167] Taunjah Bell, *Vagus Nerve Stimulation and Anxiety*. iUniverse, 2010.

the muscles of the limbs, and the sympathetic chain along the spine are highlighted; the superior cervical ganglion in the side of the neck provides access. For the social ANS branch, Cranial Nerves V, VII, IX, X and XI, observable as a group in the embryological "pharyngeal arches" structure, can be used by gently stimulating their sensory and motor components in the face and throat/neck areas.

The method for using these portals varies with different modalities. In massage, manual contact with the relevant areas, particularly the sides of the neck and the face, such as in a facial massage or lymphatic therapy, might be used. In Polarity Therapy, energy balancing and reflexology contacts could be employed. In Franklyn Sills' Craniosacral Biodynamics, the "motility of the central nervous system" and "Becker's Three-Stage Process" concepts are useful. In all cases, accurate knowledge of the anatomy is important.

Having clients participate in ANS stimulation has also proven to be supportive. For the parasympathetic nervous system, paying conscious attention to the breath and its involuntary movement of the belly is helpful. For the sympathetic system, engaging the muscles of the whole body, or, more specifically, the arms and legs for fight/flight defensive response fulfillment, followed by relaxation of the muscles and being conscious of subsequent sensation, can be effective. For the social nervous system, the approach can include recalling a favorite person or pet and using the imagination to induce the warm feelings and neurochemistry of being lovingly recognized. By stimulating the various nerve pathways of the ANS, old thwarted impulses can be fulfilled safely.

Recognition of the client's ANS state provides a blueprint for therapeutic strategy. Identifying the currently active layer, we can use the portals to guide clients in fulfilling the impulses of that layer, and support them in naturally moving through the three-part sequence. The therapeutic goal is to restore capacity to function at all three layers, but the third, the social, is the key because it is the most sophisticated tool in the stress-response repair kit.

## Applications in Pre- and Perinatal Therapy

Pre- and perinatal psychology is a rich field for application of the new ANS understanding.[168] Before birth, babies are immersed in their mother's experience yet also super-sentient on their own. The fetus definitely responds to the environment. The goal is to minimize feelings of threat and disturbance for as long as possible so a new baby has maximum time to experience security and trust, building a strong base that will serve throughout life as the ANS foundation for resiliency.

The Polyvagal Theory can transform treatment of infants as well. Among other benefits, there is now a measurable scientific basis for emphasis on ANS support as described above. Prior to Porges' work, modern anti-bonding medical practices often felt wrong to parents, observers and some primary care professionals, but clear information about the nature of the damage was lacking. Babies cannot report their experiences in normal language and the prevailing attitude was that babies are insentient and have no memory.

Now we know that newborn quarantine, anesthesia, cord cutting and circumcision affect the ANS of babies, their most important lifelong anatomical group. The practices defeat a baby's best (social) stress-response resources and force the baby to a sympathetic (fight-or-flight stress response) or, worse, to a parasympathetic (immobilization)

---

[168] See Bibliography for Ray Castellino, William Emerson, David Chamberlain and Thomas Verny.

strategy. The baby's subconscious brain[169] is imprinted with an expectation of betrayal in intimacy that may endure long into adulthood. The impact is high because of the social nervous system's top-rung place in the ANS hierarchy.

Trauma experts such as Bessel van der Kolk have noted that the two greatest determinants of "recoverability" from trauma are how early the incident occurred and whether betrayal was involved.[170] Flawed birthing beliefs create stress on both ways. An optimum birth is an excellent preventive strategy for lifelong ANS and immune system resiliency.

The discovery of the social nervous system also makes sense of the observation that humans are especially prone to post-trauma dysfunction. In the wild, other animals do not show PTSD symptoms with any frequency. There is something in human processing that engenders PTSD, and the answer is likely about our emotions. Levine and others have noted that the emotional component of a trauma, such as rage or terror, is often more overwhelmingly painful than the physical experience. In Stone's words, "A mental pain can be far more devastating than a mere physical pain."[171] The problem is particularly true in the case of betrayal trauma.[172] The experience of emotions and thoughts may be what makes humans so susceptible to being traumatized. The discussion of emotions will be continued further in Chapter 12.

Another explanation for humanity's PTSD tendencies may be modern life itself. Human biology evolved over eons

---

[169] Specifically, the amygdalae, the paired almond-size brain areas that sort our experience for threat. These brain regions are located about one inch beneath our temples and one inch behind our eyes.

170 Bessel van der Kolk, Alexander McFarlane, Lars Weiseith, *Traumatic Stress: The Effects of Overwhelming Experience on Mind, Body, and Society.* Guilford, 2006.

[171] R. Stone, *Polarity Therapy, Vol. 1.* CRCS, 1986. Book 3, p. 12.

[172] Jennifer Freyd, *Betrayal Trauma.* Harvard, 1998.

of time spent in hunter-gatherer and agrarian lifestyles. In just the last century, the challenges have changed significantly. As writer Nathan Seppa observed, "Human biology is ill-prepared for this lifestyle."[173] Some PTSD reflects a mismatch between ANS biological design and modern life's inevitable alienation, pace and pressure. This also applies to technology: humans were not constructed to experience many commonplace events of modern life. For example just one century ago the ANS dealt with a different environment. The night was dark instead of being in constant illumination. The seasons were a primary feature of experience instead of controlled central heating/cooling. The social fabric was a direct daily interpersonal process instead of through modern isolation and technological media. One century is far too short a time for evolutionary adaptation, and ANS symptoms are epidemic.

### The ANS in Large-Scale Popular Culture

Given that the large majority of human behavior is ANS-driven, any enormously popular phenomenon, including religion, entertainment and politics, must have an ANS basis or it would not become large-scale. The logic is circular but compelling. Cognitive processes alone do not explain the size of major events. Most obvious are movies and television involving ANS-centered fear (action thrillers, fright-inducing movies) or sex (romantic love stories, pornography, onscreen nudity) because these functions are at the very foundation of biological design and most fully in the domain of the ANS. The ANS is in the driver's seat of behavior: if something happens in social groups, there is likely to be an ANS explanation for who, when, where and how it manifests.

---

[173] Nathan Seppa, reviewing the book *Present Shock: When Everything Happens Now*, by Douglas Rushkof (Current, 2013). *Science News*, June 15, 2013.

An entertainment experience that has not received much commentary is the phenomenon of children's cartoons. Since television first arrived, Saturday mornings have been filled with children hypnotically watching all kinds of mayhem; "Roadrunner and Coyote" is an example. These show exaggerated crashes, collisions and falls, in the expectation that these are funny. The movie *Who Framed Roger Rabbit* (1988) addressed the topic directly and skillfully. Any laughter that appears in such a context is the ANS releasing stress, as health visionary Moshe Feldenkrais observed: "[ANS] Laughter is when we realize the danger is to someone else, not us."[174] Again, we are so surrounded and immersed in all this that we do not notice the phenomenon, an ANS disturbance hiding in plain sight.

My earliest memory of film is *Dumbo* (1941); I mainly remember the heart-wrenching separation of baby from mother. With the new understanding of the ANS, I realize how the movie had such a big impact.

Along with entertainment, advertising is the preeminent ANS pop culture application. Long ago, especially since the advent of television, commercial artists and producers figured out how to influence buyers by using subliminal messages. The craft of ANS manipulation has only become more sophisticated through the years. If there is any doubt about the supremacy of the ANS in determining behavior, commercial activity is conclusive proof. There is a wealth of information published in this topic area, so I will not dwell on it here.[175]

---

[174] Moshe Feldenkrais, *The Potent Self: A Study of Spontaneity and Compulsion.* Frog Books, 2002.

[175] Wilson Bryan Key, *Subliminal Seduction.* Signet, 1974. This gives a relatively early overview. For something more recent: Dave Lakhani, *Subliminal Persuasion: Influence & Marketing Secrets They Don't Want You To Know.* Wiley, 2008.

Major holidays reveal ANS behaviors, if we look beneath their formal titles. Pay "ANS attention" the next time you are attending a large-scale celebration, and you are likely to see subliminal processes at work, including ritualistic restoration of social engagement bonds, discharge of pent-up stress, increased financial activity and related possibilities. The time of the winter solstice is celebrated in most cultures, as is the springtime equinox with its theme of rebirth, fertility and renewal; Mardi Gras comes to mind as an ANS spectacle. At the harvest time we seem to have ancient echoes of famine during the long winter that is approaching. Perhaps most amusing from an ANS perspective is Halloween, a day given over to alter egos and frightful archetypes, ritually instilled in very young children with the odd twist of saturation bombing with sugar, a well-known hormonal toxin linked with mood changes, attention deficit disorder, diabetes and obesity. We might ask, "What are we thinking?" but there is no answer because the ANS is not about thinking.

Sports are of special interest for me, not least because I enjoy them so much. Huge crowds gather, at great expense, to don the tribal colors and join in boisterous, rhythmic Yang rituals. The spectacle comes complete with patriotic ceremonies and displays and sexually provocative sideline "entertainment," super-charged subliminal ANS practices that have no rational link to the game itself. I invite you to go to any large sporting event and watch the crowd as much as the game, viewing through ANS-colored glasses.

An ANS explanation is that modern sports, both as participatory and as spectacle, fill an important role in subconscious experience. For millennia the human ANS has evolved, and been molded by circumstances, to perform as hunter-gatherer-protector. The sympathetic branch of the ANS, the Yang Principle, has existed to mobilize with daytime alertness, to solve complex threatening situations with skillful mental and physical skills, and to experience the satisfaction of victory by hard-fought struggle.

Now, in just the last century, the human system finds itself in a far different world, in which the challenges are muted at best. At worst, a creature who is biologically designed for active engagement lives a life confined to traffic jams, office cubicles, medications and nighttime TV. The situation has been depicted frequently, making comedy or tragedy out of the futility and alienation of modern existence. *Falling Down* (1993), with Michael Douglas, and *Office Space* (1999) with Peter Gibbons, depict the situation brilliantly.

Sports give us an outlet for our ancient ANS impulses. Each sport has some quality of sympathetic ANS fulfillment, and each can be analyzed as such, with great insight. Some are about the territorial imperative, some are more about aiming a projectile toward a target, some involve sexual symbolism (sexual processes being primarily ANS events). Many create fields of action for tribal instincts that engage and exercise the social branch of the ANS.

Participants and spectators experience a momentary deployment of biologically programed physical, emotional and mental skills that otherwise would be mostly dormant in a modern life. We join with our tribe in mirror neuron gratification of super-skill performance, including dressing in the regalia of "our people," and feeling fulfillment when "our" team wins. If the team wins the top place, mob psychology can occasionally be observed, as predicted by Levine and others. The neurochemistry of these experiences is no doubt deeply nourishing for the sympathetic ANS fulfillment-starved modern participants. This is a beneficial process, an under-appreciated form of therapeutic release.

An additional level of subconscious understanding is inspired by the book *Initis*.[176] The author makes reference to a distinction between "Contraries" and "Contradictories." Contraries are the norm in daily experience, defined as anything that happens in relative "shades of gray," such as light and dark, young and old, hot and cold. Contraries can be usefully modified by "somewhat" or "relatively." Contradictories are very rare, being phenomena that are absolutely different from their complementary conditions. "Living" and "Dead" are the ultimate examples that meet the Contradictories criteria, and these are universally fascinating. The precision of science and mathematics, the celebrated winning of the big deal in commerce and the satisfaction felt by compulsive shoppers when they score a good bargain are other examples of much-enjoyed absolutist ANS satisfaction rarely available in normal daily life.

Everyone is fascinated by Contradictories, because they are a hint of the great mysteries and the infinite invisible world, which are so instinctually compelling. It seems that sports create an artificial experience of the Contradictory state, in that, unlike most of "real" life, each event has a definite outcome. The goal is scored, or not; the shot beats the clock, or not; the player is in bounds, or out; the putt is in, or out. Enormous technological sophistication is deployed to give super-slow-motion replays from every angle, with "life" and "death" hanging in metaphorical balance. Large masses of people attend these events with religious fervor, to catch a whiff of the infinite and have momentary relief from their daily grind of "maybe" relativistic experience.

In sum, sports can be seen as a much-needed field of action in a modern context, keeping the age-old sympathetic

---

[176] Andrea Ragliabati, *Initis: Congestion of the Connective Tissue.* Masterworks, 2012. This fascinating book was first published in 1910, and was brought back into print by Phil Young, www.masterworks.com.

nervous system juices flowing in a world which otherwise becomes "Yang-deficient" rather quickly.

## The ANS in Medication

The enormous popularity of intoxicants can be seen as an ANS phenomenon. Each substance has a particular neurochemical effect, either excitation or soothing, and an ANS interpretation can help make sense of otherwise inexplicable behaviors. Intoxicants of all kinds can be interpreted as form of ANS self-medication. Although these are often sub-optimum in their effects, in fact many lives are ruined in the process, the usage is still arising from an intelligent ANS intention to re-establish equilibrium in response to extremely difficult circumstances.

Selective Serotonin Re-uptake Inhibitors (SSRI-class drugs, the Prozac family) deserve more attention than they have received. Numerous experts have pointed out that these are ANS-changing, and more risky than acknowledged.[177] About five percent of users have reactions, including suicidal or homicidal ideation. Unexpected domestic violence and mass killings (such as Columbine and Virginia Tech) often coincide with SSRI usage, but news reports rarely include such information. A review of the data reveals the enormous extent of the problem.[178] In the future, investigations of these horrific events will include the question, "What medications was the perpetrator on, if any?" Patients will be much more supervised including inquiry about problematic ideation and access to weapons. ANS-distressed teenagers are a recipe for disaster if they have a set of very commonly-intersecting circumstances: a disabled social ANS, immature risk

---

[177] Peter Breggin, *Medication Madness: The Role of Psychiatric Drugs in Cases of Violence, Suicide, and Crime.* St. Martin's Griffin, 2009.

[178] See www.ssristories.com for a chilling ten-year summary of hundreds of known cases of SSRI being present in suicide and homicide events.

assessment brain areas, SSRI medications, a devotion to hypnotic "shooter" video games and access to their parents' military-grade weapons.

Additionally, the ANS effects partially account for the popularity of lotteries and gambling. The odds of winning are very low, but the players experience a temporary "what-if" euphoria before the selection of a winner. The neurochemistry of optimism surges for a time, making a lottery ticket a relatively inexpensive self-medication for anxiety or depression, with few side effects and some voluntary taxation benefits. The tax is regressive, since the buyers often are not affluent, and should be spending scarce resources on something tangible, but the analgesic effect is also significant.

## The ANS in politics

Understanding the ANS also sheds light on politics. The notion that elections are decided by thoughtful people analyzing issues and positions has been thoroughly disproven.[179] While a fraction of our mental processing does pay some attention to issues, the real action is behind the curtain, where feelings call the shots. Political persuasions generally follow ANS criteria.[180] Candidates' electability closely follows people's quick subjective impression of images of their faces.[181]

Marshall McLuhan anticipated the effect of the internet when he described how subconscious processes influenced

---

[179] Drew Western, *The Political Brain: The Role of Emotion in Deciding the Fate of the Nation*. Public Affairs, 2008.

[180] Emily Laber-Warren, "Unconscious Reactions Separate Liberals and Conservatives." *Scientific American*, Sept. 4, 2012.

[181] Kyle Mattes, Michael Spezio, Hackjin Kim, Alexander Todorov, Ralph Adolphs, and R. Michael Alvarez, *Predicting Election Outcomes from Positive and Negative Trait Assessments of Candidate Images*. Caltech 2010. http://www.hss.caltech.edu/~rma/Election Outcomes and Trait Assessments_02.pdf

behavior as new media were introduced, with print, radio and television all having specific effects.[182] Now the whole phenomenon is being magnified by the emergence of the internet, and a new science specialty is arising to interpret trends in social media traffic. Political strategists are increasingly seeking to strike the ideal emotional tone to gain advantage for their candidates, and attempting to use emotional responses to control behavior; politicians now need to be effective actors as much or more than policy visionaries.

Politics are also a playground for Yin and Yang. The modern continuum ranges between sympathy or antipathy for the poor, freedom or structure, liberty or protection, opportunity or security. All these and more can be interpreted as dualistic processes. Governments, just like families, tribes and organizations, always deal with the universal question: is it better to have a more democratic system (Yin, the periphery), which tends to be less decisive and more chaotic, or a more authoritarian system (Yang, the core), which is extremely efficient but prone to injustice and exploitation? Political parties can be characterized along these lines, and voters will align for ANS reasons more than actual policies. This can get a little strange, as some people, in acts of cognitive dissonance, may actually vote against their own best interests. The ANS perspective explains why maps of voting patterns so often resemble maps of ANS phenomena such as obesity, diabetes, poverty and education level. Even the USA political parties' blue and red color schemes match the traditional colors for Yin and Yang.

From a Yin and Yang perspective, the answer to the age-old political question, "Freedom or control?" lies in finding balance, with a gentle flow back and forth between core and periphery, and a highly functional neutral to avoid

---

[182] Marshall McLuhan, *The Gutenberg Galaxy*. University of Toronto, 2011. First published in 1962.

tendencies for fixation. The designers of the American system, with its three-part structure, were brilliant in trying to design a sustainable system for balancing between the two great polarities.[183] In the three governmental branches, Executive represents Yang principles, Legislative represents Yin and Judicial represents Neutral. Where are Goethe and Franklin (philosopher-scientist-politician-artists of their era), now that we need them?

## Applications in Groups

Because groups automatically invoke the social ANS, Porges' work has profound implications for group dynamics.[184] In a sense, the whole multi-person group is functioning as what therapist and teacher Mukara Meredith calls "one living system," with many individual cells.

In a group setting, each person's relational experience becomes expressed in a collective form. Some participants' higher faculties, namely the social nervous system layer, will be operational, but some will have experienced defeat on that level and habitually respond in older sympathetic autonomic ways (conflict or flight); more severely damaged group members will tend to use their most primitive parasympathetic responses (withdrawal).

When a group attempts to accomplish a task together, especially in a difficult or seemingly threatening context, all three layers of autonomic function will be discernible. At first, relational (social) strategies will be exhibited, except under severe conditions. These will be successful or gradually yield to sympathetic (fight/flight) tactics, and ultimately to

---

[183] The appearance of pyramids with single eyes on the back of dollar bills derives from the founding fathers being informed by their participation in Masonic ideals, which included esoteric material.

[184] For an exploration of Polyvagal Theory applications in groups, see seminar leader Mukara Meredith's http://matrixworkslivingsystems.com.

## *An ANS Terminology Note*
## *for Readers of Randolph Stone*

Writing in the period 1948-1954, Stone used the language of his era, creating a problem for modern readers. For example:

"The *sympathetic* or vegetative nervous system... repairs the body and keeps it in tune with the natural forces." *–Polarity Therapy,* Vol. 1, Book 1, p. 38.

"Sympathetic" here refers to the whole Autonomic, not just the mobilization/fight/flight subgroup, the modern meaning. In addition, the term "Vegetative" is also used to mean the whole ANS.

The reasoning behind these old terms is derived from categorizing the nervous system parts between Voluntary and Involuntary action. To repeat, the voluntary nerve groups operate for conscious volitional movements, while the involuntary nerve groups operate for actions that have little or no voluntary control, such as essential visceral functions.

In an earlier era, the voluntary groups were considered to demonstrate "antipathy" in that a separate-from-body witness consciousness is the operator. This is a Yang perspective, involving the ectodermal embryonic tissues, the brain and sense organs. The mind has to be functionally somewhat separate from the body in order to tell it what to do. Conversely, the involuntary ("autonomic") groups were considered to be in "sympathy" because there is no apparent separate control, and "vegetative" because they regulate more primitive functioning of the viscera and metabolism. This is a Yin endodermal perspective. To be in sympathy is the opposite of being in antipathy, therefore sympathetic made sense as the opposite of antipathetic (voluntary).

As discussed earlier, a third perceptual perspective, empathy, represents a mid-point Neutral (embodied in the meso tissues) and is considered by embryologist and anatomist Jaap van der Wal to be the territory of the heart.

To correct this problem, van der Wal advocates returning to the earlier language, with the divisions of the autonomic being known as parasympapthetic (Yin, baseline metabolism) and orthosympathetic (Yang, mobilization). "Para" means *along with,* and "ortho" means *straight to.*

isolation and immobility within individuals and the group. For individuals in the group, there will be a "bell curve" effect with some people exhibiting behaviors in advance of or trailing the majority. For example, as a group under stress shifts from relational to fight/flight behaviors, some participants will already be showing immobility while others will be continuing to try social engagement. This sequence sheds light on the perplexing phenomena of mob psychology, and guides us toward optimum group management.

Groups can be facilitated to "evolve" up the three-part ANS chain, using awareness and careful management. The key is to gently re-establish full range of motion in the ANS, by intentionally invoking the highest function, the social nervous system, while also acknowledging, de-pathologizing and safely fulfilling the impulses of the older ANS branches. For example in a classroom dealing with challenging material, teachers can splice in social nervous system activities (having students interact with allies), encourage movement (sympathetic ANS fulfillment) and provide snacks (parasympathetic fulfillment). Similar to the effects of the "Roots of Empathy" program, such strategies can be expected to lead to enhanced learning, less anxiety, more creativity and higher and more integrated functionality.

Similarly, groups can be managed to maintain functionality in the collective social nervous system layer by carefully noting when individuals, or the group as a whole, start to slip down to a lower base. For optimum functionality, the critical mass majority should be maintained at the social ANS level. Group participation can help individuals by pulling them up to function at a social level, even though their individual systems may be habitually more inclined to lower levels. Properly conducted, a group experience can be healing for an individual with an ANS problem, rather than making it worse, as is often the case.

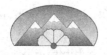

## PART TWO: Applications
### Performing the Dance

### Chapter 7

# Practitioner Skills

This chapter begins to apply the theories of the previous sections of the book. The foundation for Yin and Yang applications is a set of inner disciplines that we call "practitioner skills, Step-By-Step." The practitioner skills support not only counseling but other therapeutic practices and life management as well.

Yin and Yang awareness is based on subtle perception, requiring extra sensitivity and attunement on the part of the practitioner. Practitioner skills are a way to systematize and manage the progression of events in a therapeutic encounter. This method has been time-tested and well-proven: learning to perform each step in the sequence is a reliable way to set the stage for effective and safe therapies of all kinds. Mindfulness is enhanced throughout the whole experience.

Practitioner skills are built incrementally; they are not "all-or-nothing." Acquiring a little bit of one skill sets the stage for acquiring a little bit of the next, and so on. Opportunities for constant refinement and improvement are infinite. If we feel insecure at any one step, we can just go back to the previous step or the one before that, and re-build the sequence again.

### #1: The Skill of Being or Presence

The skill of being, also called the skill of presence, means creating a calm state in which we are sensitive enough to detect expressions of subtle phenomena. In a loud and fast-paced world, this is no small task. Micro-movements and similar subtleties are often unseen by our normal consciousness; modern life tends to routinely generate sense-dulling noise. With the practitioner skill of being, the "noise" inside ourselves is reduced and subtle perceptions become more available. These practices create a basis for access to information that might otherwise be below the

---

## Practitioner Skills Summary

### 1. *Skills of Being and Presence*
Centering & Grounding, Midline and Settling
Neutral; nonjudgmental and non-pathological attitude
Not "better than" or "less than"
Ability to witness both internal and external phenomena
Inner stillness

### 2. *Skills of Relationship*
Presence & Contact, proximity is not too close or too far
Wide perspective viewing, not tunnel vision
Compassionate; not enmeshing or abandoning

### 3. *Skills of Listening*
Listening generally in an open, receptive way
Helping the other person "feel heard" as if saying "I See You"

### 4. *Skills of Recognition*
Recognizing the qualities of Health, ANS states, Yin & Yang indicators
Body reading the Three Principles and Five Elements

### 5. *Skills of Conversation*
Recurrent feedback loop processing
Asking about what was happening before the symptoms appeared
Managing ANS states: "Body-Low-Slow-Loop"
Two-chair process (Chapter 10)
Life Coaching to avoid Yin and Yang dysfunctions

---

threshold of awareness. As Stone inquired, "Can man go from the rim of this wheel of speed to the center, and find rest?" [185]

A body-centered, meditative stillness is the essence of this first skill. By bringing our awareness into the body, slowing down the pace of awareness, and learning to notice subtle phenomena, we can gradually expand our range of perception. Events that were once seemingly invisible become evident, just as an accomplished musician can detect subtleties in sound that are imperceptible to a beginner. There may be an anatomical component for increased range of perception, in the form of increased neural network proliferation in selected areas of the brain. [186] For example, in the motor cortex brain region controlling a violinist's fingering, increased signaling activity and more dense neural network pathways are found after more experience. Through repeated concentrated practice, we can develop a comparable increase of sensitivity and hypothetically grow more network connections in the relevant brain areas. By consistently practicing the skill of being, the brain may actually adapt for greater sensitivity and equanimity.

The skill of presence can be developed through repeated steps of mental and physical focus. First, we bring attention into our own bodies. It may be helpful to scan the sensation data flow, surveying what messages are coming from the whole sensorium including body, feelings and thoughts.

As described earlier, body sensations are most useful because they are fully in the present and much less vast in terms of content and speed. Thoughts and feelings are much more complicated, but denial of them does not seem to yield

---

[185] R. Stone, *Polarity Therapy, Vol. 1.* CRCS, 1986. Book 1, p. 19.

[186] Marian Diamond, *The Brain: Use it or Lose It.* Mindshift Connection (vol. 1, no.1), Zephyr Press, edited by Dee Dickinson.

good results. When setting a base for practice, it is better to acknowledge thoughts and feelings and mentally make a note to attend to them later, when the time is appropriate.

The skill of being includes exploring how to be *centered*, *grounded* and *neutral*. These all refer to states that may heighten perceptual sensitivity. All can be developed to become accessible quite efficiently, even in the first few minutes of a therapy session. All can be refined, probably to unlimited degrees, and therefore they can serve as lifelong projects for professional practice, self-healing, personal growth and ANS resiliency.

## *Centering*

Centering refers to using awareness to find the energetic balance point of the body. Centering gathers attention from the periphery of awareness to the core. Esoteric anatomy holds that there is an energetic middle in the vertical axis of the body approximately located along the spine. This non-physical channel is thought to carry the original energy flow that organized the body in its earliest days, represented by the embryological primitive streak. By visualizing and sensing this earliest ordering phenomenon, we can access a state of being that precedes imprinting, adaptations and history. Centering enables practitioners to experience a steady neutral place to anchor awareness, so that clients can have the benefit of a stable reflective presence in which to observe their patterns. Centering also supports us in differentiating and maintaining our own identity and coherence during inquiry into another person's experience. This practice can therefore protect against caregiver burnout.

Each practitioner will discover a unique formula or practice for centering. Visualizing a central line of the body, similar to practices in the martial arts in which a red thread is imagined extending up into the sky and deep into the earth, is a proven approach. Some imagine a space instead of a line, a sort of pipe or channel with a rising airy flow. Some have described a tone or sound, such as Stone's description of the "ultrasonic core."[187] Yogic practices describe the *shushumna*, a central canal linking the chakras. Ancient Greeks and Egyptians referred to the Caduceus or Staff of Hermes. Tibetan Yoga calls this midline the "Central Channel." All of these models share the idea of a non-physical location that helps organize the rest of the body. By meditatively imagining this centerline, we inevitably gain a measure of peace and stillness, creating an effective platform for enhanced perception.

In sensing our centers, it may be helpful to shift the attention outward, to the periphery or horizon, then return inwardly, back to the middle. This gives us a sense of "not center" as a contrasting perception, creating a "That" vs. "Not That" experience, a repeated theme in ANS self-regulation.[188] Shifting between the periphery and the core also echoes our earliest weeks of life, when the primitive streak (a primordial centerline) was preceded by signaling and nourishment from the trophoblast (the embryonic periphery), suggesting that the ordering forces originate in the field, not the center.

## *Grounding*

In martial arts or in everyday life, the word "grounded" normally implies being "earthy" and practical. Symbolically interpreted, it can also refer to our interface with gravity, such as our feet on the floor or our seat in the chair. Here the meaning is expanded to include the whole idea of lowering the locus of awareness, increasing the range of perceptual activity so that we are not always "in our heads." More

---

[187] R. Stone, *Polarity Therapy, Vol. 1.* CRCS, 1986. Book 2, Chart 03.

[188] The phrase comes from Zen practice: for an example of the context, see Sensei Janet Jiryu Abels, *The Stepping Stones of Zen.* http://stillmindzendo.org/talks-publications/the-stepping-stones-of-zen/

information may be available from lower "listening stations," such as the throat, heart or belly.

A lower center of awareness is helpful in many situations. Each station has its own tone, similar to the lenses of different kinds of sunglasses. Just as skiers use amber for overcast, gray for bright sunlight, we might listen from the head for insight, from the heart for compassion and from the belly for sympathy. Being able to adjust the location of attention along the vertical axis increases our capabilities in terms of being able to find the appropriate optimum perceptual base for interacting with any client.

### Neutral

The third component of the skills of being is known as neutral. A state of neutrality creates a stable platform for any session work. Neutral implies that we are neither too ambitious nor too dispassionate, and not over-committed to either direct or indirect methods. Neutral means quieting the mind and reducing the natural impulse to overcome perceptual limitations by trying harder. A paradox of subtle listening is that trying harder usually does not lead to better sensitivity. Instead, relaxation, trust and "soft" neutrality make a better foundation for subtle perception.

Achieving neutrality is difficult; for many, it is a lifelong learning project. We can be easily pulled from neutrality by many factors:

• Sympathy for clients in their suffering; as osteopathic physician James Jealous put it, "The hardest barrier is wanting to fix the client."[189] Our inner desire to help people in need creates a natural bind, like Ulysses wanting to hear the Sirens in *The Odyssey*; we need to "bind ourselves to the mast" of neutrality and close off our crew's ears with wax to

---

[189] James Jealous, DO, *Rebalancing and Side Effects #1*. Audio CD #5 in series "The Biodynamics of Osteopathy." James Jealous, 2005.

make it through the narrow strait where so many have run aground.

- Needing to feel good about ourselves; feelings of inadequacy (or in some cases, feelings of over-confidence).

- Distractions in our own lives, including the financial pressure of needing to satisfy customers in order to have a successful practice.

Inadequate neutrality distorts both our perceptual process and our relationship with the client. We tend to try too hard. Physician and author Paul Lee describes it this way:

> If we attempt to use <u>active</u> pursuit of the thought process to achieve knowledge about the unmanifest, we get blocked or confused... just as thought cannot perceive the greater thought of the unmanifest. But the <u>passive</u> reception of information about the unmanifest routinely occurs through reflection, contemplation and meditation.[190]

Perhaps the greatest obstacle to neutrality is comparative thinking, or the "better than/less than" bias. Most people think comparatively, as when school children are given grades on their projects, which they then inevitably compare with the grades of their friends. Similarly, sports competitions, beauty contests and celebrity publicity all conspire to make us compare ourselves with others. These ways of thinking become so habitual that they are no longer even noticed. Comparative thinking has to be curbed or at least managed if we are to enter into the realm of subtle perception to support Yin and Yang practice.

No two practitioners can really be compared, although obviously one may have more education, experience or confidence than another. We bring our unique entire life experience to the session encounter, and subtle factors

---

190 Paul Lee, *Interface*. Stillness Press, 2007, p. 103.

determine the outcome. A novice practitioner may have just the right profile of life experience to strategically match a particular client, perhaps even more than a veteran practitioner would. There may be special circumstances relating to having a common history in some way. I like the saying, "Karma beats talent every time." If we are destined to be helpful it will happen whether we are supposedly "better than" or "less than."

This approach, going beyond comparison, relieves our burden to "fix" the client. We can show up, be as prepared as possible, and sincerely make our genuine effort, but ultimately the full responsibility for the outcome is not all in our hands. The session process will unfold more naturally if we maintain this attitude of neutrality.

The philosopher Gurdjieff was fond of the phrase, "not my will but thine, O Lord."[191] This attitude, that the client will get better or not depending on a higher order of action, can be a great comfort as we try to maintain neutrality in the presence of suffering. This phrase may be helpful as a silent mantra or self-reminder when the session is starting. If this particular phrase does not work, perhaps an alternative can be identified from within your own belief system; anything that feels right for you and conveys a sense of yielding to larger forces could be effective for the purpose of strengthening neutrality.

"Better than/less than" thoughts will naturally arise in sessions, especially at the start. We can protect neutrality by acknowledging and naming a thought instead of trying to push it away or ignore it. We can notice the thought, name it, find some way to appreciate it (or at least normalize it by recalling its origins), and invite it into consciousness. After a

---

[191] Numerous sources have versions of this, starting with the Bible's New Testament (Matthew 26:36-46; Mark 14:32-42; Luke 22:39-46). Edgar Cayce and G. I. Gurdjieff also used the same phrase.

few moments, when the time feels right, it can be mentally marked for future processing and temporarily put aside.

Neutrality benefits both practitioner and client. For the practitioner, the capacity to find and be steady in a neutral state is another protection against "caregiver burnout," supporting longevity in the profession. Without neutrality, we may try too hard, expend our own internal reserves and reach a state of professional exhaustion. The whole therapeutic equation is changed by neutrality.

## A Note on the Term "Healer"

In the context of neutrality, the use of the term "healer" is problematic. "Healer" implies responsibility for changing the client's condition in an active, Yang way. An indirect, Yin method sees healing as coming from within the client, not externally from the practitioner. Neutrality is about having equal access to both sides. Descriptive words such as "facilitator" and "practitioner" have advantages over "healer," because they represent a more neutral positioning, leave space for Yin and avoid disempowerment of the client.

Also as a side note, Stone generally excluded psychic healing.[192] His objections included:

• There are probably sufficient resources in the present physical body for many therapeutic processes.

• Psychic interventions may be disadvantageous for some practitioners, who may be unintentionally drawn into deeper invisible world responsibilities for the client than they intended. This may lead to fatigue or longevity problems.

• Using a psychic approach can make us vulnerable to prideful or grandiose delusions and to over-estimating our powers. This can be another obstacle to stability and durability in the health care profession.

---

[192] R. Stone, *Polarity Therapy, Vol. 1*. CRCS, 1986. Book 1, pp. 2, 55, 66.

## Other Considerations with Neutral

A neutral state is also protection against "counter-transference," in which we get confused and buy in to our clients' projections. By cultivating the capacity for neutral we have a better chance to be aware of counter-transference when it happens, instead of being dominated by it.

Neutral may seem to be somewhat uncaring at first glance, but that characterization is not accurate: Neutral is a basis for effectiveness. People who are called to the health care professions are likely to have more empathy, not less. But the Yin and Yang approach calls for steadiness, not going too low with the observation of distress or experience of therapeutic failures, nor too high with our successes. For best results, neutral is a key factor. When I am feeling drawn in to clients' problems, the last words of poet William Butler Yeats serve as a reminder:

> Cast a cold eye
> On life, on death.
> Horseman, pass by![193]

There is an art to manifesting neutral in a style that also conveys sincere caring. Ideally, we are perceived by clients as a friendly mirror: empathic and well-informed but not predisposed to any particular characterization. To get an accurate reflection, the client needs a true surface with minimal distortion or agitation. It is difficult to comb our hair using a reflection of the visor mirror in a pickup truck going down a bumpy road. Neutral extends to every aspect of practice. Even our appearance can be made relatively nondescript so that new clients' propensity for assumptions is further minimized.

---

[193] W.B. Yeats, *Under Ben Bulban* in *Collected Poems of W. B. Yeats.* MacMillan, 1956. These words are also engraved on his tombstone. "Horseman" refers to the mythical four horsemen of the apocalypse, an archetypal image of suffering.

Moving into a state of "centered, grounded and neutral" has huge benefits for every practitioner. Repeatedly going through such a routine during each day, with every session, is similar to having a regular meditation or martial arts practice. As increasing equanimity is developed, the rest of life becomes smoother. Minor neurotic habits gradually diminish. A special attraction of this particular vocation is that the service we provide can also be so beneficial for us.

The skills of being are more a process than a destination. Even on the first day of training, we can shift awareness a notch or two in the direction of center-ground-neutral. Years later, the same will still be true.

## #2: The Skill of Relationship

The skill of relationship is about finding a way to create rapport with another person. This idea is also known as "reciprocal equanimity." The practitioner skill of relationship has great significance in all forms of therapy, directly stimulating the social branch of the ANS.

At its simplest, skills of relationship begin with experimenting to find what spatial or energetic proximity feels right for each client. All people have "comfort zones," arising from prior life experience, especially their maternal relationship history. Some clients need more contact, some need more space. If we come too close to a person who needs space, the client will subtly move away in self-protection; if we are too distant with people who desire contact, they will energetically reach out and pursue, or appear as if they do not care. The optimum relational proximity can be thought of as a "sweet spot" that optimizes authentic communication between client and practitioner.

If we are trying to detect subtle phenomena when our client is cringing in self-protection, we could erroneously conclude that the client has particular stress patterns and problems when in fact, the client may simply be responding to our being too close. This situation can create great confusion and can even become self-perpetuating: we create a problem by being invasive or abandoning, and then diagnose the problem as being a character flaw of the client. We then go about trying to help the client with the problem, which was partially a reflection of wrong relationship, in addition to other factors from the client's history. This can become a repetitive cycle, and go on for a long time.

By taking some time to track our own internal state, we can create a safer and more supportive basis for therapy. In a larger sense, anyone can practice this with anyone else, in any situation, with good effect. In a relationship, people seeking to shift disturbing dynamics can simply take a moment and

## Practitioner-Client Interactions

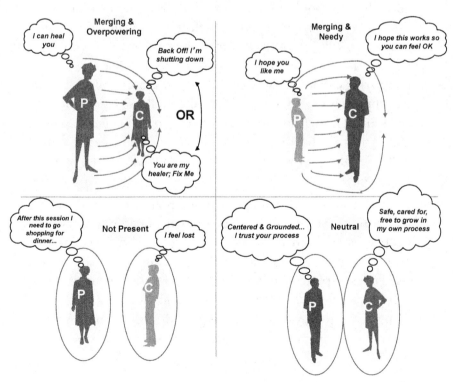

reconsider their energetic proximity to the other person, on all levels, including physical, emotional and mental. They can consider giving the other person more space or more contact. After making an adjustment, a minute or two should be given for the effects to unfold. This can be a revelation for many people in moving away from conflict and toward more communication. Even in business or casual contexts, skill in relationship proximity can minimize interference and promote effective communication.

Relationship generally implies Yin and Yang principles. Any meeting of two or more people represents a temporary energetic unity, a paired field. Communication of any kind constitutes a recurrent feedback loop in the field. Finding the right relationship can induce movement. Conversely, being either too crowded or too distant can create fixation.

The art of relationship is to be in the right proximity, and also to hold appreciative and/or neutral thoughts. Thoughts can have a significant effect on a relationship. The same physical proximity can feel quite different if we have intentions about doing something, if we are distracted and not paying attention, or especially if we are thinking critical (or appreciative) thoughts. With the first two practitioner skills in place, clients are more likely to relax and express their situation and needs much more clearly and authentically as a result of not feeling crowded, abandoned or criticized.

The power of exuding appreciation is enormous and has a huge impact on the therapeutic relationship. Most people have a finely tuned radar for when someone is thinking critical or judgmental thoughts, and naturally there will be a self-protective impulse to manage, defend against or repel a judgmental person. We can create a strong basis for therapeutic progress by noticing and appreciating some characteristic of the client: a particular part of the story, the palpable presence of life force in the body or even something seemingly trivial such as a choice of clothing or ornamentation. The old business-coaching adage, "Catch the person [client or employee] doing something right," serves well in practitioner skill #2.[194] Hakomi Therapy founder Ron Kurtz taught his students to find at least one thing to appreciate in every client, in every session.[195]

Right relationship also extends to other aspects of the client-practitioner dynamic, and it is an influence toward highest conduct in ethics, business practices, confidentiality, non-exploitation and respect. The practitioner occupies a place of power in the therapeutic relationship, and attention to this practitioner skill is excellent protection against error and accidental abuse of that power.

Building rapport is valued and emphasized in varying degrees in different psychotherapy systems.[196] In a Yin and Yang model, finding some mutually common ground, such as a place or life experience, increases the flow of information because the speaker feels recognized at a deeper level.

### Dual Relationships between Client and Practitioner

Practitioner skill #2 invites a precautionary statement on the subject of "dual relationships," when therapists and clients have more than one shared field of action, such as social interactions in addition to their therapeutic meetings, especially if they live in a small town and contact is unavoidable. Various experts have taken positions for and against dual relationships (they all agree that any sexual

---

[194] Kenneth Blanchard and Spencer Johnson, *The One Minute Manager*. Morrow, 1982.

[195] Ron Kurtz, *Body-Centered Psychotherapy: The Hakomi Method*. LifeRhythms, 2007.

[196] For example, see Robin Dreeke, *It's Not All About Me: The Top Ten Techniques for Building Rapport with Anyone*. Robin Dreeke, 2011. Dreeke's work experience is in security and defense institutions.

contact is totally unacceptable), generating an interesting scholarly debate.[197]

From a Yin and Yang perspective, the counselor is in the Yang role relationally, so our top priority is about conduct according to the archetypes. Just as a parent (Yang) is responsible for the conduct of a child (Yin), a practitioner holds responsibility for ensuring that the practitioner/client relationship is always protected. By guarding the Yin and Yang balance within the therapeutic environment, we create a safe space for the healing process to unfold.

## #3: The Skill of Listening

The practitioner skill of listening builds upon the prior skills of being and relationship. If we can become quiet and find the sweet spot of right relationship, what will we hear? Common practice places great emphasis on our being able to assess the client's condition and project some diagnostic hypothesis to see if it fits. But a key preparatory step might be left out: the step of more open, receptive, appreciative listening. We may move to diagnosis and treatment strategies too quickly, thereby missing very important information.

The normal way to relate to and interact with another person is often by an outward gesture of attention. In the listening phase, the impulse to analyze or even inquire is postponed. Instead, the first focus is on just receiving, using an inward signal emphasis. We create a momentary perceptual one-way street. Clients generate a steady flow of signals about their current states. They do this in many ways, obviously including the content of their words, but also using subtle body language and facial micro-movements. In the

---

[197] Ofer Zur, "The Conversation Continues... Notable Shifts in the Debate of Therapeutic Boundaries," in *California Psychologist,* 2008. Vol. 41, No. 1, pp. 6-9.

listening phase, these signals are allowed to just flow in, unimpeded by premature analysis or judgment.

In this phase we serve the client as an attentive audience and a recurrent feedback loop is likely to be initiated. Many people do not often have the experience of being heard in a fully-attentive, non-judgmental, receptive way. Taking adequate time to simply listen creates a basis for relationship that will be conducive to restoring movement in the form of increased sensitivity for both self-awareness and ability to attend to another person. I think feeling heard is also stimulating to the social ANS, thereby elevating the highest resource of the whole system.

A useful resource for intentional listening comes from biofeedback research, explained at length in *The Open-Focus Brain* by Les Fehmi and Jim Robbins.[198] This book explains the difference between narrow-focus tunnel vision and a wide visual perspective. Cultivating "open-focus" skills can be inherently supportive of the practitioner skill of listening, because the normally predominant left-brain perceptual process is subtly softened and whole brain integration appears.

For a listening phase, we take some time to switch off the outgoing perceptual process, and let the incoming process take over for a time. Osteopath James Jealous refers to these two as efferent and afferent, or sensory and motor faculties of perceptual process. Instead of going out searching for information, we sit back and let the information offered by the client stream in, without much differentiation, naming or judgment. A minute or so may be all that is necessary to create a sense of relational balance. The listening phase inevitably transforms into the next practitioner skill,

---

[198] Les Fehmi and Jim Robbins, *The Open-Focus Brain: Harnessing the Power of Attention to Heal Mind and Body.* Trumpeter Press, 2007.

recognition, by its own natural progression. With some practice, this phase becomes second nature and also has benefits in other relationships outside the therapy setting.

The listening skill is not passive. "Active listening" refers to the process of reflecting back what clients said in a way that deepens their process and elicits their own insights and wisdom. Questions for the listening phase are often open-ended, such as, "Is there anything you would like me to know for our session today?" or even just, "Tell me a story..."

### #4: The Skill of Recognition

The practitioner skill of recognition arises naturally and organically from effective listening. In this stage we begin to identify information coming from the client. This can be very simple, such as noticing a particular gesture or emotion, identifying something that fits in a theoretical system, or naming a symptom or ANS state. The therapeutic benefit can

---

### A Listening Vignette

As a 12-year old boy scout, my buddies and I went on bird-watching outings with a professor from the local college. We would go out into the woods and sit quietly in the pre-dawn darkness near a bird hotspot such as a quiet, isolated pond.

When light started to appear, the birds would become active, and the professor would help us find the different varieties so that we could mark them on our merit badge cards.

Repeatedly he would point at a tree and identify the species, but we could not see it. Looking through our binoculars, we had tunnel vision. He would instruct us to put down the binoculars and just look at the whole tree, and let the bird's movement come to us, instead of looking for it so intently. The method, not trying so hard, worked every time.

The phase of listening is similar: a gentle pause allows more information with less judgment and premature jumping to conclusions.

---

be enormous; naming anything shifts the experience from "participant" (a monopole, undifferentiated) to "observer" (a dipole, with dualistic perspective and possibility of movement).

Recognition has endless possibilities, depending on the practitioner's knowledge and skills. An anatomy expert recognizes physical details, whereas a Freudian psychologist recognizes instinctual drives. Cross training, for example, a psychotherapist who learns anatomy, or a medical doctor who learns about psychological trauma effects, can be very beneficial, since recognition of the client is always about the

---

### About Monopoles and Dipoles

These terms from physics, chemistry and cell biology are also found in applications such as audio system design. "Monopole" means a magnetic pole considered in isolation, with one effect (attraction or repulsion) and no direct relationship; monopoles are mainly just theoretical. "Dipole" means a pair of oppositely charged poles, separated by a space, that together create a dynamic electromagnetic field in between.

In a Yin and Yang perspective, a dipole is much more interesting because it implies relationship. In nature, monopoles are hard to find, whereas the water molecule is an omnipresent example of a dipole.

A theme in Yin and Yang therapy is to reestablish flow. A client or couple who has become fixated and lost the capacity for dancing between Yin and Yang could be said to be functioning as a monopole. As practitioners we engage with our clients and thereby establish a dipole. The dipole configuration is much more conducive to flow and therefore health. The dipole action of practitioner-client stimulates renewed polarized flow action within the client. The client or couple can then see situations in a new light and gain freedom from being limited to just the same habitual responses.

---

whole person, including mental, emotional and physical experience.

Recognition does not necessarily have to be verbalized. The benefits of recognition can be gained to varying degrees with or without actual spoken naming. When the client feels recognized, the relationship is strengthened and the practitioner is more accepted, leading to a more robust feedback loop.

Meeting a dear friend from childhood is a good analogy for this experience. Instead of having a normal, shallow conversation, old friends immediately go to a much deeper sharing of more personal information, because each speaker feels truly recognized by the other.

For recognition, knowledge of subtle anatomy is helpful in the Yin and Yang approach. Clients reveal their stories not only with their narratives but also with their body language, which can give a reliable indicator about their status within the Three Principles and Five Elements model. Body reading is discussed further in Chapter 13.

In the recognition phase, we strive to identify phenomena without pathologizing, and to remember that all actions of the body serve the biological imperative of survival. Even inefficient, problem-causing strategies have at their core a kernel of the impulse to survive. Carefully recognizing and appreciating the intelligence behind the symptoms, more than the pathology of their potential side effects, allows us to maintain the neutrality of the relationship so that the feedback process can continue to unfold.

## #5: The Skill of Conversation

The skill of conversation is the fifth component of the foundation for Yin and Yang practice. Effective conversation benefits from the prior four skills being in place and well-established. In the therapeutic conversation, we begin a more active role: questions may be posed, verbally, or, if the practice includes contact, non-verbally using sensitive touch. The client may answer, also verbally or non-verbally. With every loop of the process, the information becomes richer and more useful.

An analogy for conversation is the recurrent feedback loop of a playground swing. In this analogy, the practitioner is the adult, and the client is the young child. The conversation begins with the first push of the swing; the child's response is either "Push more!" or "Too much!" Based on the feedback, the adult modifies the force and direction of pushing, the child responds again, and so on, to continually refine the experience in a recurrent feedback loop process. The information builds up as the play continues.

For example in the case of a client with a sore neck, we might ask the obvious question, "When did this condition first arise?" The answer might hold important information about the origin of the condition in some part of the person's experience, including cues for Three Principles/Five Elements experience. Verbal responses are obviously very useful, but we may also recognize valuable information in non-verbal responses such as tone of voice, posture, facial micro-movements or gestures.

The skill of conversation includes unlimited possibilities; here are a few samples of conversation starters, their rationale and an example or two:

• **Open-ended questions**, to stimulate information and jump-start recurrent feedback. Examples: "Tell me a story." "How are you today?" "What would you like me to know for today's session?"

• **Contact statements**, to deepen clients' process by recognizing particular expressions, gestures, emotions and other signals. Examples: "I notice you just shifted breathing."

"You just swallowed, can you describe what you notice in your throat area just now?"

• **Probes**, to move the conversation along. Examples: "How old do you feel just now?" "Where in your body does that thought or emotion reside?"

• **Appreciation**, to elevate the ANS. Examples: "That's great, you handled a difficult situation very well." "You made it." "That last statement was very well put."

• **Body reading**, to increase self-awareness. Examples: "I observe that you are gesturing with your right hand at chest level; that could be Yang Principle and Air Element." "Could you speak a sentence with the words, 'I want _____' and fill in the blank?"

The skill of conversation is a reminder about the spectrum spanning all health care modalities, discussed above in Chapter 1. With the skill of conversation, the goal is to be able to work in the full range, including direct (advice and interpretation) and indirect (supporting corrections that arise from within the client) methods.

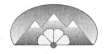

# Chapter 8

# Values

*It is far easier and safer to prevent illness by observance of the laws of health than to set about curing illness that has been brought on by our own ignorance and carelessness.*[199]

–Mahatma Gandhi

The Yin and Yang approach offers specific lifestyle values that can help clients build coherent and healthful lives. If we have guidelines for living, we can have a frame of reference to guide choices during times of stress. Having values means, "When in doubt, I'll go this way."

Values also represent a form of preventive care, in the sense that by bypassing errors, we avoid issues that later would need treatment. We intuitively know that prevention is more cost-effective than treatment, even though economic comparisons are not available. Perhaps the medicine of the future will make a stronger effort to quantify the value of prevention compared to treatment.

An orientation to particular values is included in most traditional health systems as well as most religions and philosophies. However, the modern era has become much less inclined to promote particular values, for several good reasons.

---

[199] M. Gandhi, *Gandhi's Health Guide.* Crossing Press, 2000. p. 1.

The first reason relates to modern globalization. As cultures mix together and we are exposed to new beliefs, we have more ability to re-evaluate the assumptions of our native culture. The result is an "anything goes" era and as a result, we feel more free to experiment with life decisions, using trial-and-error to figure out what feels right. The benefit is new possibilities, but the risk is "throwing the baby out with the bath water," as highly beneficial knowledge based on substantial experience may be discarded. As a rebellious teenager of the 1960s, I thought there were no limits to my ability to reinvent life. As the years passed, I grew to appreciate the validity of some of my parents' values, which I had previously scorned.

In an "anything goes" era, many feel a reluctance to take a stand on controversial topics. We fear being politically incorrect or offending anyone, so we are more likely to keep our opinions to ourselves. Again, there are benefits and risks for this attitude as well.

The question of whether we should represent certain values or be relatively value-free is a matter of some debate in the general psychotherapy community. Should behaviors be judged by some standard, or is anything permissible as long as the adult participants are consenting? If a client smokes tobacco, harming self and others while also self-medicating for anxiety, should we point this out with an intention of influencing the client to stop, or should we wait for that impulse to arise from within? Strong arguments exist for either approach, reflecting the validity of both sides of the health-care spectrum spanning the two principal modes, direct (intervention) and indirect (wait and let our clients find their own ways).

When we adopt certain values, we are already putting some weight on the direct side of the scales. After that, it is an open question as to when and how much to make values a part of our practice. I personally tend to be more values-oriented than average, and apparently I also seem to use direct methods more liberally than some of my colleagues.

Lifestyle factors, as well as our response and flexibility toward change, all shift as we get older. A young child needs firm support and clear direction, whereas a mature adult may find lifestyle suggestions inappropriate or unwelcome. As they age, seniors become more Yang in terms of world experience, and many are unreceptive to advice.

Various religious and spiritual systems often include guidance about values; we avoid aligning with any one system but we become curious when many sources give the same advice. The method resembles a principle of scientific inquiry which regards duplicate results from independent sources as a form of confirmation.

Taoism offers detailed practices for longevity, also advocating studious attention to ethical living including close attention to "what you think, what you say and what you do." Yoga systems espouse an *ahimsa* (non-violent) lifestyle. Buddhism has its "basic precepts."[200] Buddhism also offers the "Four Immeasurables" of loving kindness, compassion, joyful empathy and equanimity.[201] In Christianity, the "Golden Rule" serves a similar purpose. Stone taught values such as self-awareness, love, compassion and forgiveness.

Stone's default advice for all purposes is about attuning to nature. According to him, the more we stray from nature, the more complicated our situations will become. Stone

---

[200] See www.Buddhism.about.com for a simplified summary. This same site is a source for basic details about the other health practices discussed in this chapter.

[201] David Tuffley, *The Four Sublime States: The Brahmaviharas.* Altiora, 2012. Also: B. Alan Wallace, *The Four Immeasurables: Practices To Open The Heart.* Snow Lion, 2010.

advised us to re-establish natural rhythms and processes as much as possible. In his words, "It is best for man to work with Nature and to be in tune with Nature..."[202]

Beyond that, Stone was opinionated about his clients and how they conducted their lives. He was apparently not shy about pointing out a dietary error, a behavior that was subtly damaging, or what he considered to be an unrealistic attitude or expectation that was leading to suffering. Consistent with this approach, the Yin and Yang therapist may well advocate for particular values in the sessions and take on a "life-coaching" role in addition to other functions.

Values for the Three Principles and Five Elements were already introduced, so a quick summary of key values is provided below.

We can use these values to guide clients when they are facing difficult situations. Clients in either Yang or Yin roles can be reminded of the appropriate main values for that role. For example, a Yang role player may be feeling ambivalent about a decision; a reminder about the importance of being decisive may be helpful to nudge the process along and thereby avoid prolonged side effects such as becoming more Yang deficient (the wimp archetype). The Elements also benefit from having clear values. A client with Air Element symptoms can pay close attention to desires, optimism and idealism, thereby reducing further complications.

### The "Polarity Lifestyle Values"

Stone's teaching proposes that eating a vegetarian diet, abstaining from promiscuity and avoiding intoxicants can be significant contributors to overall functionality, reducing turbulence of the three levels of experience (body, emotions and mind). These can be protective lifestyle habits that

---

[202] R. Stone, *Polarity Therapy, Vol. 1.* CRCS, 1986. Book 3, p. 114.

support high-functioning and maximum awareness in each of the three levels of life. Together they suggest a lifestyle that reduces physical, emotional and mental disturbance.

I refer to Stone on this topic because his writing represents a fresh start that is not encumbered by particular cultural or religious belief systems. Many people resist being asked to change their cultural foundation, especially when it comes to making personal decisions about how to conduct their lives. Stone borrowed freely from everything he could find, and the result is a composite that serves as an umbrella

| Principles | Values |
|---|---|
| Yang | Responsibility, commitment, decisiveness, reliability, consistency and creativity |
| Yin | Contentment, discrimination, nurturing, reflection, attunement to natural rhythms and adaptability |
| Neutral | Stillness, calmness, insight, aesthetic beauty, harmonious sound and inspiration |

| Elements | Values |
|---|---|
| Ether | Sense of self-esteem, expressiveness, spiritual impulses, capacity for making choices, discrimination and appreciation for beauty |
| Air | Expressiveness, optimism, idealism, hope, lightness of being and heart-felt caring |
| Fire | Will power, forcefulness, muscular strength and determination |
| Water | Loyalty, discipline, mutually respectful sexuality and strong relationships, especially with significant other and family |
| Earth | Stability, security and courage under stress |

encompassing many local belief systems and cultural contexts.

## *A Health Practice for the Physical Level: Vegetarian Diet*

> *We cannot kill for the sake of our palate without it having*
> *a profoundly destructive effect on our mental health...* [203]

It can be argued that a vegetarian diet supports the value of non-violence in the physical body, specifically by avoiding the neurochemical after-effects of slaughter in the meat that is consumed. In this line of thinking, the animal's last experience before slaughter includes a surge of stress chemicals in its sympathetic ANS, leaving the cells suffused with adrenaline and related stress response chemicals. In theory, this leads to an elevated sympathetic autonomic state in the person who consumes neurologically-active chemical residues in the meat.

Another, more esoteric argument relates "non-violence" based on vegetarian diet to the concept of karma. Stone describes this in several places, for example:

> Besides such physical reactions as the toxins produced in our body when we eat the flesh of slaughtered animals, fish and fowl, there is also the factor of karma, that we inevitably reap what we have sown. We are responsible for all our actions, past and present, and experience the consequences in our physical, mental and emotional state of health. [204]

> Naturally, he curtails his animal nature and lessens his karmic burden by following the strict instructions not to eat anything that must be killed

---

[203] R. Stone, *Health Building*, CRCS, 1986. p. 26.
[204] *ibid*, p. 5.

or stopped in its progress of development, like eggs, meat, fish and fowl, or anything containing them. [205]

Theravada Buddhism also embraces "not killing" in its "five basic precepts." In Buddhism, precepts are considered to be lines of inquiry more than direct commandments, but the language is unequivocal. Similarly in the Ten Commandments, "Thou shalt not kill," seems to be a clear statement, although obviously the interpretations are very diverse.

Dr. Julian Johnson, a student of Himalayan mysticism in the 1940s, was taught about a "ladder of life" of increasingly sophisticated consciousness, in five elemental stages. [206] All five elements are present on all rungs of the Five Elements model, but the elements are supposedly "awakened" incrementally. In this Himalayan tradition, plants have one element active, insects and reptiles have two, birds and fish have three, mammals have four, and humans have all five elements active. "Life feeds on life," so some reaction is inevitable at every step. But the subtle impact grows as higher levels of the ladder are accessed.

For an analogy from the same tradition, imagine someone crossing the yard of a homeowner. If some grass is trampled, it is not even noticed. If some insects are stepped on, the impact is still minimal. However, if a pet bird is harmed by the trespasser, the owner will at least be angry, and if a mammal such as a pet dog or cat is injured, the consequences are likely to be more substantial. If a human is hurt, severe effects will follow, including imprisonment or even capital punishment. The reaction grows in proportion to

---

[205] R. Stone, *Mystic Bible*. RSSB, 1956. p. 14.

[206] Julian Johnson, *Path of the Masters (Abridged)*. RSSB, 1940. pp. 104-105.

the consciousness of the injured creature. Using this esoteric line of thinking, a plant diet minimizes the reactivity.

Support for the non-violence of vegetarianism began long before other reasons for a plant-based diet came into public consciousness. As author John Robbins has eloquently described, dietary choices represent an intersection of modern environmental, economic, political and ethical debates.[207]

Dietary choices are extremely personal and the conversation gets complicated quickly, such as in meditation retreats that have a vegan diet just for the days of the event. Also, some people seem to have a hard time not eating meat, based on blood type or other factors, and an anti-vegetarian position has also been articulated.[208] For this discussion, these kinds of details are left to individuals to decide on their own, following their own personal and medical guidance.

### A Health Practice for the Emotional Level: Moderation in Sexual Activity

Minimizing sexual promiscuity can support non-violence in the emotional layer of the system. Promiscuity here means sexual interaction without mutual agreement about intention. If the activity is frivolous, it should at least be mutually frivolous.

Realistically, "free love" is rare because the intensity of sexual intimacy invokes strong emotional feelings, and true mutuality of the emotional experience is unlikely. One partner may hope for a deeper relationship while the other simply seeks pleasure. Often this mismatch falls along Yin and Yang lines because the two have different agendas. As Stone said, "Creation has an outward purpose [Yang] for the

---

[207] John Robbins, *Diet for a New America.* Kramer, 2012. First published in 1988.

[208] Lierre Keith, *The Vegetarian Myth: Food, Justice, and Sustainability.* PM Press, 2009.

body and an inward purpose [Yin] for the soul."[209] The intensity causes this mismatch to reach deeply into the level of feelings, and the effects can reverberate for a long time. Emotional continuity and coherence can become fragmented. From a Yin and Yang perspective, a client engaged in a tumultuous private life may start to show ANS stress because overall coherence is being undermined.

In monastic Buddhism, attention is also paid to sexual activity, with a precept about "sexual misconduct." The phrasing could be interpreted in many ways, starting with extremely strict celibacy rules for monks and nuns. In my interpretation, the teaching is the same because I interpret "misconduct" to mean lack of mutual intentionality.

Sexual intimacy benefits from being "contained" safely by common agreement in order to avoid feelings of exploitation, betrayal or other emotional stress. Containment is created by self-awareness and discipline, not an easy task because the impulses arise primarily from involuntary autonomic levels.

### A Health Practice for the Mental Level: Minimizing Drugs and Alcohol

In Stone's opinion, intoxicants are considered to be a form of violence in the mind. The problem with intoxicants is that they disrupt mental coherence. In Stone's language:

> Alcoholic beverages of any kind are definitely to be avoided because they dull the mind and senses, and stimulate the nervous system and the earthy *pranas* [energy currents] which have a downward material tendency and result in deterioration.[210]

---

[209] R. Stone, *Health Building*. CRCS, 1986. p. 21.

[210] R. Stone, *Mystic Bible*. RSSB, 1956. p. 14.

Mahatma Gandhi had a similar opinion: "Alcohol makes a man forget himself."[211]

Monastic Buddhism also excludes intoxication in its most basic precepts, using straightforward language: "Abstain from fermented and distilled intoxicants which are the basis for heedlessness." Heedlessness, for our purposes, means careless, thoughtless and unmindful behaviors. Again Buddhism is consistent with Stone's health practice ideas, for the same reasons.

To deal with life's complex challenges, which seem to be only increasing, we need all the perceptual sensitivity and mental clarity that we can muster.[212] Intoxication tends to prompt us to think and behave in ways we didn't really intend. These actions have consequences, and life gets more confusing.

There is a distinction between moderate usage and behavior-altering intoxication. Usage leading to regrettable thoughts, words or actions is the real focus here. Unfortunately the alcohol or drug user will be unreliable for judging the difference.

Different intoxicants have different effects and energetic signatures that can be quite unique. The addictive and destructive qualities of alcohol, "uppers" and "downers," cocaine and heroin are well-known, but "softer" substances can also be quite problematic.

For example, marijuana is popular and effective for reducing anxiety and pain. However, it seems to have the effect of reducing Yang mobilization and increasing disengagement from life. Peter Levine has spoken eloquently

---

[211] M. Gandhi, *Gandhi's Health Guide*, Crossing Press, 2000. p. 61.

[212] Douglas Rushkof, *Present Shock: When Everything Happens Now.* Current hardcover, 2013. The author describes how human biology is not designed for current circumstances.

about the problem, noting that the effectiveness of his trauma resolution methods goes down significantly if marijuana is being used.

The usage of some intoxicants for ceremonial experiences deserves to be in a separate category because the whole intention and supportive understanding is so different; indeed, the effect can be to increase coherence. Many authors have described therapeutic benefits, with some of the more compelling examples arising from indigenous shamanic rituals.[213]

Milder psychoactive substances such as caffeine, nicotine and sugar, as described in the book, *Sugar Blues*, all deserve further reflection and self-inquiry as well.[214]

The argument here applies to the more common and casual use of alcohol and similar recreational and social intoxicants. In particular, combining intoxication and promiscuity, a typical scenario on college campuses, can lead to major mental and emotional chaos. I have seen many clients in their early thirties who are still trying to resolve events, particularly with intimate relationships, that happened under the influence of intoxicants over a decade earlier.

### *The Three Health Practices Over Time*

The three health practices constitute a form of indirect psychotherapy. If clients work with these practices for an extended period of time, autonomic disturbances and emotional swings are likely to gradually recede. However, many people are not able to voluntarily stop intoxication, promiscuity or a meat diet because the underlying motives are compulsive in some way. As with any compulsive

---

[213] Jeremy Narby, *The Cosmic Serpent*. Tarcher/Putnam, 1998.

[214] William Duffy, *The Sugar Blues*. Grand Central, 1986.

behavior, these situations would be opportunities for further inquiry into the functioning of the client's ANS.

A true sense of health is generally accompanied by a feeling of choice, and in compulsive behavior there is little or no sense of choice. We can feel enslaved by our habitual lifestyles, caught in a repeating pattern of harm to ourselves and others, and a feeling of "no choice" in the matter. Stone viewed this feeling of "no choice" as a central psychological sign of disease.

In therapeutic practice, offering the lifestyle values as an option can gently make clients aware that these have been advanced as practices by Taoist, Yogic and many other related traditions. This awareness may be helpful in opening a new line of self-inquiry and perhaps some needed restraint in helping clients move their lives into a more orderly state. However, any value is greatly compromised if the client feels coerced or if the overall session environment becomes tilted away from neutrality. A judgmental or critical attitude is not part of the equation here.

Some clients are attracted to philosophies or spiritual groups that promote or enable behaviors that are directly contrary to the health practices outlined above. While it is important to respect belief systems, it may also be useful to explore whether the approach is actually working in the person's life. The debate between paths to insight and liberation is not new: in ancient Greece the extremes were represented by hyper-rational Apollo and pleasure-seeking Dionysius. The Yin and Yang approach would lean more to Apollo's ideal, with consciousness as the primary basis, but without its excessive asceticism; the Buddhist concept of a "middle way" applies. However, there is also a certain simplicity in making just one rule and applying it uniformly, so that we do not have to decide again and again, any time we are offered a drink or a tasty treat, or tempted by a prospective sexual partner.

These health practices are also helpful for therapeutic practitioners themselves. Practitioners will have a more difficult time with the "skill of being" if they have been out drinking the night before, or if they are engaged in casual romantic action on the side. The presence of stillness and neutrality are less likely to be readily accessible to us in these conditions.

The three "health practices" advocated by Stone and so many others is not a definitive requirement for using Yin and Yang principles in psychotherapy. Practitioners may want to experiment with adding or taking away various elements to experience the effects on their practitioner skills. The baseline should be to minimize materials or behaviors that disturb perception.

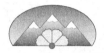

# Chapter 9

# Self-Care Practices

A top priority in therapy is to re-establish a client's self-regulating autonomy as soon as possible; self-care practices support empowerment and helping people become their own health managers. Similar to physical exercises such as weight or cardiovascular training for the physical body, these exercises are simple, quick and inexpensive ways to cultivate mental and emotional ANS wellness on our own. These practices have also proven to be effective for self-balancing.

All of the strategies given here have at least one of the three main actions:
- **Increasing ANS balance and resiliency**
- **Encouraging self-discovery and empowerment**
- **Amplifying flow between Yin and Yang**

Peter Levine has several words for the third of these, including "pendulation" and "titration." Here the word "loop" is used because it is shorter, simpler and easier to remember than the alternatives. I also like it because of its usage in the physical sciences.

The Self-Care practices are often "prescribed" for clients as "homework" at the end of a session. I often give homework assignments because it gives clients something to do on their own behalf and thereby subtly transfers some responsibility for their healing back to them, where it belongs.

It is a little sneaky and a bit manipulative, as giving homework represents a bit of direct (Yang) therapeutic intervention.

### Body-Low-Slow-Loop Practice (BLSL)

*Anna Chitty had the original insight to create this practice, after her study of Somatic Experiencing. BLSL has become one of our most useful methods in both classes and private sessions.*

This practice provides ANS first aid in the simplest possible way. It helps clients get started in self-regulation, and introduces the body-centered approach to people who have not studied trauma resolution. BLSL is a simple exercise that anyone can learn and apply safely and effectively with minimal training. It is not a cure-all for solving autonomic distress or a substitute for more substantial therapy; instead it

---

### Body-Low-Slow-Loop Summary

**Body**

- Direct the attention into the body to notice a sensation.
- *This effectively means present-tense orientation, countering trauma's past-future tendency.*

**Low**

- Direct the attention to the lower border of the sensation, or downward generally.
- *This effectively counters the upward effect of trauma (alarm & orienting responses).*

**Slow**

- Ask about the details of the sensation.
- *This effectively slows down the awareness, countering trauma's tendency to speed things up.*

**Loop**

- Direct the attention somewhere else for a minute or so, then back to the first site. Repeat as needed, slowly and gently.
- *This effectively re-establishes polarized movement and counters trauma's tendency toward fixation.*

---

is a first-aid method that can be learned for general soothing, and then deployed in a time of high stress when other resources are not available.

Regularly performing BLSL daily for ten to fifteen minutes can help gradually overcome the residual effects of trauma without having to go into the details of what happened. This practice has been very effective for many people in restoring the ANS back to an approximation of its original design. It seems to take about six weeks of regular practice to get the full benefits.

Each word in the phrase Body-Low-Slow-Loop is one stage of the process:

### Body

In this first step, we direct clients to bring their attention into the body and to notice the sensations. Bringing the attention into the body, instead of the thoughts or feelings that may be present, can be a revelation in itself. The mind becomes the audience, the body the performer. The sensations that initially attract attention could be caused simply by sensory nerves detecting contact with surfaces due to gravity, or just the movement of breath.[215] We all have these basic sensations, all the time.

In addition to the ever-present normal sensations, the initial primary (or "loudest") sensations could also be after-effects of recent or old experiences, for example a sore joint from a recent injury or a chronic stomach ache.

Tracking the body's sensations effectively pulls the client into present time, rather than the traumatic past or the

---

[215] Breath is particularly interesting because it is one of the few body functions with fully overlapping voluntary and involuntary control, an always-present interface between the conscious mind and the ANS. This partially accounts for attention to breathing as such a popular meditation and self-healing application.

anxiety-inducing future. When the physical body is observed in this mindful way, its unique processing capabilities are heightened. Instead of thinking about dire consequences or being buffeted by strong emotions, a client learns to convert awareness to a simple curiosity about the physicality of the experience. By shifting the attention to the more manageable physical level, the problematic emotional and mental dimensions may be temporarily set aside.

## Low

Next, attention is directed downward to the lower border of the area being considered in Step One, or the "southern" body areas such as feet or seat. This could consist of focusing on the lower edge of a problematic area or noticing the body's contact with the chair or floor. It does not need to be forced; if curiosity does not naturally lead to a lower perceptual target, we can just move on to the next step.

When we are startled or afraid, the body tends to elevate our center of gravity, for a host of physiological reasons, including heightened sensory sensitivity in the head, protection of peripheral limbs by reducing the circulation, and activation of some of the most powerful stress response tools in the heart and brain. Guiding the attention downward effectively counters this upward effect of stress or fear.

## Slow

The third step is to inquire about the details of the sensation. Detailed questions are posed, such as, "Is this more on the left or the right?" "Is it shallow or deep?" "Is it moving or still?" "Is it hard or soft?" There is no limit to the variety of these questions. The purpose is not about getting the information; it is about what happens when detailed questions are asked. The client could be guided to detect the texture of clothing, the temperature in the room, the border of the sensation, or any number of focusing possibilities. One possibility is to ask the client to imagine having a felt-tip marker, and to visualize using it to trace the border of the body area that has become the focus of attention due to sensations. Another possibility is to ask the client to compare one side of the target area to the other side.

Often clients will use their hand to indicate which body area feeling sensation. I have found that it is better to have them point to the area but not actually touch it. Touching can introduce new, different sensations and alter the natural awareness process.

Detailed questions cause our awareness to become more specific. When clients are asked these kinds of questions, they invariably pause, to try to figure out an answer. Their curiosity about their own sensation is heightened, causing a corresponding transfer of attention away from mental or emotional processes that may be overwhelming. Curiosity is a gesture of witness consciousness, automatically pulling us away from fixation.

Stress and trauma are notorious for their time-bending effects; time seems to speed up under stress. This step effectively slows down awareness processing, countering trauma's tendency to accelerate. By holding a curiosity about the sensation's specific attributes, the whole system starts to slow down.

## Loop

The final step is derived from the great innovation developed by Peter Levine.[216] In the Loop phase, the client is directed to shift the attention somewhere else for a minute or so, then back to the first site. This is repeated once or twice as needed, slowly and gently. The key is to induce perceptual movement from pole to pole, a form of "That" (initial

---

[216] Peter Levine, *In an Unspoken Voice*. North Atlantic, 2010.

foreground sensation) and "Not That" (elsewhere in the body). Any second location can do the trick: noticing the feet or hands is a common choice because they are rarely the site of ANS activation, unless they were the main site of an injury. Under attack, we would naturally use our hands and feet to protect our more vulnerable torso and face, so the ANS seems to consider them to be less mission-critical or worthy of priority attention.

If the first area of attention has been uncomfortable or activated in any way, it is better to find a second site that is not experiencing unpleasant sensations, to establish a pole-to-pole process. The Loop part of BLSL sets up a temporary dipole in the awareness to facilitate or induce movement.

If clients are in pain or feel overwhelmed, they may report that they can't find another place to use for the second target. For such occurrences, we can induce sensation by touching their feet or some other contact, thereby creating increased sensory activity while asking the client to report what can be noticed. When doing the practice without a

---

### "That and Not That"

A foundation of perception is differentiation. In BLSL, the phrase "That and Not That" is shorthand for shifting sensory attention from one target to another. The focus is not so important as the shifting back and forth. Generally the various dimensions of the body are useful (top-bottom, left-right, front-back, core-periphery). Frequently "that" is a part that hurts in some way, and "not that" is another part that does not hurt.

In a larger sense, "That and Not That" means the action of a pendulum or recurrent feedback loop, in any form. Self-Other, Present-Past, Speaker-Listener are all examples. The two-chair method discussed in Chapter 10 owes much of its effectiveness to its ability to induce "That and Not That" action.

---

facilitator, we can lightly move our fingertips or toes against each other or whatever other surface we are touching, to amplify sensory nerve stimulation and signaling.

After a minute or two of focusing on the second location, the attention is brought back to the first view of the body, whichever area was being focused upon, and we begin again at the start of the Body-Low-Slow-Loop process. The first locale is often different, perhaps more diffuse, less painful or entirely uninteresting, due to the effect of restoring awareness movement.

Levine describes how dwelling for too long on a painful sensation or situation can deepen the problem, making us become more fixed in whatever painful state was initially created by the response to an incident. The Loop phase of the BLSL process effectively re-establishes pole-to-pole movement and counters trauma's tendency toward fixation.

### Using BLSL as a Supportive Practice for Health

The BLSL practice can be done without any particular context or specific pain being present. Once a person has become familiar with it in stress-free times, it can be used when there is an upsetting situation, compulsion of any kind, heightened emotions such as fear or anger, or other such ANS situations. Consistent practice seems to gradually strengthen autonomic functioning, as if the non-cognitive intelligence begins to trust that beneficial movement is the new normal, instead of harmful fixation. As discussed earlier, neuroscience has clearly demonstrated that repetition can lead to the formation of new neural circuits; if true, the benefits of BLSL repatterning could be long-lasting.

For example, a female client who was extremely fearful about air travel was encouraged to try Body-Low-Slow-Loop starting about eight weeks before an unavoidable trip, at least once daily for about fifteen minutes at a time. After the first two weeks of practicing without imagining any particular context, she began to visualize going to the airport as a prelude to the practice. Then in the next two weeks, she imagined waiting at the gate, then in the next two weeks, walking onto the plane, continuously repeating the same BLSL sequence. In the sixth week, she actually got in her car and drove a few blocks toward the airport, then did the practice. By the time the actual trip arrived, there was very little fear left, and she was able to travel without complications. She also reported many other benefits, including a decrease in general anxiety, better sleep and increased patience.

Bedtime is a good time to practice BLSL, using contact with the sheets and blankets as a sensory stimulus. By settling the system down just before sleeping, we can optimize the restorative powers of dreamtime. A few minutes of BLSL before sleep may also help a person integrate the day's experiences and re-train stress responses. BLSL has also been used effectively as a remedy for insomnia.

Body-Low-Slow-Loop offers a simple practice that anyone can learn, and it can be quite transformative. However, it seems to be out of range for some clients, for example those who are in a deep depression or state of parasympathetic shock. These clients seem to be unable to remember the practice, or to stay with it for very long. In these cases, they need someone to coach them through the process, reminding them, and even stimulating sensation (for example by rubbing the feet) in order to create a second pole for oscillation of awareness. A BLSL audio recording has been created specifically for the benefit of these clients who need a boost to get started at home.[217]

---

[217] John Chitty, *Body-Low-Slow-Loop*. www.energyschool.com. 2009.

In another example, a client who suffered an auto accident was having panic attacks when driving to work, to the point of considering resigning from work to avoid the commute. She learned the BLSL method and experienced relief very quickly. In addition to symptom relief, she gained the great benefit of feeling less trapped. Instead of feeling helpless if a surge of anxiety started to appear, she knew she had a method to cope with the situation, and her fear did not escalate as it had before. She kept her job and did not need further sessions.

Similarly, a high school student was having panic attacks and learned BLSL in one session. She applied it in class and felt a reduced urgency in her anxiety. She was able to avoid a host of impending negative consequences and had a full recovery, without the expense of additional sessions.

BLSL is not a substitute for full-scale trauma resolution therapy. It is a first-aid strategy that belongs in our toolkit with other methods. It is easy to learn for all ages, applicable in diverse circumstances, self-empowering and free of cost. It could be a useful part of training for anyone who is in a potentially traumatic professional environment, such as law enforcement or the military. In addition, it offers emergency caregivers such as medical staff, police, ambulance drivers and school health personnel a valuable tool to use in difficult situations where ANS disturbances are common.

## Forgiveness Practice

*Inspiration for this practice comes from Buddhist teachings and from Tao Master and doctor Zhi Gang Sha.*[218]

In this self-help practice, clients are instructed to rest in a sitting or reclining meditative state and to use their awareness of the breath to cultivate equanimity. During

---

[218] Zhi Gang Sha, www.DrSha.com. This extensive website has downloadable Tao mantras for forgiveness and many other purposes.

*inhalation,* the thought "Acceptance" is silently repeated; during *exhalation* the thought "Forgiveness" is repeated.

The imagined recipient for these thoughts is not necessarily an antagonist, such as an estranged partner, it can also be God or one's personal sense of a higher power. Equanimity ultimately arises from a relationship with the larger forces that organize life; our inner well-being is too important to be dependent on another individual's performance.

Used as a mantra, "I forgive, and I am forgiven" and "I release, and I am released" are variations on the theme, and can be self-guided as a meditative practice and also offered to clients as a therapeutic process. Note that forgiveness can be healing in both outward (forgiving those who offended) and inward (self-forgiveness to lighten the burden of regrets).

Using the Forgiveness Practice regularly for a period of time can be very helpful in reducing pressures from interpersonal binds. A typical prescription might be once a day for ten minutes, until the next session.

### Resonance Practice

*This practice was developed by Anna Chitty, combining aspects of several sources including mindfulness meditation.*

This practice usually involves two people.[219] Sitting in chairs, facing each other, both take turns reporting their sensory experience, for about two or three minutes at a time. The first report is about describing places of contact, such as seat on the chair and feet on the floor. The report then continues with any other sensations that are being noticed.

When one is talking, the other is in Yang observer mode, listening hyper-attentively and noticing every detail

---

[219] It can also be used individually, although the effect may not be as deep.

about the speaker's expressions and movements. The speaker's eyes can be closed, to heighten the self-sensing Yin process, while the listener's eyes can be open, to heighten powers of observation.

At some point, during the two or three minutes spent listening, the listener should think an appreciative thought. This can be anything about the speaker, perhaps something about the story the person is telling. The appreciation could also be about appearance, gestures, sincerity, observation skills, tone of voice or any other attribute. The topic of appreciation can be profound or trivial, whatever feels appropriate. It does not have to be spoken; merely thinking the thought seems to be sufficient to boost the pole-to-pole flow of reciprocal Yin and Yang action.

The two continue for about fifteen minutes, until each one has had two or three turns in each role. By alternating reporting our inner state then observing our partner's report, our awareness is pushed to movement from self to other. The "self-other continuum" is a foundation of social experience. We are encouraged into being fully aware of our own inner experience and then we shift to also fully experience the other person in a rhythmic body-centered process. In Attachment Theory, the capability of full range of motion from self to other and back is a key measure of health and resiliency.[220] This practice builds that capability in a direct way with minimal risk of activation or distress of any kind.

Couples can use this practice as a way to reset their relationship. With couples, a more verbal variation can be used as one person reports thoughts or feelings, not just sensations. The partner still listens and thinks an appreciative thought, as before. The practice can also be useful in a private

---

[220] Kim Bartholomew, *Attachment Categories*. From J.A. Simpson & W. S. Rholes (Eds.), *Attachment Theory and Close Relationships*. Guilford, 1998. pp. 25-45.

setting, to deepen coherence between partners and reduce ANS tension (such as sexual dysfunction) before intimacy.

## Boundary Practice

In this practice, clients are instructed in a three-step process to imagine a surrounding "shell" that can protect them from intrusive events. Ideally this shell is about arm's length from the body, in all directions, forming an invisible egg shape that defines an energetic boundary. The concept is similar to artists' depictions of the human aura. The boundary practice is another example of a mind-body healing interchange between conscious and subconscious processes: we consciously go through the practice, and repetitively doing it subtly changes our subconscious reality.

The boundary shell is analogous to the function of the immune system, which protects the inside of the body from the outside environment. Boundary-challenged individuals may be considered to have a weakened ANS immune system, and the boundary practice can be a general remedy when we feel susceptible to upsets from outside ourselves, such as with other people who are irritating or threatening us in some way.

### Three Steps: Inspect, Repair and Rest

The first step is to imagine and visualize a shell surrounding the whole body and to mentally examine its condition. Clients often report specific observations when they do this for the first time, such as having a boundary that is too close, missing in some areas, discolored or damaged; the imagined right-front-upper area may be quite different from the left-rear-lower area. The location of the boundary problem may have some relationship to real events in the past (for example a car accident from the left may come into memory when the left side is imagined), but the focus here is not on events. Here the boundary visualization is our present-time sensing process, unrelated to any one specific context.

In Step One, we sweep our attention from front-center to right, then right to rear, then rear to left, then left to front, forming an imaginal sense about the condition of the boundary or shell. Some areas may seem missing entirely, fragmented, too close, too far, or any other variation.

In Step Two, we scan again, using the findings from Step One to imagine repairing the boundary in each quadrant. Any imaginary repair materials can be used: plaster, plexiglass, bricks and wood have all been conjured up by clients. The circular sweep of all four quadrants is conducted again, "doing" the repairs (in the imagination) as needed. The repair can also include re-setting the distance of the boundary, pushing it further out if it is too close and pulling it in if it is too far, with the intent to create a uniform distance from the body. There can be an imagined fortification of the shell, or a change in its color or texture. It can be imagined to have changed from opaque to transparent, so that approaching events can be seen. At the end of Step Two, we should be able to imagine a complete shell, with no holes or cracks, all at a consistent distance from the body. Far-fetched though it may seem, clients usually manage to create a sense of boundary repair.

Step Three is taking time to settle and rest within the newly restored boundary, feeling the effect of having our own secure, protected space. Within the shell, we have full choice about all interactions; no one else can enter without permission. This settling phase can be enjoyed for an extended period of time. Having a restored boundary can be quite a novelty for a person with chronic anxiety.

Some people have very disturbed boundaries, especially as echoes of early childhood when there may have been a high level of helplessness and intrusion. The boundary practice is extra useful for these people, but more repetition may be needed to really arrive at a felt sense of safety and protection within the energetic shield. It takes time and repetition for the felt sense of safety to become familiar and then habitual. Once again we are attempting to take advantage of how repetitive thought processes can re-wire the brain, in this case to a state of feeling safe.

In a variation of the practice, to make it more tangible, the client can sit on the floor and rolled blankets or towels can be placed in a surrounding circle, representing the boundary's ideal distance.

### "Teflon" and "Velcro" Practice

Similar to the Boundary Practice, this practice involves bringing awareness to the energetic boundary and imagining that the outer shell is made of Teflon (nothing sticks to it) or Velcro (everything sticks to it). Each imagined surface usually yields a specific sensory experience. Once the visualization has become established, we imagine that a particular context is present, for example, imagining that an antagonist (a person with whom there is conflict) is actually in the room. By using the imagination to alternate between the two kinds of surfaces, useful insights may arise and new strategies for dealing with problematic situations may emerge. The process of alternating between two states is deployed again as a way to restore movement where fixation may have taken hold.

For example, a client was having a problem with an ex-partner who was very angry. The client was susceptible to reactive responses that consistently made the situation worse. By practicing between the two states, and getting a feeling of being impermeable like Teflon, the client became able to be more "immune" to the interactions and less reactive to the ex-partner, and her anxiety receded. There was a secondary benefit in real life because her ex-partner actually became less aggressive, hypothetically because she no longer had "receptor sites" for his anger in her boundary shell.

With a non-stick outer shell surface, we are much less likely to take personally the insults being created by an outside disturbance. This is not a long-term solution to underlying relationship and communication issues, but rather a way to cultivate a sense of being protected and loosen up fixation so that new insights may arise, reducing emotional stress in the process.

### Left-Right Body Practice

Similar to the Body-Low-Slow-Loop practice, the left-right body practice is a simple way to settle the ANS. The three main physical dimensions (top-bottom, left-right, front-back) of the body are all potentially useful for alternating focus from one area to another. However, left-right and top-bottom seem to be more effective than front-back. This may be due to the relatively small sensory nerve supply on the back side of the body, with its large muscles and corresponding preponderance of motor nerves.

According to Stone, the dimensions of the body are directly correlated with Yin and Yang, so oscillation of attention between two poles is effectively undoing fixation in the basic flow patterns of the body:

| Yang | Yin |
|------|------|
| Right | Left |
| Top | Bottom |
| Back | Front |

The two sides of any of these pairs are often very different. One may feel more dense and the other more airy or spacious, or one may have movement and the other not. While different states may have meaning, it is useful to avoid over-thinking the observations or judging one as better than the other. For the most ANS benefit, letting the sensations simply stand on their own merits is a better approach.

The left-right practice involves bringing awareness to one side of the body. Lying down, the left elbow touching the floor or other surface may be the strongest, most leftward sensory nerve signal. We then expand our sensation inquiry from just the left elbow to other points of signaling, such as the shoulder and hip contact with the surface. The goal is to sense what is present, including density, texture, temperature, contact and any other attribute on one side.

After one or two minutes, we transfer attention to the other side and repeat the survey. The client can be guided to loop back and forth one more time, then repeat the next day. Doing this continually, it is likely that the two sides will gradually start to even out, and the ANS will recover some of its original flexibility.

For a top-bottom version, the torso can be very useful, often more so than the head and feet. Above and below the respiratory diaphragm in the solar plexus, the throat or heart areas can be used for "above," and the belly being moved by the breath can be used for "below." Top-bottom awareness can be helpful with clients who have become habitually top-heavy due to chronic ANS activation.

The same method can be very useful at the beginning of a touch therapy session to help the client settle into a more relaxed and self-aware state. Often this practice engenders client curiosity about what factors are present in the asymmetry, a first step in self-discovery.

### "Walking Toward" Exercise

This is another way to cultivate sensitivity to the subtle boundary that exists around the body. Becoming sensitive to boundaries is a way to facilitate relationships and reduce conflict, especially for people who had a maternal bonding experience that was invasive, abandoning or distracting. This practice is often used in classes to develop the second practitioner skill, the skill of relationship (Chapter 7), and it can also be combined with the Boundary Practice.

For this exercise, participants stand quite distant from each other, as far as the space allows. The pair take turns playing either the active or passive role. The active individual slowly starts to walk toward the partner, watching closely for micro-expressions that indicate when a pause would be appropriate. Whenever there is any indication that the other person is reacting, the first person stops and waits, noticing responses and observing closely the subtle signals coming from the second person. The exercise can include approaching too quickly, being too close, or any other combination, in order to cultivate sensitivity and create information for discussion.

Many people have layers in which autonomic proximity adjustments are being made, after which further advance is allowed. Moving closer or further can reveal habitual relationship patterns and boundary issues that would otherwise go unnoticed, even though they are important factors in a person's experience of contact.

Trying this with different people can also be illuminating, because proximity preferences are greatly affected by many variables such as gender, age, height, appearance, degree of eye contact, personal history with one another and more. Practicing this exercise can make the participants much more sensitive to spatial dynamics in intimacy, as well as any social or business situation, including work environments.

A solo simulation of this is to use an object for the other person. The "fitness ball," a large sphere used for sitting and exercising, is excellent because it can so easily be moved closer or further, to experiment with the effects.

## Shaking and Stamping Practice

In this practice, the client alternates between vigorous movement and stillness. This exercise is useful when clients are dealing with pent-up frustration, from the recent or distant past. It is also remedial for parasympathetic (hypotonic) states. Ceremonial rituals among indigenous peoples, in which a tribe uses group dancing or movement to periodically clear its collective being from old stress, have some similarity to this exercise.[221] Stone described it well:

> ...rhythmic expressions of song and dance, which use all the bodily forces and muscles for expression, free the emotions by naturally liberating the energy blocks, suppressions, frustrations and stagnations.[222]

This practice should be performed when there is no concern about sound because it can become quite loud.

Either standing or lying down, make a fist with each hand and press inward. Then let that muscular contraction spread throughout the body. This part is similar to the defensive response gestures used in Somatic Experiencing, bodywork[223] and other therapies. The fist is squeezed, then released, with ample time for mindful awareness of sensations in each state.

The next progression is to vigorously shake the whole body and even stamp the feet on the floor, for a minute or so; vocalizing can also be used. Then we bring the body to complete rest and bring our attention to sensations arising subsequent to all the motion. The resting/listening part of

---

[221] Bradford Keeney, *Shaking Medicine: The Healing Power of Ecstatic Movement*. Guilford, 2007.

[222] R. Stone, *Health Building*. CRCS, 1986. p. 18.

[223] Franklyn Sills, *Foundations in Craniosacral Biodynamics Volume Two*. North Atlantic, 2012. See page p. 539 within chapter 20, "The Polyvagal Concept" for specific instructions.

this practice is as important as the active part, and I recommend dedicating about the same amount of time for each process. This exercise can be done periodically as a way to release the inevitable accumulations of daily stress. Body-Low-Slow-Loop can then be used to help digest the liberated charge released by the movement.

Shaking and stamping can be observed in concerts, sporting events and sometimes even in religious services. These are modern-day, highly beneficial ANS subconscious self-corrections for the participants, comparable to the ritual practices observed in indigenous tribes.

### Hyper-Mobile Face Practice

This practice exercises the social ANS. Any sensory-motor action that fires the circuits of the social ANS will probably be beneficial for the whole ANS because the social ANS is at the top of hierarchical phylogenic sequence.

Psychologist Paul Ekman has provided excellent material in linking facial expression and ANS processing:

> To learn the mechanics of facial expression – which muscles produce which expression – my colleagues and I systematically made thousands of facial expressions, filming and then analyzing how each combination of muscle movements change experience. To our surprise, when we did the muscle changes that relate to emotions, we would suddenly feel changes in our bodies, changes due to ANS activity. We had no reason to suspect that deliberately moving facial muscles could produce involuntary ANS changes, but it happened again and again.[224]

---

224 Paul Ekman, *Telling Lies*. Norton, 2009. (First published in 1985). p. 118. The first three episodes of the television series *Lie to Me*, based on the work of Ekman and his colleagues (the "Truth Wizards") provide a great primer in interpreting micro-movement to get to ANS reality.

Resting comfortably, we begin this practice by simply listening to our inner state, including sensations, feelings and thoughts, but with particular attention to sensations. There need be no particular context or narrative. After a few minutes of mindfulness, we take a minute or two to mobilize the facial muscles, with spontaneous exaggerated expressions of smiling, joy, sadness, fear or any other emotion. This is done in a playful way, and in a group it can be quite amusing. It may be hard for some people in any group, for good ANS reasons, so we never apply pressure in any form. After a few minutes, we return to the baseline state and track the responses of the body.

Similar exercises can be developed around vocalization, based on the rhythm and musical quality in the voice epitomized by a mother's instinctual cooing sounds with her newborn baby. Touch can also be used, such as massaging the sides of the neck, jaw, and throat, to stimulate the ANS circuits repeatedly. After the stimulation, we return to deep listening. The social ANS neurochemistry filters through the system to reset the whole ANS, softening habitual states of sympathetic (fight or flight) or parasympathetic (immobilization and dissociation) stress responses.

### Expectations and Intentions Practice for Couples

This practice helps couples probe into subtle aspects of their mutual experience. It can be combined with Body-Low-Slow-Loop or Resonance practices, sharing similarities to both, but it is more aggressive and provocative, and is appropriate for couples who have sufficient resources to stretch and nourish their relationship. For volatile relationships and couples who are in acute stress, this practice is not as immediately useful unless they have skilled support.

In this exercise, the couple or two individuals start by each establishing a felt sense of the other's presence, similar to the "Walking Toward" or Resonance practice. Then, each

person takes a turn repeatedly saying, "I expect _____,"
filling in the blank with whatever arises and feels authentic. A
particular topic can be pre-agreed or the inquiry can be
open-ended. While one person talks, continuing for two or
three minutes in a type of monologue, the other person listens
attentively and, at some point, thinks an appreciative
thought. After the first monologue, the second person may
ask a question or two, in order to clarify what was meant, but
there should be no criticism or reactivity in this process. If
there is activation (if either person feels threatened or
agitated), suspend the exercise and use Body-Low-Slow-Loop
to re-establish a fresh ANS base. Each person has a turn in the
exercise, using the same fill-in-the-blank prompt.

Moving to the second part of the practice, the second
person then takes a turn, speaking about intentions in the
same way, "I intend _____" either relating to a certain
context or as a general expression of one's life experience.

Stone placed great emphasis on attitudes and
expectations, both of which have enormous power
throughout life. Frequently beyond conscious awareness,
attitudes and expectations are rarely actually spoken or
expressed. Many people are unable to articulate what they
expect and intend with each other, setting the stage for
confusion and mental unease or worse. Even if they can come
up with words for their thoughts, they may be too abstract,
complex or vague for their partner.

This practice is similar to therapies and personal
growth practices relating to setting intentions. As many have
observed, articulated and written-down plans have a higher
probability of success than unrecorded daydreams.

## Exaggerated Yang/Yin Exercise

For couples, this practice is a way to stimulate
resistances and ancestral patterns so that they can be

processed in the present and, perhaps, brought to greater balance. The effect may be to create movement where there has been stagnant fixation. It is particularly useful for couples with very young children who are showing signs of anxiety, to re-establish a polarized field for the children's felt sense of security, while also cultivating mutual self-awareness and compassion in the parents. It is also useful when a couple has lost relational vitality. "Loss of spark" can happen for many reasons, including feeling overwhelmed in life, one person's irritability or the distraction of children. This phenomenon is called "de-polarization" and it can sneak up on a couple that is too busy to identify the symptoms.

In this practice, two people in an intimate relationship agree with each other prior to engaging this exercise, to experiment with re-polarization, one by acting more Yang and the other, more Yin. The effect is to stimulate energetic movement and flow in a relationship, and to evoke resistances as a felt-sense experience so that those resistances can be addressed consciously.

These do not have to be statements that would ever actually be spoken; they are just to give the energetic field a

**Exaggerated Yin and Yang Exercise Options**

| Yang Possibilities | Yin Possibilities |
|---|---|
| "I show my love by doing things for you." | "I show my love by inspiring you and reminding you of spirit." |
| "I am the benevolent king of this space." | "I am content and supportive about what is happening." |
| "My intention is _____ and I am totally commited to achieving this goal." | "That is wonderful and I really appreciate _____ [insert any compliment here, particularly a physical attribute]." |
| Leaning slightly forward, using firm voice quality. | Leaning slightly rearward, using melodious soft voice quality. |

stimulus. Ideally this can be done with some humor, and the couple can find amusing ways to "ham it up," to further enhance the effect.

The exercise is likely to induce various interesting body processes, emotions, memories, interpretations and other phenomena. It is helpful to view these experiences as the data from the experiment; they are usually well worth follow-up discussion and consideration.

By exaggerating the polarized positioning of Yin and Yang, the fundamental dynamics of a relationship are often exposed. It can be most provocative and confounding. The earlier discussion of archetypes is pulled into full focus as they are experienced in the exercise.

In addition to the activity itself, a point of the experiment is to get to what happens after the words have been spoken. These kinds of statements will often engender complex sequences, including physical sensations and emotions, even to the extent of creating a mini-crisis if the dyad has been de-polarized, off-balance, or reversed for some time. These effects can then be studied mutually to good effect. As with most of this chapter's exercises, the intention is to give the Yin and Yang pendulum a push.

When young children are showing signs of insecurity, engaging this play-acting in front of them can be a revelation. The parents do the practice, then closely observe how the children respond, including how male and female children may respond differently. If there has been longstanding stress between the parents that has been affecting the children, this practice done daily for a few weeks can gently re-establish the young child's equilibrium and sense of security.

This exaggeration practice can create discord, but with positive benefits. One male client tried this exercise with his wife and thought it did not go well because she seemed to be offended. However, he noticed the relationship seemed to shift favorably as a result, so he continued periodically just doing it silently in the presence of his wife and their two young children. A few months later he reported that the emotional tone of the home was much different, and he thought his solo silent practice had been a key factor. He had been re-polarizing his own process relative to his family without them knowing it, and they were responding, without knowing why.

### "Potted Plant" Practice

In an age where everyone is on the go and moving back and forth across the planet, the natural instinct for having a true home has often been misplaced. Human evolution is a different story; for millennia humans lived their lives in one setting, with familiar family and tribe, and they became accustomed to the local seasons, weather, terrain, food and dangers. Now, just in the past few generations (hardly any time at all from an evolutionary biological perspective), many of us are more like potted plants: we live where our jobs pull us, but we don't really put down roots. This exercise is a way to soften the situation, for the benefit of the ANS. It is best done outdoors, with bare feet on soft grass, but it can be done anywhere, using the imagination. This practice can also be done as part of touch therapy, with the client resting on a massage table as the practitioner guides the visualization.

In this practice we bring our attention into the body and scan for sensations. As this semi-meditative process unfolds, we look to see if we can detect a downward flow pattern, from the head moving down into the torso, and then progressing to the legs and feet. This flow is visualized and imaginary; it does not have to be tangible.

Once there is a sense of downward flow, the practice is to extend that downward current further into the earth below, as if we are a plant sending down new rootlets. There may be a sense of a root-bound potted plant being moved to the garden, with a loosening of the root fibers and a spreading into unconstrained nourishing space. Some clients have reported that they can feel the loosening in the hips and pelvis. The downward expansion can also include envisioning finding water and minerals deep in the earth.

When the time is right, a reverse upward flow is imagined. Now the imagined roots are conduits for nourishment from deep underground. There might be a sense of relief, comparable to how a former house plant might feel when it is finally allowed to be in its true permanent home.

If in real life we are not settled where we are, this practice can seem to contradict current events, but the sense of settling/nourishment still provides an ANS resource. We are replacing an actual experience with an artificial mental one, but the effects can still be profound. No matter how far from "home" we may be, even in a hotel in a faraway foreign city, this practice can help us tap into instinctual expectations.

## Supervised Self-Help Practices

Additional practices have been developed for use in sessions. Unlike the self-care exercises above, these are more complicated and potentially more strenuous. These are appropriate when there is a practitioner present to manage the process and help clients keep from feeling overwhelmed. As a solo exercise, these would be appropriate only for more advanced individuals who have built up a good immunity to the presence of overwhelming feelings and who have a strong base in equanimity.

## Idealized Mom Practice

This ten-minute practice involves resting comfortably and recalling memories in which our mothers were "at their very best," such as a particular time in childhood when they were serving the family and providing for us most optimally.

The memory, once identified, is then embellished with as much sensory detail as possible: season of the year, time of day, location, details of the space, nature of the occasion, who else was present, what sights, sounds and whatever other sensory memory information can be accessed or imagined. The objective is to have a complete body-centered experience of what happens when the memory's "mind picture" is as detailed as possible. In the presence of the memory of one's mother performing in her most loving way toward us, the attention is then turned to body sensation, including a "Body-Low-Slow-Loop" process.

There are limitations to the "Idealized Mom" practice, such as when no such memories are available, or when the imagination turns too quickly to a betrayal or disappointment memory that is hooked to the initial search for an event. In these cases, it is suggested that the practice not be used, or used only with skilled guidance.

If appropriate, the client may use a purely imaginary scenario instead of memories of the actual mother. A fictional character such as the "perfect mother" can be conjured up to get the felt sense to start appearing. We are all instinctually programmed for an optimum mother experience, whether or not it actually happened. The autonomic responses relating to maternal bonding are always present throughout life. This practice is a gentle way to re-program the ANS in accordance with its original expectation.

The same practice can be done with an idealized father, or any other important relationship. We can be creative and experiment with different possibilities as long as the process does not become overwhelming.

### Defensive Response Exercise

As described earlier, thwarted defensive responses are ANS impulses or actual gestures that would have been appropriate in a threatening situation. They have also been called "Acts of Completion" as a way to heighten the positive interpretation.

For example, a child may have had an impulse to run away or fight back in the presence of an abusive adult. Because the abuser was physically larger, completing an impulse to counter-attack might have made the situation worse, and running away was not an option. Therefore the natural impulses were blocked by circumstances.

This exercise does not try to establish any particular context; for that, the support of a skilled counselor is important. Here the process is just about the felt sense unrelated to any particular story. It can be done in any position, but seated is perhaps the better option.

Resting comfortably, we put our hands against a strong surface, that barely yields to pressure, such as a large piece of furniture. Then we push firmly against the resistance with hands and arms, or legs, and then release. After a practice round or two, we can add a vocal component by also saying "No!" while pushing.

After pushing and saying, "No!" for a short time, there is a time for rest and mindful inquiry into the body about what sensations arose after the pushing ended. Often, a reorganization and release of tension somewhere in the system will manifest as a sense of streaming or an increased feeling of flow, power and embodiment. Emotions may also come to the surface, and Body-Low-Slow-Loop can be used to digest those feelings.

If the client feels at all overwhelmed with this exercise, it should be discontinued and later discussed with a therapist who is knowledgeable about trauma resolution methods. It can also be done as part of a bodywork session, effectively discharging pent-up tension. In bodywork, the client can press against the hand of the practitioner, who gradually yields. It is important for us to be located not directly facing the client but rather off to the side, to avoid having the client subconsciously get us mixed up with an earlier antagonist.

After this exercise is completed, we allow time to notice the effects. There may be streaming, tingling and similar body sensations, in addition to emotions, memories and any number of other possibilities. During this time, just after such a practice, the ANS is re-adjusting itself, reducing parasympathetic immobilization symptoms and moving held sympathetic charge. Meanwhile the subconscious is also re-establishing boundaries for itself.

## Other Supportive Methods

Deserving brief mention, practitioner skills, values, bodywork, diet and exercise can all be effective self-care components of Yin and Yang care.

• The practitioner skills (Chapter 7) are an effective self-care method alone.

• Bodywork can support psycho-emotional processes generally, but can also be applied directly within a session, circumstances permitting. In craniosacral therapy, "CV4" (compression of the fourth ventricle) helps Yang (hyper-) states while "EV4" (expansion of the fourth ventricle) is excellent for Yin (hypo-) states.[225] Stone's touch methods for the ANS include pelvic work, five-pointed star and autonomic balance; for Yang support, path of fire, umbilical contacts, and autonomic balance are helpful.[226]

---

[225] Franklyn. Sills, *Craniosacral Biodynamics Vol. 2*, p. 273 ff. Also, Michael Kern, *Wisdom in the Body*, North Atlantic, 2003, pp. 177-8.

[226] R. Stone, *Polarity Therapy, Vol. 1*. CRCS, 1986; Pelvic work: Book 1, page 82 ff. and Book 2, charts 31 & 32; Five-pointed star: Book 2, Charts 9 & 10; Autonomic balance: Book 2, Charts 29 & 30; Path of fire: Book 3, Chart 8; Umbilical contacts: *Vol. 2*, Book 6, charts 2 & 18

• Diet coaching can also be an effective support for Yin and Yang therapy. Clients using optimum diets usually feel lighter, healthier and more empowered, supporting greater insight and improved vitality. A time of focused Yin and Yang therapy is a good time to use an optimum diet, and a time of optimum diet is a good time to use counseling to heighten the effects, letting go of outworn mental/emotional patterns.

Similarly, natural cleansing practices such as those for colon, lymph and liver are highly supportive of ANS function. Special care can also be given to the gums, as the oral cavity is the first line of defense for the immune system; infections from old dental work or other gum problems preoccupy immune system resources, to the detriment of other needs elsewhere in the body. Another hidden factor that is worthy of attention is the possibility of parasite infection; natural remedies here can be supportive of ANS health.

• Polarity Yoga is a useful adjunct in counseling.[227] Postures can be recommended as homework after a counseling session, effectively increasing clients' self-empowerment. Poses and movements that open up the Yin (lower) aspect of the body are the focus, as Stone constantly emphasized:

> In the pelvic basin, at the bottom, is the sum total force accumulation of sensory tension and emotional frustration.[228]

Examples of postures for this purpose include the squat (in *Energy Exercises*, p. 54), pyramid (p. 52) and scissors kicks (p. 59). In some cases an energy-balancing posture might be used within the counseling session, to support movement and flow.

---

[227] John Chitty and Mary Louise Muller, *Energy Exercises*. Polarity Press, 1990.

[228] R. Stone, *Polarity Therapy, Vol. 1*. CRCS, 1986. Book 2, Chart 9.

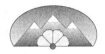

# Chapter 10

# The Two-Chair Process

The two-chair method, made famous by Fritz Perls[229] in the late 1960s as part of his Gestalt Therapy, is definitely the superstar of Yin and Yang psychotherapy. The Yin and Yang version of the two-chair method is basically Perls' concept augmented by mindfulness, body-centered trauma resolution, Yin and Yang archetypes, relationship dynamics, Polarity cosmology and energy anatomy.

In the two-chair method, we facilitate the client's exploration of a dualistic situation. Clients are guided through changing perspectives while also practicing mindfulness and ANS self-regulation, most often within some context of their life experiences. By creating and supporting a "conversation" between two perspectives, emphasizing sensation awareness throughout the process, a natural oscillation begins, safely and quickly reducing energy fixation and creating movement, often with dramatic benefits.

The effectiveness of the method derives from inducing a change of perspective, revealing the inherently dualistic nature of experience. Normally, the world is seen through one habitual primary lens, and the system can gradually become fixated. The more fixated our perspective, the more we are

---

[229] Several film clips of Perls doing the two-chair method in about 1970 can be viewed in YouTube, using "Fritz Perls" as search terms.

prone to disease and dysfunction in physical, emotional and mental dimensions, as well as in our relationships.

The setup is simple. Two chairs are placed to face each other, with the client in one chair, opposite the other empty chair, and the practitioner sitting off to one side, equidistant between the two client chairs. With this arrangement, the Three Principles are represented by Yin and Yang as the two chairs, and Neutral represented as the space between the chairs. The practitioner's position also represents Neutral.

In a Yin and Yang two-chair session, we listen and observe carefully as a story is told, often arriving at an assessment of which Principle and Element seem to be in

---

## A Brief History of the Two-Chair Method

The two-chair concept originated in the 1950s within the practice of psychodrama (Carstenson, 1955), and has been adapted by many other psychology subgroups. In a 2004 article, Scott Kellogg, Rockefeller University, gave a useful history noting five different therapy schools using some form of the method: Gestalt (Perls, 1969), Process-Experiential Therapy (Elliot, 1993 and Greenberg, 1979, *et al.*), Redecision Therapy (Goulding, 1972), Cognitive-Behavioral Therapy (Goldfried, 1988, *et al.*) and Schema Therapy (Young, 2003, *et al.*).

The range of applications described by Kellogg is vast. Included are direct/indirect, imaginal/realistic, before/after, present/past or present/future, inner-self dialogues and self/other dialogues, private sessions/group settings, and more. The possibilities are unlimited. Repeatedly the article cites therapists talking about remarkably fast, solid results. From a Yin and Yang perspective, Kellogg's article confirms the idea that the two-chair method is tapping into larger forces, which are bigger than any one psychotherapy model.

Scott Kellogg, "Dialogical Encounters: Contemporary Perspectives on "Chairwork" in Psychotherapy." *Psychotherapy: Theory, Research, Practice, Training,* 2004, Vol. 41, No. 3, pp. 310-320.

---

play. If the client is agitated, a round of Body-Low-Slow-Loop may be conducted. Repeatedly, we invite the client to return to observing physical sensations first and foremost, more than the thoughts and emotions that are inevitably also present.

After a few minutes of these preliminaries, the client is invited to imagine that someone or something else is in the other chair. Usually this leads to a new configuration of sensations in the body, and as these are reported, the client tracks these with interest. If the client feels overwhelmed, the Body-Low-Slow-Loop process can be repeated as necessary. There is always a safety valve release pathway. If an extremely overwhelming moment arises, we just say, "Switch to the other chair," and a new ANS configuration usually appears.

Then we invite the client to say something out loud to the imaginary occupant of the other chair. This can lead to yet another set of sensations, and these are again followed with great interest. After the sensing of self has progressed a bit, we invite the client to switch chairs.

## Two-Chair Setup & Logistics

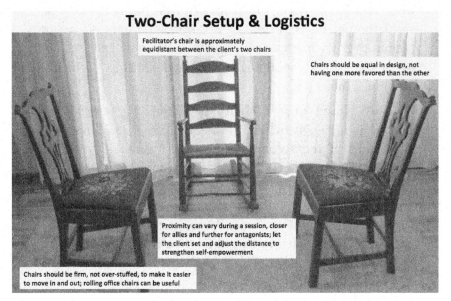

Facilitator's chair is approximately equidistant between the client's two chairs

Chairs should be equal in design, not having one more favored than the other

Proximity can vary during a session, closer for allies and further for antagonists; let the client set and adjust the distance to strengthen self-empowerment

Chairs should be firm, not over-stuffed, to make it easier to move in and out; rolling office chairs can be useful

Sitting in the second chair is often an immediate revelation in itself, including a change of sensations, patterns, thoughts and feelings. Clients are often amazed to experience how one state instantly falls away and another configuration appears, seemingly out of nowhere. This is persuasive in helping clients experientially understand that their habitual, dominant state of being is not so fixed. It becomes obvious that there are also other states that may have been forgotten, sometimes for decades.

A dialogue ensues between the client and the imagined person in the other chair. The details of the conversation are obviously important, but the underlying basis for the method is also the changing of positions. In time, switching back and forth between chairs, the ANS fixation of the client loosens up, new insights arise and new strategies emerge. Subsequently, we may ask the client to write down a summary of what happened, to maximize the effects of the process.

### Switching Chairs

The movement from chair to chair gives us a reliable and low-risk way to help clients explore issues, de-pathologize conditions, create self-awareness, avoid feeling overwhelmed, solve problems, add new insights and explanations for conditions, resolve relationship problems, and much more.

By sitting in one chair and imagining some other perspective, then switching to the other chair and having an experience of the second perspective, "walking a mile in another person's shoes," flow is re-introduced between the two poles. Some reviving of flow happens simply by the back-and-forth physical movement, the switching back and forth, from "State A" to "State B,"no matter who is imagined to be in the other chair, or what is actually said. The content of the dialogue adds value and further grist for the transformation mill. Any change of state, properly managed, will probably lead to an improvement in conditions simply because movement is being introduced. Pendulation or oscillation of sensation-oriented experience is inherently healing.

The two-chair method has unlimited possibilities. The rest of this chapter describes it in detail, not least because there are few other descriptions in print, and apparently none from a Yin and Yang perspective.

### Background of the Two-Chair Method

The two-chair technique was observed by first-generation Polarity students when both Perls and Stone were teaching in California in the late 1960s. Psychiatrist Robert Hall was the key synthesis-maker, apprenticing with both Perls and Stone for three years each (first with Perls starting around 1967, then with Stone starting around 1970). Hall astutely recognized that what Perls was doing was a profound application of Stone's theory.

There is no record of Stone and Perls ever meeting each other or collaborating, although they may have crossed paths at the Esalen Institute. Perls died in 1971 and Stone retired in 1974, followed by a move to India where he died in 1981, so Hall caught the wave of innovation at its peak. There are few written descriptions of that era from anyone involved. But throughout the 1970s and 1980s, Hall and other Polarity students, particularly those who later created the "Alive Polarity" school, where I studied starting in 1979, continued to refine and develop the method. Alive Polarity referred to the hybrid method as an "Awareness" session.

Perls' Gestalt Therapy went on to become a major movement within psychotherapy. The German term Gestalt roughly translates to mean "all of it," or the whole multi-layered context of any situation, including the idea that the whole is more than the sum of the parts. As a body of work, Gestalt stands on its own, and Polarity's adoption of the two-chair process by no means presumes to represent the entire Perls legacy. Stone was a liberal adopter of key concepts from many traditions, and his students' borrowing of the two-chair method can be seen in that light, nothing more. The two systems should not be seen as too closely connected. However, as the accompanying commentary indicates, the affiliation of the two systems is theoretically reciprocal. Yontef's description of Gestalt clearly references Polarity ideas just as much as Polarity refers to Gestalt.

## Two-Chair, Polarity and Somatic Experiencing

In the 1990s, Peter Levine's work became popular with those practicing Polarity Therapy, adding new support for Yin and Yang applications. Levine presented his ideas at Polarity Therapy conferences (recall Levine's lengthy comment on pages 42-43), giving an insightful explanation for why the two-chair method was so effective. The two-chair method can readily be combined with Levine's approach for a very efficient body-centered therapy.

Somatic Experiencing® (SE) is a complete system with a comprehensive scope for healing the effects of trauma. For example, Levine's remarkable chapter "From Paralysis to Transformation: Basic Building Blocks"[230] is a state-of-the-art summary of trauma therapy, and required reading for all two-chair method students. The two-chair method's borrowing of several of Levine's points does not imply that the whole of Levine's SE is represented. The situation is similar to how some Gestalt portions were adopted, without attempting to represent the whole of Gestalt Therapy. There is a wealth of additional material within SE that goes far beyond the parts that are borrowed for the two-chair process.

---

[230] Peter Levine, *In an Unspoken Voice*. North Atlantic, 2010. p. 73.

# About Gestalt Therapy

From Gary Yontef, PhD, *Gestalt Therapy, An Introduction*

*Differentiation of the Field: Polarities vs. Dichotomies*

A dichotomy is a split whereby the field is considered not as a whole differentiated into different and interlocking parts, but rather as an assortment of competing (either/or) and unrelated forces. Dichotomous thinking interferes with organismic self-regulation. Dichotomous thinking tends to be intolerant of diversity among persons and of paradoxical truths about a single person.

Organismic self-regulation leads to integrating parts with each other and into a whole that encompasses the parts. The field is often differentiated into polarities: parts that are opposites that complement or explicate each other. The positive and negative poles of an electrical field are the prototypical mode for this differentiation in a field theoretical way. **The concept of polarities treats opposites as part of one whole, as yin and yang.**

With this polar view of the field, differences are accepted and integrated. Lack of genuine integration creates splits, such as body-mind, self-external, infantile-mature, biological-cultural, and unconscious-conscious. **Through dialogue there can be an integration of parts, into a new whole in which there is a differentiated unity.** Dichotomies such as the self-ideal and the needy self, thought and impulse, and social requirements and personal needs can be healed by integrating into a whole differentiated into natural polarities (Perls, 1947).

Gestalt holds that **the polarity of individual and field is a significant universal factor.** Whatever a person is doing, or feeling, it is all in relationship to a wider set of factors. Awareness of the individuality and the field and **re-gaining the ability to oscillate one's awareness between the two**, is a therapeutic strategy, and is accomplished in many ways within Gestalt.

Of particular interest among Gestalt's many methods and styles, is the two-chair technique associated with Gestalt Therapy. Again, this technique is not the whole of Gestalt. It is mentioned in the literature, but not at the top of any descriptions. *(Bold text emphasis by John Chitty)*

*Example #1*

A male client, age 55, came to a session with a physical problem: a chronically sore right knee. He'd had two surgeries in the past and was scheduled for a third a few weeks later. He also reported a history of neck pain, particularly on the right side.

The session began with a short interview, starting with probing questions. Meanwhile, I silently double-checked the initial practitioner skills (center-ground-neutral, right relationship) to create a strong foundation for the session. My first question was, "When was the first appearance of the knee problem, and what was happening in your life at that time?" As the client told his story, I observed closely to see what Principle and Element seemed to be momentarily in the foreground.

The client proceeded to tell a story about a high school soccer injury to the knee, forty years earlier, which happened at a time of great stress in the family. Asked for more information about the family stress, he described how his father was domineering (the tyrant archetype) and his mother was overly passive (the doormat archetype), and how he had strongly wished to protect his mother from his father's verbal and physical abuse. Being just a child, he was unable to do much; as he got older, he became more frustrated. He added that he was also afraid for his own well-being, adding a story about how his place at the family dinner table was to his father's immediate right. Unpredictably, his father would often hit him during dinner, and he had a constant, thwarted impulse to somehow protect himself or evade the blow.

We set up two chairs and I invited him to choose one and take a seat. I guided him to begin with a body scan for sensations and report whatever he noticed. Having just talked about a very difficult time in his childhood, he already had activation present in the form of heat particularly on the left side of his head, and an absence of sensation signals from the rest of the body. I guided him in a round of Body-Low-Slow-Loop to reduce the activation and shift awareness of sensation more widely through the body.

When the time felt right, I suggested, "Imagine that your father is in the other chair." Immediately a new set of strong sensations arose, including heat and tension in the right shoulder and right leg. Emotions of rage and fear came to the surface. I acknowledged the validity of these and let the wave of emotions pass before guiding back to sensation. I

## Somatic Experiencing meets Yin and Yang

Peter Levine's Somatic Experiencing (SE) methods are profoundly effective in treating the effects of trauma. SE combines autonomic nervous system knowledge, understanding of micro-movements, body-centered awareness and pendulation to achieve excellent results. The SE organization (http://www.traumahealing.com), has trained trauma therapists worldwide and has influenced many other subgroups.

Somatic Experiencing, Yin and Yang psychotherapy and Polarity Therapy overlap significantly:

• The Yin and Yang approach borrows SE's idea of shifting between two locations in the body or states of autonomic tone. While SE tends to do this with the client stationary, alternating detailed attention to states and locations, the two-chair version is based on a similar concept but changes location to another physical placement (actually moving to the other chair) to heighten the effect and also give the client an easy way to avoid feeling overwhelmed.

• Yin and Yang ideas and SE can be combined with touch therapies; possibilities are described later in this chapter.

• SE and Yin and Yang systems also both rely on close attention to micro-movements and subtle gestures, in order to recognize autonomic states and thereby know how to precisely guide clients out of trauma-based conditions. In SE, the focus is more on autonomic states, whereas in a Yin and Yang approach the inquiry includes consideration of the Three Principles and Five Elements, including "energy anatomy" (see Chapter 13).

then invited the client to speak to his father who, in actuality, had been dead for decades. The first spoken words consisted of a report, "Dad, I am noticing _____ just now," with the blank being the physical sensations that were present. Then I said, "Okay, good. Switch chairs."

When the client arrived in the other chair, a completely different posture and set of sensations spontaneously appeared. I guided him into an enhanced curiosity about the new state's physical manifestations. The "father" then was asked to respond to what the son had said. What emerged was a statement of the father's extreme frustration and despair about his own life, arising from severe abuse and difficult conditions of his own childhood. Sensations flooded in, and another wave of emotions. Again I waited for an auspicious moment to switch chairs. As stated earlier, with the two-chair method there is always a fail-safe way to guard against overwhelming feelings or re-traumatization, because every switch instantly shifts the person to a different mind-body configuration.

Back in the first chair, he once again became his familiar primary self. The heat and locations were much different, and micro-movements started as his system started to mobilize for action. These were short twitches, especially in the legs. I asked, "What would the legs like to do just now?" The answer was something about a strong movement to the right. This might be the gesture and direction of escape from his father's rage at the dinner table, among other possibilities. This was encouraged to continue, using Body-Low-Slow-Loop again to drain away some of the charge.

The session continued through four more chair position changes, lasting about thirty minutes. Anger was gradually replaced by grief and some vigorous shaking came and went. Fibrillation or body shaping is often a good sign indicating that the previously held charge is dissipating. At the end there was a bit of a reconciliation between the father, who was very remorseful to observe the effects of his behavior, and the son, who was biologically "wired for love" for his parents.[231] After the session, the client was asked to write down as much as he could remember of the process, as if writing a screenplay, to help secure the awareness insights in his mind.

This client noticed such immediate improvement in his knee symptoms that he canceled the surgery and went on a European vacation instead. In theory, the knee problems were echoes of the thwarted impulses of the sympathetic ANS bind that had been a major theme throughout his life. When pendulation was exercised, reversing decades of fixation, the symptoms started to recede.

In this example, I chose the client's father as the occupant of the second chair because the knee symptoms were on the right (Yang) side. I suspected that fear, surrender and flight impulses might arise, because the knee and neck are both earth element locations, and in energy anatomy the earth element manages experiences relating to security, including fear. These were just "soft guesses;" it was not necessary to be exactly correct because cause-and-effect is questionable at best and not a primary concern. Using body reading just helps get to the main action efficiently.

In theory, the benefits of changing chairs and gaining another perspective are only partially about the content of the conversation. As stated earlier, the physical act of moving from one vantage point to another will revive movement where there has been fixation. Clients in great distress can be so consumed in their miserable feelings that their body-minds are cycling around just one state, and no longer oscillating to

---

[231] Stan Tatkin and Harville Hendrix, *Wired for Love: How Understanding Your Partner's Brain and Attachment Style Can Help You Defuse Conflict and Build a Secure Relationship.* New Harbinger, 2012.

## Robert K. Hall, MD

Robert Hall (born 1934) is an expert in-person witness to the intersecting life arcs of Fritz Perls and Randolph Stone (as well as Ida Rolf and Peter Levine). He is known in Polarity Therapy for writing the Foreword in Stone's *Health Building*. In his illustrious career he was a co-founder of the Lomi School and faculty member at Naropa Institute, then director of El Dharma meditation center in Baja Mexico. In 2013, he was still using the two-chair method in his retreats.

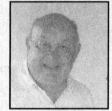

Hall hosted Dr. Stone for the California retreats that elevated Stone to a new audience in the late 1960s. Prior to that, Hall had apprenticed with Dr. Perls and studied extensively with Ida Rolf. He introduced Peter Levine to Stone in 1970 in Los Angeles. He taught Perls' work to the people who taught me, beginning in the 1970s.

**Dr. Hall in 2013**
*Photo by Alvaro Colindres*

Describing his practice in group settings in a magazine interview (*Inquiring Mind*, Fall 2012), Hall commented:

"[In the 1970s] there was a general dismissal of emotions in the whole body-mind community....One exception was Fritz Perls....I think his contribution was to make it possible for people to feel and name their emotions. He developed techniques for the purpose, such as the empty chair conversation, where you...explore your projections on to other people....I make use of what I have learned in Gestalt over the years by bringing forth the conflicts within the personality, the polarities....When the work is really successful, [the clients] realize all the conflict is taking place within their own minds.

"Fritz Perls was always looking for the point where the two sides of the ego, the polarities, would come to a stalemate. He called that place 'the impasse.' At that point, a kind of transcendence could occur, an awakening out of duality...

"Essentially, our consciousness is split: we see the world through a lens of opposites. Fritz saw that split occurring within each of us, in the ego structure. He called the two polarities 'the top dog' and 'the underdog.' There is always the dominator and the passive one, and they are in constant conflict with each other. Emotions arise out of those conflicts. Gestalt is a way of isolating the conflicts within the ego and then working toward the integration of the two sides. It's brilliant..."

anything else. They have become a monopole instead of a dipole or, in Yousef's terms, a dichotomy instead of a polarity.

The two-chair method's easy access to oscillation provides a solution to some difficult situations in trauma recovery therapy. For example, it has been noted that mindfulness and meditation practices, which are so beneficial for so many people, can be problematic in post-traumatic stress disorder unless there is close supervision. The peacefulness of a meditative state and the "playing possum" affect of dissociation are very similar; one may lead to the other, or they may become confused. In a deep resting stillness, a PTSD client can feel drawn into a vortex of overwhelming feelings, ending up in dissociation. This is highly unlikely in the two-chair method because changing chairs provides immediate relief. In addition to being pulled out of the problematic state, the client's non-cognitive intelligence is learning that instead of being trapped, there is always a way out of an overwhelming emotional state.

The two-chair method also offers a solution to a common problem in couples counseling. Instead of talking to each other face-to-face, which can lead to intense emotions and increasing fixation within entrenched, habitual positions, the partners take turns talking to the imagined presence of the other in the empty chair, while the other observes from a distance. After the client expresses whatever needs to be spoken, he or she goes to the other chair and experiences the statement from the other side of the Yin and Yang equation. Instead of an endless, unproductive ping-pong game of blame and defensiveness, which is so common in couples counseling, the two-chair method offers an easy way to move to a much more productive interaction.

Archetypes are ever-present in two-chair work. Inevitably, one chair expresses the role of Yin and the other becomes the role of Yang. Knowledge of these archetypes can hugely enrich the client's process. Parental imprints can be revealed very efficiently, particularly as they express the four great archetypal dysfunctions (too much or too little of Yin and Yang).

Two-chair processing can be entirely non-verbal and still quite effective. The client can be coached to have a "felt-sense,"[232] complete experience of his or her initial state, and then some other person or situation can be imagined to be in the other chair. Without words being spoken at all, the configuration is likely to manifest in contrasting ways in each chair. By switching back and forth a few times, even with no narrative or context at all, there can often be a profound softening of habitual fixation, with many benefits.

The two-chair method also addresses another common problem in psychotherapy, in which attachment styles become habits. The classic is an "Avoidant" man discussing issues with an "Ambivalent" woman. Some of what is interpreted as attachment styles is also just the archetypal expression of Sun and Moon. Talking to each other directly in person, the situation will often seem hopeless. However, by talking to the imagined presence of the other person and then switching places, the attachment styles loosen up and relationships are often pulled into new and more functional territory. The couple can "feel" what they have been doing, with a fresh perspective. Having both partners present and taking turns in the two chairs is an efficient way to move beyond the habitual patterns and to differentiate between the various factors. A man who is being pushed into a wimp

---

[232] Eugene Gendlin, *Focusing.* Everest House, 1978. The term "felt sense" derives from Gendlin's Focusing method. It means awareness of an embodied state, often perceived just prior to the naming of the state. Gendlin showed that awareness of physical sensation and close attention to bodily sequences, is the common factor in most effective therapies. Gendlin (born 1926) is a key pioneer in the field that later became body-centered psychotherapy.

## A Yin and Yang View of "Attachment Styles"

The study of attachment styles is a foundation for therapy with couples. From my perspective, author and therapist Diane Heller's work is the "state of the art" in applying attachment theory in therapy.

While Stone had no comment on the subject, which was not yet discussed in his era, Yin and Yang principles are quite discernible in attachment styles, and we can use this information to excellent advantage in practice, particularly when combined with the two-chair method.

The basic premise of Attachment Theory is that the adult's relationship style is subconsciously derived from maternal bonding experiences in early childhood. If the mother was "good enough" in her parenting skills (nurturing, predictable, affirming, consistent), the child will be more or less *Secure*. In adult life, the person will have equal awareness access to Self and Other, will be able to transfer attention easily and accurately to monitor both, and will be less susceptible to fixation in autonomic states.

If the mother is insecure herself, the child is more likely to become either *Avoidant* or *Ambivalent*, and this will still be present in adulthood. The Avoidant style is more distancing and might track others well but may be limited in terms of self-awareness. This coincides with Yang attributes, so there may be a tendency for males to go this way in dealing with a stressful parental environment. It also may tend toward a more sympathetic ANS (fight or flight) habit until it eventually reaches exhaustion.

Meanwhile an Ambivalent person responds to a mother's stress by trying to merge with her, or by flipping back and forth with love/hate, approach/escape cycles. This echoes the Yin archetypal story of inherent paradox. Ambivalent gives mixed signals, does not track the other very well, may not be able to articulate needs, and may appear to be self-centered. It is also somewhat sympathetic ANS in nature. The psychological terms "Codependent" (Other-centered) and "Narcissistic" (Self-centered) can overlap with Attachment Style language.

If the childhood environment is even more severe, the *Disorganized* Attachment style can be the result. This is a more disabled condition, in which neither Self nor Other is readily accessible. It may resemble parasympathetic autonomic shock, and involve harsh destructive behaviors with self or others in an effort to self-regulate and re-vivify experience. In Yin and Yang terms, Disorganized represents a loss of polarized functioning, leading to chaos.

archetype will start to behave in ways that could easily be interpreted as "avoidant," but the whole dynamic can be observed to shift when he sits in the other chair, and he can start to feel much less pathologized and more validated as a result.

## Who is in the Other Chair?

There are multiple possibilities relating to the empty chair. At the simplest level, the imagined occupant of the other chair is actually a secondary perspective of the client. As Robert Hall described in his article above, Perls taught that coexisting within everyone there is always a "top dog" (the primary, habitual consciousness and ANS state) and an "underdog." Most people are so habitually immersed in their primary perspective that they do not even realize that another perspective exists. This is unfortunate because often the secondary perspective holds great insight.

For example, a mother was worried about her child in his mid-twenties who was not flourishing after finishing college. In the two-chair process, she put the son in the other chair and switched roles. Doing so she realized, through a much bigger perspective, what her son was going through. Later she reported that the relationship had improved significantly from just that one session. Of course, the real son was not in the room, it was her own secondary perspective having a clear opportunity to express itself. It is as if the needle gets stuck on an old LP record and the person is in a Yin or Yang state instead of being able to dance back and forth, seeing situations in a more complete light. This induced oscillation from chair to chair, literally from Yin states to Yang states and back, is at the core of the method's effectiveness.

In another example, a couple was fighting about how time was being spent. He was always working, and she wanted a playful vacation, but their positions were entrenched. When he stated his familiar priorities in one chair, we could observe the habitual position. But when he changed to the other chair and really felt into her experience, he "got it" in a way that was previously inaccessible for him.

At another level, the empty chair often may contain a valid representation of another person. This is because the imprinting is fairly accurate. What is spoken from the second chair, and even more, what is expressed in posture and gesture, are often reliable when the conversation is played out in reality. For example, a client was troubled by her husband's seeming lack of consistency. When she imagined her husband in the empty chair and switched roles, "he" immediately started to sag into a posture of resignation and defeat. The indications were clearly appropriate for a wimp-critic dynamic, and after a few more switches, she could see the effects, with compassion instead of anger, and she could experientially realize her part in the process.

---

### In their own words...
#### Clients describe their two-chair experiences

*The two-chair process was exceptionally helpful. Through this process, you helped me access insight and understanding that I was not previously consciously aware I held. In the process, not only was an abundance of guidance available, but it was simple and easy to approach. The information I received came quickly and felt obvious, even though the problems I was facing had been feeling insurmountable.*

*My own insight was more credible to my mind than anything another person could have explained to me, because it came from me. In the past I have been given advice, and have found it hard to really "get it" on a deep level. This advice came out of a deep place, and as soon as I spoke it out loud, I felt as though I already got it. The information permeated my being to a much greater degree than if it had come through another person such as a friend or counselor, and I was able to translate it into my life experience easily and effectively."*

---

Additionally, the other chair may represent the client's alternative autonomic states. This can be a little different from just a different perspective, because the body itself manifests the physiology of the state: the "person" in one chair can be agitated with eyes darting around and sweat appearing on the forehead, while the "person" in the other chair may be tranquil and highly self-aware, even though both chairs are actually being occupied alternately by the same person. From an autonomic perspective, just changing chairs alone, regardless of the content of the conversation, can be valuable because subconsciously the system is "learning" through experience that there are options. It is liberating to have a felt-sense of a different state, when one particular configuration has been predominant for a long time. The client begins to understand that the primary habitual state is actually not quite so all-pervasive and unavoidable as originally thought; movement and change are possible.

Any situation can be explored using the two chairs, because all phenomena exist in multiple dualistic relationships. As a general baseline, anyone can experience stimulation and increased self-awareness by putting the mother or father in the other chair, having a complete experience of the perspective on both sides, and changing chairs back and forth a few times in conversation. The most universal other-chair occupant is probably the client's mother; this reflects the basic reality of maternal bonding as the key formative process in our lives. Fathers are almost as common as other-chair occupants, for similar reasons. Casting a wider net for other-chair options, we find spouses or significant others, bosses and employees, states of being, God, parts of the body, departed loved ones, unborn children, historical figures; all of these and more can all be useful "two-chair conversation" imaginary partners. There is no limit to the helpful possibilities when we use the two-chair process.

## Yin and Yang Two-Chair Possibilities

| Chair #1 | Chair #2 | Purpose |
|---|---|---|
| Self | Mother | To explore Yin |
| Self | Father | To explore Yang |
| Spouse/Partner #1 | Spouse/Partner #2 | To assess and resolve conflict |
| Self in ANS state #1 | Self in ANS state #2 | To loosen ANS fixation |
| Parent or Self | Prenate, baby, child | To "rescue" the child from a bad situation or gain insight about behaviors |
| Self | Ancestors in any combination | To soften blaming and increase compassion |
| Self | Departed loved one | To resolve unfinished business, receive guidance |
| Self | God, "Guru" or "higher power" | To address deep anger at life, receive guidance |
| Self | Former partner with whom there is still attachment | To become free of old impressions, "filaments" & "hooks" |
| Self | Boss, co-worker | To solve vocational problems |
| Uninjured self | Injury, condition, disease | To discover meaning of the condition and restore connection to health |
| Self | Impending difficult conversation subject | To discover the most workable approach |
| Self | Desired or undesired attribute | To discover blocks to optimum functioning |
| Self | Antagonist, perpetrator | To get past stuck places in previous life events |
| Self in the present | Past self "before the disturbance" | To pick up a "dropped stitch" in normal development |

These encounters are imaginary, but reality is also present in the two-chair encounter. No matter who we imagine is sitting in the other chair, or what the topic may be, when the client moves to the other chair and feels what arises, speaking the thoughts and experiencing the emotions, the results are usually revealing. A person having overwhelming and unpleasant sensations relating to a recent life event is often astonished to experience a state in which what had seemed unavoidable, overwhelming and terrible just a moment earlier in one chair is instantly transformed in the other chair. Puzzling situations, such as a partner's behavior or feelings, suddenly make sense and are experienced as a whole-body process, not just a thought or emotion.

## Putting the "True Nature" in the Other Chair

The True Nature, Essential Self, "Higher Power" or "God," can be a very useful occupant of the second chair, because no matter what the term means to a given person (even an atheist or agnostic), it is likely that some version of a higher power or idealized intelligence will materialize as we switch. By switching to the "God" chair, we are likely to experience a quite different state of being, often being able to offer profound advice and insight about some current life problem.

There is a great advantage in having life advice come from the client, instead of the practitioner, because the credibility is so much stronger. Surrogates for "God" can also include a highly respected person in the client's life, such as an elder, a counselor, a guru, a positive childhood influence (a favorite pastor perhaps), or any other embodiment of the person's sense of wisdom. Clients have used Jesus, Buddha, Kwan Yin and Moses, as well as modern day teachers, both living and dead. Even archetypal heroes can be put into the chair. For example, we may suggest to a client who feels very weak and victimized, "Put Superman in the other chair."

Switching to the other chair engenders a different felt-sense state, that the client may not have experienced in a long time. Switching back and forth a few times, the client can become more self-aware of an alternative state of being. Obviously, Superman is not really in the chair, it is just a side of the client that he or she cannot usually access or articulate. The archetypal hero may provide a felt sense of mastery and safety, an experience that is enormously empowering.

We all have an inner duality between our "higher selves" and our "lower selves" (also known as bigger/smaller or true self/egoic self) and these two sides can engage in a useful dialogue. Often the higher self feels dominated by the lower, while the lower feels despair at the state of chaos but also feels unable to relinquish the driver's seat and yield control. By switching back and forth, the rigidity of habitual positioning can be softened and new options will naturally arise. The two aspects of the mind can even negotiate a settlement and a peaceful transfer of power.

### Visiting the Time Before the Problem Started

The client's own experience as a child, fetus, embryo or even pre-conception consciousness can also be put in the other chair. We are programmed for certain sequences of biological events, and we all have a continuing thread of that original guiding intention. If clients are suffering from a serious problem, there can be great benefit in finding a time before the problem started.[233] This can be recent, such as before a car accident, or earlier, such as before the divorce of one's parents. It may need to be very early in life, as the problem may have been within the mother, even at the

---

[233] Nassim Haramein, *Crossing the Event Horizon* DVD. The Resonance Project, 2009. Haramein describes just such a sequence of reconnecting our present state to a time before the trauma, but from the perspective of theoretical physics. This DVD set has wonderful material touching multiple other subjects as well, and is highly recommended.

moment of conception, in the case of a chaotic personal life, or shortly thereafter, in the case of a mother who smoked, drank or lived in a toxic emotional state. By switching between the current experience and the hypothetical much-younger state, the system begins to oscillate between a much better condition and the present, gently re-establishing movement and flow where fixation had become habitual. The healing process takes on the feel of repairing a tapestry by picking up the broken thread and bringing it into the present.

With very young "before" situations, I often suggest that the adult might offer a place of refuge for the infant, such as a gentle space in the heart area. The process then takes on a quality of rescuing the child and thereby re-uniting parts that have been separated for a long time.

In addition, I often ask, "How old do you feel?" in one chair or the other; often the client will have a felt-sense of a time in life when there was great stress. Switching back and forth between "then" and "now" can begin to soften the fixation about a certain age-state, with the possibility of "updating the files" to present-time circumstances.

### Using Before-and-After with Accidents

Another two-chair experience can involve the times just before and just after a major event. Diane Heller gives excellent instructions for "before-and-after trauma resolution" in her book *Crash Course*; the Yin and Yang approach can be viewed as a two-chair version of Heller's work.[234] With a known incident such as a car accident, there was a moment right before the problem started and a moment right after the person realized that survival was probable. In a car accident, the "before" would be the moment when the very first warning appeared, for example a

---

[234] Diane Heller and Laurence Heller, *Crash Course: A Self-Healing Guide to Auto Accident Trauma and Recovery*. North Atlantic, 2001.

peripheral movement perceived in the corner of the eye, and the "after" could be when the accident or medical treatment is over and a self-survey reveals no life-threatening injuries. The two chairs can initiate a before-and-after body-centered oscillation, with excellent results.

Before-and-after can also work with other situations, including any major disappointment or betrayal; after these experiences the ANS may have created invulnerability, as if to say "closed for business" in that particular field of action. A particular area for this is, again, intimate relationships. If we have suffered a major disappointment in love, we may subconsciously "decide" to protect against a recurrence. For example, obesity (including compulsive overeating) can be an effective protection against new relationships. The two-chair method can reveal the dynamics efficiently with a before-weight gain and after-weight gain dialogue. Many people in their late twenties or early thirties are paralyzed about intimacy and commitment because of disappointments and betrayals in their "anything goes" teenage or college days; the two-chair method is an excellent remedy for this situation.

### Mr. or Ms. Right

Some clients experience a repeated inability to find a partner. Cognitively they may think that they want to be in a relationship, but reality finds them not putting themselves in social situations, not attracting appropriate partners, being totally preoccupied with other fields of action such as career, or similar processes that are effective relationship show-stoppers.

A two-chair approach for such a situation is to put a hypothetical "Mr. Right" or "Ms. Right" in the other chair and closely observe what the body does. Many ANS phenomena may appear, such as avoidance, fear, sadness or other emotional states. These can be digested with

Body-Low-Slow-Loop or other methods. Then, when the time feels right, switching chairs can be a revelation. Often, in the other chair, there will be direct accurate feedback about the whole situation, including "why" Mr. or Ms. Right is not being attracted.

A client in her mid-fifties was feeling lonely and sought support for exploring whether subtle factors might be in play. Through a two-chair process, she discovered that she was still cycling around her disappointment with a failed marriage many years earlier; her husband had drifted into the wimp archetype after the birth of their three children (see "husband lost in space" in Chapter 11). The fixation was compounded in her next relationship when her boyfriend of many years died. The effect was that on a subtle level she was "closed for business" regarding new relationships. The first half of the session addressed reducing the charge with her former partners. One at a time, she put each one in the other chair, switching back and forth to discuss their experiences while also using Body-Low-Slow-Loop to release emotions and physical tension. After reducing the old charge with her other partners, she put "Mr. Right" in the other chair and switched back-and-forth, engaging in a very insightful conversation. The effect was to shift to "open for business" instead of being "closed."

Within a few months, supported by a much more self-aware perspective and intention to recognize and work through the old resistance pattern, she met someone new. She had a much higher chance for success in the new relationship because the system was no longer in fixation from the previous disappointments. In addition, the sessions included education about relationships and she had new resources to apply to the whole situation.

*Working with Antagonists*

The two-chair approach can be an effective way to work with antagonists, including people who have abused the client, attackers or people with whom there are active conflicts. The process often includes the victim's gaining access to defensive responses that could not be used at the time of the attack. Putting the offending person or situation in

## Literature sample: Two-Chair Options (Kellogg, 2004)

| Chair #1 | Chair #2 | Sources & authors |
|---|---|---|
| Self | Person with whom there is unfinished business from the past, especially family | Process-Experiential Therapy (Greenberg, 1993; Paivo, 1995) |
| Self | Idealized person from the past | Schema Therapy (Young, 2003) |
| Self in the present | Self as abused child | Redecision Therapy (Goulding & Goulding, 1997) |
| Self as a child in the past | Abuser | Gouldings, 1997) |
| Dreamer | Dreamed entities | Gestalt Therapy (Perls, 1969) |
| Habitual argument | New counter-argument | Schema Therapy (Young, 2003) |
| Realistic | Unrealistic | Cognitive-Behavioral Therapy (Gottfried, 1988) |
| Inner critic | Defiant anti-critic | Anthetic Therapy (Elliotts, 1992) |
| Future outcome | Present decider | Gouldings, 1997 |
| Disease condition | Rest of self | Young, 2003 |
| Pre-exercise a difficult conversation | The other person | Greenberg, 1993 |
| Conflict between 2 values | Value #2 | Mode Therapy (Fabry, 1988) |
| Saying goodbye | Person who has gone | Tobin, 1976 |
| Imagined witness to an incident | Self or perpetrator in the incident | Redecision Therapy (Massé, 1997) |

the other chair may be highly charged emotionally, but the two-chair method has built-in protection because switching chairs is always available. Before the encounter with the antagonist, the client can be supported in building resources such as putting an ally in the other chair, or imagining an earlier time when there was harmony in the relationship. Then later the current-time conflict can be approached from a position of less fixation.

For example, a woman had suffered childhood sexual abuse at the hands of her father, who had died many years earlier, without reconciliation. The first two-chair session was between her adult self and her child self, to "rescue" the child. In a second session, there was a process with her adult self and her imagined husband as an ally who was highly motivated to be a protector. She was able to share what had happened, and "he" was very sympathetic. In real life he had been mystified about some of her aversion behaviors in their intimacy; the process between the two was illuminating what had previously been secret. In a third session, the opposing chair was occupied by her father, long deceased. Understandably, this was very emotional at first, with immense anger and then grief on her side, and shame and regret on his. In her chair, she practiced defensive responses and experienced intense shaking. In her father's position, him being "on the other side," there was extreme regret, and the imagined father repeatedly said, "I'm sorry, I'm sorry..."

When one side tries to apologize, I insert an additional phrase, "What can I do to make up?" An apology alone does not really bridge the gap; repair is needed as well for full resolution and healing. The principle is true in real life as well as two-chair processing because there is true "restorative" power in repair, whereas apologies alone can become empty, habitual and meaningless. An action of compensation is needed. In this example, the action to make up was to bring support from the invisible world for a problem in current time.

A fourth session took the reconciliation with father and explored its relevance with her husband. She had a limited capacity for intimacy in the relationship, which is common and quite understandable in such situations. For the client, being in each chair furnished a felt-sense experience of gradually softening the barriers that had been present for a long time. Insights about her husband's own history also arose from within, and she could relate to him with a compassion that had previously been unavailable.

Antagonists present special challenges due to the potential for acute emotional states in view of the real damage that has been done. I prefer to dip slowly into such waters, spending more time than usual with building healing

---

### In their own words...
#### Clients describe their two-chair experiences

*The most effective aspect of the two-chair method for me is that it has been multilayered. On the most superficial (but still extremely potent) level, I gained a deep understanding from another person's perspective, meaning I have the strong sense of what it is like to "be in the other person's shoes," so to speak. This feeling is not just an intellectual understanding, but a visceral feeling in my physical and emotional body– a feeling as if I know what it is like to be them from the inside, especially in regard to the topic at hand. This allowed for a level of empathy and understanding which I hadn't experienced before and thus altered the way I viewed these people (and behaved with them) in my life from then on.*

*Then, on a deeper level, there is also a realization that the "person" in the other chair is just me, and that these polarities exist within me. This has led to some deeper insights and shifts. In comparison to talk therapy, I find this method gets straight to the heart of the issues more quickly, without the wasted (or even counterproductive) time whining about my story.*

---

or supportive resources, such as having an ally in the other chair first, rescuing the child, bringing in an imagined protector to sit in an additional chair right by the client, and similar strategies. Generally, less time will be spent in the antagonist's chair until the charge has partially drained away. Antagonists were themselves victims, and this can emerge as a way for the client to re-frame the experience. It is not helpful to try to rush to forgiveness; the defensive responses and resource-building processes are necessary first. However, forgiveness is a valid eventual destination, if it can arise from within the client.

### "Filaments"

Old relationships, especially troubled relationships like those of a victim and an abuser, or a love relationship that went sour, often present a phenomenon called "filaments." This is a situation where something is holding the client and a former antagonist or lost love together, often many years later. Invisible lines seem to connect the two in a spiderweb effect, and the client cannot feel full freedom in the present to be in a healthy relationship. A new potential partner will feel subtle interference patterns without knowing what is the problem, and a new relationship might face major obstacles.

Encountering this situation, I get out the chairs. Putting the other person in the empty chair, the client can work through some of the history by making statements and asking questions, then switching to the other chair to experience what naturally arises as a response. Then at a certain point, I ask questions such as, "How do you still feel connected?" and "Where in your body is the continuing connection?" Many people report they sense something like a tiny invisible fishhook holding a thin line stretching over to the other person, in one or more places. There can be dozens of filaments, and the locations are often precisely where there have been physical problems in real life. One strategy is for the client to imagine removing the hooks one by one. Shifting to the other chair, the imagined other person can feel the unbinding effect; typically both sides have been feeling constrained. The unhooking process has to be done in both chairs to get the full effect. Often the breathing changes to a more expansive pattern when the imaginary filaments are released.

Working with filaments also has relevance when using the two-chair with a departed person, especially when there was trouble such as in the antagonist example above. The abuser and the victim may be still linked by the anger, fear, guilt and shame regarding the situation. After the emotions have been cleared, an "unhooking of filaments" can be tried. Often abusers are just as glad to be liberated from the trauma bond, because they have been held back from "moving on," even after death. I don't know the physiological mechanism for the filaments phenomenon, but the method has been repeatedly effective.

### Reconciliation with Departed Loved Ones

Two-chair therapy can be very healing for unresolved feelings relating to a departed loved one. Not only are there often unspoken messages energetically pent-up in either side, but also the "departed one" often can offer very good advice about current-time situations. Often clients have unfinished communication with family members who died, and who now seem to somehow still exist as consciousness in another dimension. Switching back and forth between the consciousness of the client and that of the symbol of the departed individual can be rich with resolution, forgiveness and insight. Hypothetically this is because the imagined departed one is now viewing circumstances from a more expansive perspective. The widened awareness emerges naturally from the client by putting the deceased in the other chair and switching. Even if the client does not believe in consciousness surviving death, switching to the other chair usually leads to spontaneous dialogue as if the belief were fully present. When the switch happens, the first impulse that arises often simply bypasses whatever belief system has been present, and an alternative, useful perspective just appears directly, with accompanying physical sensations.

For example, an agnostic scientist was grieving the loss of his elderly mother, with whom he had a long history of estrangement. He told his story and was invited to shift the attention to his own physical body sensations, which were not part of his normal primary awareness process. The body sensations and posture began to gather around the heart, feelings began to appear, and a cycle of Body-Low-Slow-Loop was used to digest and release the non-cognitive stress patterns. When this seemed to be complete for the moment, I invited him to imagine that his mother was in the other chair.

Immediately a new wave of feelings and sensations arose and was processed, again using BLSL. Then he was invited to make a statement to his mother; this was well outside of his belief system, but because he had been through such clear preparatory sensory processes he did not hesitate. He asked her, "Are you OK?" and switched chairs. Arriving in the other chair, a completely different configuration and ANS state appeared. He was amazed, to say the least, and another round of BLSL processing was used. Then, in the second chair, as his mother, he was asked to respond to the question. Without hesitation, a narrative from her perspective flowed spontaneously, complete with physical and emotional components, as if she were really there, speaking from beyond the grave. Through four more shifts the "two" profoundly worked out their problematic patterns and he began to comprehend the depth of her childhood suffering. A spirit of forgiveness and reconciliation replaced the alienation and anger he held at the start of the session.

*In their own words...*
*Clients describe their two-chair experiences*

*I am delighted to comment on a process I have found so useful. Initially I thought it was going to be like what I would experience with a Gestalt process which I have found is limited to sorting out thoughts, which can be helpful.*

*The two-chair process goes much deeper. When using it to help illuminate and clarify conflicts I was having with a housemate, I found I could access a "body sense" of my own deeper sensations, and also get a deeper understanding of the sensations and feelings my friend must be having in trying to relate to me. I did feel validated in my position to some extent, but could also experience that there was more truth beyond my narrow perspective. That in turn freed me from the confines of my emotions and limited focus enough to get outside my story. As a result there has been a subtle but significant shift in our relationship. I enjoy her more and generally feel less threatened. I stand my ground more easily when we have our more difficult interactions, and to her credit I would say she allows this more too.*

*In terms of the effectiveness of this process as a technique, the skill of the facilitator is vital. I think it is a way to go back through nervous system reactions slowly and with support that was lacking originally. When the client gets to places where there was a panic reaction, the facilitator can guide a kind of "re-experiencing," helping the client in the following ways (the ones that I have experienced or can see that I could):*

- *Body-sense more of the full reality and truth of the experience*

- *Release charged energy that has been held in tissues*

- *Realize how bias and pattern has crept into current experience from these past reactions and not only see other options, but both in session and in life, experiment with new responses (best done while the re-experiencing is fresh)*

*In my experience [as a counselor] working with people, mental insight is rarely enough to alter or release patterns. That requires a bodily experience below the pattern so that the client knows the pattern is not who they are. Even then it is quite a trick to get the pattern dismantled because it is so automatized in the nervous system. I think this two-chair process has great potential to help in this way, and I am very eager to learn more about it.*

Two-chair processing with the departed is not limited to unhappy relationships, of course. Some people felt loving and supportive, but simply did not get a chance to say good-bye when the one they loved died, due to distance or temporary alienation of some kind. In the two chairs, the final communication can be offered and received, often in heart-touching ways.

The loss or deliberate termination of a pregnancy can leave a residue of long-lasting feelings, in some cases creating severe unconscious emotional fixation that affects later relationships in many ways. The effects can be greatly relieved by the two-chair method. Embryos and fetuses were never just "a clump of cells," as some people seem to think. Switching back and forth between the two chairs, rich territories of subconscious, highly-charged, undigested experience are often revealed and resolved. There can be significant physical changes following the resolution of these kinds of old experiences, including resolution of physical problems with pelvic and lower-back areas.

## Working with Health Conditions in the Other Chair

It can be productive to put an actual health condition in the other chair. For example, a client with chronic headaches could use the method. The first chair would be the person in the normal headache state, while the second chair is "everything else," a "that-and-not-that" setup for the process. By switching back and forth between the two chairs, tracking sensations along the way, remarkable processes and insights may arise. An actual physical headache may appear when the client is in one chair and disappear in the other. The physiology for these kinds of fast changes is a mystery, but they happen frequently and the experiences are very useful for clients.

With one headache client, every time there was a switch, the separation between the two states was softened, and other changes began to be expressed including gurgling in the abdomen, indicating visceral movement. Meanwhile, the "headache chair" was able to give the "headache-free" chair insight into the problem. The problem was a severe bind in the woman's life between wanting to further her very successful career, while she also wanted to give full attention to her two young children. Switching back and forth, she devised a compromise solution for herself and felt much better.

Another client, who had survived breast cancer, complained of tightness in the chest, specifically around the heart, which she described as numb. I suggested that she put the numb aspect of her heart in the other chair, while she, in the first chair, was everything else. Observing the second chair, she described what she saw as dark and dense. Switching to the second chair, she felt overcome by a great weight and a guarded feeling that was quite unpleasant. I asked the second chair occupant, "How old do you feel?" The answer was spontaneous, "Five years old."

As a five-year-old girl, she had experienced serious stress in her family, and her heart and chest had gone into a protective mode. Switching back and forth a few times, with guided body awareness throughout, the darkness started to lift, and eventually the "adult" offered "the child" a safe space in her chest, in an imaginary miniature cave-like space. I gave her a small pillow to hold to her chest, to have the felt-sense experience of reunion. Interestingly, the second chair "heart-child" still felt a little guarded during and after the reunion. The guardedness had served an intelligent function under the circumstances and we "de-pathologized" the response. I expected that the darkness would lift in time, after the process had a chance to gently integrate at its own pace. Trust comes only from experience, so I never rush anyone to make changes, discard strategies or prematurely resolve conflicts. The effect will be better and more stable if the gentle pace of nature is respected and allowed.

As discussed above in relation to a "before and after" scenario, being overweight can derive from a person's experience in previous or current relationships. The individual who is suffering may perceive being in a relationship as dangerous, due to being invaded during childhood, having some trauma during puberty or being disappointed or betrayed in love as an adult. The two-chair method can be a way to sort out the history, with the overweight consciousness in one chair, and a hypothetical receptive-to-relationships consciousness in the other. Switching back and forth, the observation can be offered that the overweight state is serving as protection from vulnerability, and the person's strategy can be de-pathologized.

### Surrogate Processing

In another mysterious sequence, the two-chair process has been effective with people who are not even present. Sometimes a client will be concerned about something that is happening with a family member far away, who is in a bind of some kind, but who does not have resources or even a belief system to get help locally. A person can try the two-chair as a remote stand-in for a loved one and occasionally this leads to good outcomes.

The person who is present can start the session in one chair, then put the missing person in the other chair. Each time, we take care to have a complete kinesthetic experience. Once in the other chair, the first chair occupant can be changed to someone in the absent person's life, and the switching back and forth process begins with the client as a surrogate for the real person or people far away.

For example, a woman was very worried about her sister, who was having great trouble with her teenage son. They lived in another region, and therapy was not perceived as being available to them. Being much more familiar with the benefits of counseling, she had a strong impulse to help but did not have a way to participate; she did not know what to do. The two-chair process provided a possibility.

The session started with her in the first chair, processing her own state of being, using Body-Low-Slow-Loop for about ten minutes to create a general foundation. Then, when the time seemed appropriate, I directed her to imagine her sister being in the other chair. The two switched back and forth twice, as the sister explained the situation. Next, when she was in the second chair, now as her "sister," she was directed to imagine that the "son" (the actual client's nephew) was in the other chair. A conversation about their issues ensued, with switching back and forth accompanied by emotional releases in both chairs as each person (the client's sister and her son) aired their concerns and responded to each other's statements.

I repeatedly reminded the client that there was no obligation to reality within the process; nothing that is said has to be anything that would ever really be said. The intention is purely about expressing whatever naturally floats to the surface in the moment.

Back and forth she went through several stages of her sister's and nephew's emotion, regret, history and autonomic states. With each switch we took time to really digest the physicality of the experiences in each chair, more than the thoughts or feelings. After some time there was a reconciliation and new insight about what the son really needed from the mom, which was some degree of resolution about his mother's earlier divorce from his father. Divorce is often devastating for children, but almost always denied or trivialized by the parents, who are usually preoccupied with a host of feelings and issues of their own.

The session came to completion, and a week later she called to report that there had been positive and unmistakable changes across the country with her sister, and the crisis seemed to have passed. Again, there is no clear explanation for how the faraway change happened; my personal opinion is that it is a confirmation of Rupert Sheldrake's "morphogenic field" theory.[235] Additionally I sometimes find myself curious about the "entanglement" and "non-locality" effects of quantum physics as a possible explanation.[236]

Similarly, when one person switches to the chair of an absent partner and has a complete felt-sense experience of that other person's perspective, a subtle wave seems to go out through the field and actually affect the other person. When one partner does the two-chair process, has insights into the experience of the other, and then goes back home, the other often notices and comments that something is different; positions start to soften and shift as a result. This has been confirmed repeatedly in my private practice throughout my career. In another "synchronicity" variation, a client might have a two-chair process with an estranged family member who lives far away, and later that day an unexpected, conciliatory telephone call from the faraway person might be received.

---

[235] Rupert Sheldrake, *Morphic Resonance: The Nature of Formative Causation.* New Park, 2009.

[236] Dean Radin, *Entangled Minds: Extrasensory Experiences in a Quantum Reality.* Paraview Pocket Books, 2006. Other highly recommended authors in this genre include Lynne McTaggart and Russell Targ.

## Multi-Generational Awareness

Switching back and forth between parents, or even between generations, can be very helpful. Often the family tree can be explored with excellent results, as each generation gains insight and perhaps forgiveness or compassion for the previous or subsequent generations. Clients often discover that aspects of their behavior were used by their ancestors, either identically or sometimes in reverse. This can also be very helpful in couples therapy situations, with one partner watching while the other is in the chairs. When working with couples, the effect is to create a larger vantage point of origins for patterns and, usually, introducing more forgiveness in the relationship. Skipping around with different figures in the family tree, the process can resemble Constellation Therapy, but with additional resources.[237]

In another example, a couple was very distressed and the husband was close to seeking a divorce out of frustration with his wife's tension level. They both attended the session, with him taking the first turn while she watched from a distance. In the first exchange, him talking with "her," the conversation was quite volatile. So instead of him talking to her, I changed the second chair's imaginary occupant to be his own mother.

Commonly the spouse and the same gender parent have similar or reversed archetypal positions. He and his "mother" had a brief exchange, and in the second chair we shifted the identity again, to his mother's father. Back and forth through three generations, it was revealed that the same painful patterns were being repeated. This was astonishing and enlightening to his wife, observing at a distance. In real

---

[237] Joy Manne and Bert Hellinger, *Family Constellations: A Practical Guide to Uncovering the Origins of Family Conflict.* North Atlantic, 2009. Constellation Therapy has many similarities to the two-chair method, and the two can be used together very effectively.

life she began to cry and feel compassion for the whole picture, whereas before she had been mainly angry.

In time the couple switched places: now she was in the chairs and he was observing from a distance. Some multi-generational two-chair processing helped him see a bigger picture for her tension as well. This couple also benefitted from education about the "marriage triangle" (Chapter 11) so that there could be less pressure to resolve all the past generations' undigested material.

Clients who were adopted are likely to have attachment disorders of some kind because the blueprint for maternal bonding was not fulfilled as evolutionarily programmed.[238] Switching back and forth between the adopted (the client) and the original birth mother can be very liberating and emotional, leading to profound changes in state as the "maternal bonding files" are being "updated."

Adoptive parents may gain insights into how they might help their new adopted baby overcome the bonding interruption by putting the adopted child in the other chair and switching back and forth a few times. By expressing the concerns, such as "Baby, I am concerned about bonding," or "I am feeling insecure about how to approach our relationship," and then switching chairs, the tension is often reduced. There is frequently and spontaneously an expression of valuable direct advice by the "baby in the chair," who may have ideas about what remedial strategies will be effective. In some cases, there are palpable changes later in the day as some kind of unexplained after-effect begins to manifest.

---

[238] I have learned to be cautious with the word "programmed" because it can be antagonistic for some clients who are not comfortable with computers or software development.

## Undoing Hypnotic Trances

Clients who were raised by critical or demeaning parents may have been effectively "hypnotized" to believe the messages that they heard as children. The effect is total in infancy, then somewhat softened but still present in childhood; *delta* and *theta* brain frequencies predominate and make the child susceptible to hypnotic suggestion.[239] Children may become fixated in a debilitating belief system, as described by Pia Mellody (Chapter 13). Many clients are basically hypnotized children walking around in adult bodies, with no way to recognize, much less undo, the spell. The two-chair process can be an effective remedy.

---

### In their own words...
### Clients describe their two-chair experiences

*I have found the two-chair process to be one of the best benefits from my training in Polarity Therapy. As a Somatic Experiencing therapist, I have found this method to be very effective and very safe for clients and myself as well.*

*Recently a woman came to see me for anxiety. She settled in this country about 12 years ago, from Central America. Her uncle, with whom she was very close as a child, died this past spring. She was unable to return for the funeral and was feeling the hardship of the distance from family, most of whom are still there. We brought in three family members, one at a time, for two-chair conversations. It was truly the "next best thing" to being at the funeral.*

*She received tremendous comfort from her relatives and many words of wisdom, which helped reassure her that it is all right for her to be in the U.S. and not be present at the funeral. Her love for her uncle was seen and appreciated and she felt a sense of completion. She later reported she was less anxious, able to sleep better and move on with her life. She had not realized how much the feeling of being in a bind was affecting her.*

---

[239] Bruce Lipton, *The Honeymoon Effect.* Hay House, 2013.

In a hypnotism-ending scenario, the client talks with the imaginary more critical parent. After switching a few times, perhaps discovering how the parent also suffered in his or her childhood, the imagined parent may show regret for the damage that was inflicted. Even extremely abusive parents have a thread of goodness still present, or life could not continue. When the parental regret becomes accessible, there can be a "breaking of the trance." Sitting in the second chair as the parent, once that person is motivated to do something about the situation, the client can be instructed to "break the spell" by making a gesture and sound, such as loudly clapping the hands or snapping the fingers, saying something like, "I release you from this message."

Switching to the first chair, the client can then be on the receiving end of a de-hypnotizing process, tracking sensation through really hearing the parent's statement, especially the sound that was given. In addition to hearing the content of the message, the experience of receiving can be helpful, including a question such as, "Where in your body does this message seem to land?"

The sharp sound is important because it is non-cognitive, processed in the deep layers where hypnotic trances reside. In hypnotherapy this is known as "bypassing the critical factor."[240] To help the therapeutic changes deepen and become long-lasting, we seek visual, auditory and kinesthetic cues that are more memorable for the ANS than mere words and concepts. A token of the release can also be

---

[240] James Russell, *Psychosemantic Parenthetics*. IHTR, 1988. Russell defines critical factor as "the filtering system of the mind, screening conscious directives to the subconscious mind."

offered, as an "anchor"[241] for the experience. Later the client may find a representation of the anchor that was used in the session. For example, one client reached a truce with an antagonist. In the antagonist's chair, she imagined a smooth pink oval quartz crystal appearing in her hand to give as a symbolic compensation for the injuries caused. Later she reported finding just such a gemstone in a shop, buying it and keeping it with her as a constant reminder of the new perspective.

As with many two-chair sessions, "homework" for the client to do as a follow-up can be very empowering. Homework for de-hypnosis sessions can include taking a few minutes each day for the next week or two to recall the experience of switching back to the first chair after the "parent" has made the releasing sound and statement. The sound itself can resonate very deeply and may become quite memorable. Another useful homework practice for the post-trance client might be the Forgiveness practice described in Chapter 9, as the parent and child release each other and withdraw filaments of resentment, blame, shame and guilt. As another form of empowering homework, writing down what happened in a de-hypnosis session can be supportive of the process taking hold and having a lasting effect.

---

[241] In this context, "anchor" means a tangible representation of a mental or emotional experience. The concept is well-developed in hypnotherapy and Neuro-Linguistic Programming. People unconsciously use anchors frequently, such as wearing something inherited from a loved one, to give a comforting experience of their presence. In the two-chair process, an anchor can be an imaginary token of the meaning of the moment, given from one chair occupant and received by the other, to deepen and establish the message of the moment. For more on NLP and anchors: Lisa Wake, *NLP: Principles in Practice*. Ecademy, 2012.

## *Boundary Practice*

A variation of the Boundary practice (Chapter 9) can be done with the two-chair method. Here the clients take time to do the Boundary practice as described above, then imagine that they are also in the other chair, but without the same boundary. In switching to the other chair, great insight may arise about what happens to the ANS when the boundary situation is changed. The capacity for holding a boundary can be greatly enhanced by this alternating "that" and "not that" practice, as clients increase their sensitivity to the condition of their boundary.

---

### About Strong Emotional Expression

Feelings and tears are helpful in the two-chair process, to discharge held emotions. Through discharge, energy being used to encapsulate an indigestible experience becomes available for dealing with the present-time challenges of living our lives. As Anna Chitty says, "E-motion means energy in motion." However, strong expressions should not be allowed to become overwhelming. Of course, "overwhelming" is a relative and subjective term. A modest amount of emotional discharge is good, but it should not move into uncontrolled sustained expression, or it might become re-traumatizing. I prefer to use a series of small sequences rather than one big cathartic process, for the reasons described in Chapter 1.

Many of us are afraid of feelings, not least out of fear that they may become overwhelming and permanent; here we can help clients by explaining that feelings tend to come in waves, with peaks and valleys, and that body-centered processing can be very helpful in riding the wave through a cycle. Once the client comprehends that an intense body experience is a temporary state, the appearance of strong emotion becomes less terrifying. Indeed, it can be a revelation for clients to discover that feelings can be experienced as peaks and valleys, instead of steady, unmanageable states.

---

## *More Examples of Two-Chair Processes*

### *Example #2*

A client had recently experienced an ectopic pregnancy, leading to emergency surgery in a life-threatening situation. The baby would have been her first child, and she was devastated by the sense of loss. Her plight was compounded by the trauma of medical procedures coupled with a sense of guilt, not knowing whether she could have done anything differently. She showed signs of being in parasympathetic autonomic shock, describing horrific events with a detached, vacant look. First we used BLSL to discharge some of the emotions, and then there was a brief interlude for education about the ANS, to reduce her self-assessment that she must surely have a deep character flaw. Then I set up two chairs and she took a seat in one of them.

After a few minutes of BLSL, I suggested that she imagine that the baby was in the other chair. There was an immediate surge of tears and feelings.

After settling with BLSL, I then encouraged her to begin communicating with the baby. Any question or comment can serve the purpose. For maximum initial effect, I use only open-ended questions, so that the wording and tone come from the client, not from me. The client asked the baby, "What happened? Where are you? Are you OK?" Switching to the second chair, the physical agitation was immediately replaced by quite a different configuration, and a conversation ensued in which the "baby" told the mom about how the mom's safety was most important, how the baby had given her warnings through subtle intuitive thoughts that something was not right, and how it was not the mom's fault but rather a destined sequence with much larger forces at work.

Switching back to the first chair, the mother experienced enormous relief and began to show signs of coming back into her body. I saw that she was recovering from the parasympathetic ANS stress response because her attention was now more focused. She was beginning to digest the experience of the whole loss and emergency sequence. There were several more shifts between the two chairs, with the baby's comments being consistently full of wise insight and the mother's relaxation progressing to deeper and deeper levels of settling and integration. Only one session was needed; the client felt better and her parasympathetic shock symptoms did not return.

### Example #3

A female client sought help with high blood pressure. After a few open-ended questions, during which I had an opportunity to assess which Principle and Element were in play, the two chairs were set up. The process was initiated by one round of Body-Low-Slow-Loop to educate her in the exact method while also demonstrating its value. After one pass from tension in the chest to the feet, and then back to the chest, the tension was noticeably reduced. Then I offered the suggestion, "Put the high blood pressure condition in the other chair." Upon switching, the client looked back at the first chair and began to laugh, saying that the tension was so evident it seemed like a cartoon. Switching back to the first chair, there was a major shift of state; the laughter softened the ANS fixation, as discussed in Chapter 6.

Then I suggested a progression of the process to explore a possible context. Using the hierarchy of action fields model (Chapter 5), the client's relationship with her boyfriend emerged as a fruitful topic. At first, the client had talked about the stress of her job, expecting that to be the source of the high blood pressure. But vocational stress is lower in the hierarchy of action fields, and therefore the higher fields of action (Self, Intimate Partner) needed to be checked first. After the client's boyfriend was put in the other chair, a series of previously unrecognized insights began to emerge. The client expressed a desire for more connection, and upon switching chairs the "boyfriend" demonstrated a physical avoidance/withdrawal pattern of leaning back and rotating the body to one side. The imagined boyfriend was showing an "Avoidant" attachment style. This gradually began to dissipate, and a new set of impulses became visible.

Switching back and forth two more times, the client ended up having an experience of being in a bind with her boyfriend. She realized that she herself was unconsciously ambivalent about commitment, contributing to his avoidant behaviors; previously she had thought it was all his fault. She began to take more responsibility for the whole situation, instead of blaming him and feeling victimized. She also felt a clearing physically in the upper chest area, and had a clear sense of how tension in the heart and throat areas from the emotional bind could relate to her high blood pressure.

After shifting between chairs twice more, re-negotiating the relationship and taking responsibility for the hidden dynamics, she felt much better and became determined to work on solving the relationship stress. I advised her to write down what she could remember of what was said in each chair, as a way to solidify her understanding, also adding more power to her newly discovered resources and how she was processing them. Later she reported that the high blood-pressure situation was reduced and that whenever she felt tense all she had to do was remember the laughter and cartoonish perception that had appeared in the second chair. One session seemed to be sufficient at the time; later perhaps more exploration might be helpful for releasing ancestral and earlier-life history that contributed to the pattern.

### Example #4

A client was feeling abandoned and guilty because her new husband had left her for another woman. Before leaving he had told her it was all her fault, because he could not tolerate her emotionality subsequent to a series of very stressful events. She believed this and was distraught at having ruined the relationship; she was still dedicated to her marriage.

In the first chair, she took some time, with guidance, to have a complete experience of her current state, including sensations, feelings and thoughts. She practiced Body-Low-Slow-Loop when the experience became unpleasant. With guidance she learned to break up the flooding of grief and anger into sets of two-to-three minutes of experiencing the sensations and feelings of the primary state, then one-to-two minutes of experiencing some other part of the body (in this case, her feet) that was not a primary location of sensation.

After two or three Body-Low-Slow-Loop cycles, I directed her to change chairs. In the second chair, as her "husband," the set of experiences that had been so strong suddenly disappeared. In their place she experienced a sort of distracted dreaminess. There was no initial comment or response to what had been said in the first chair, just a state of dissociation, a parasympathetic ANS stress response. She explored this experientially for several minutes, again using Body-Low-Slow-Loop as needed to induce polarity movement within the state. She could feel a quality of separation that she recognized in her husband's behavior, but had not named.

Switching back to the first chair, she experienced quite a different state. The overwhelming feelings of anguish, anger and guilt were noticeably softer. Instead of believing that it was all her fault, she could identify the previously invisible part that her husband had been playing. She had been the "identified patient," but he had been a factor with a more socially acceptable detachment that was actually evading responsibility as a full participant in very difficult, commonly-shared experiences. She realized that this had been going on for a long time with him, before they had even met, and that it was therefore clearly not all her fault. She had a great sense of relief and the awakening of new resources. Her feeling of fixation, being stuck in a victim role, was greatly relieved, and she felt compassion for her husband's situation.

In retrospect, this marriage probably could have been saved with some follow-up two-chair processing, but the divorce was already far along and the husband was not interested in counseling. Lack of interest in counseling often accompanies a parasympathetic ANS stress response. When a person is becoming immobilized and resigned, engaging in therapy is not on the menu of options. It is an unfortunate situation, because the two-chair method could actually have been helpful.

*Example #5*

A client complained that she had many great creative ideas but could not overcome her tendency to procrastinate. There was little movement in her career as a result. She was encouraged to take a complete physical inventory of the present state. Then we moved the process along, by imagining that the other chair held all the creativity while the chair she was currently in held everything else, including all her inertia and distraction.

When the creativity was isolated and imagined to be in the other chair, her posture immediately began to change, leaning and sagging to the left (Yin) side. Then she switched to the second chair, which held all the creativity unrestrained by her procrastination tendencies. The whole posture and sense of self was immediately very different. She became authentically fascinated by the dramatic change in sensation, posture and sense of self. The two sides conversed about her life for two turns: first, one spoke of the creativity, then the other responded describing immobilization. With each shift the difference was less: the polarity was being stabilized, and she felt better. She was so used to the procrastination tendency being in control that it was a great relief to understand that the creative aspects were still available.

I coached the two sides to negotiate with each other, with the fearful part expressing its concerns and the bold part becoming more respectful of the valid role fear had played earlier in her life. The two sides performed a transfer of authority from one side to the other, as if the procrastinator yielded a car's driver's side and steering wheel to the more mobilized part of her consciousness. The session was completed, as many are, by me coming up with some form of homework to help her feel more empowered. In this case the homework was to write down the two-chair conversation and do Body-Low-Slow-Loop once a day for a week or two.

## Useful Details for the Two-Chair Method

• It is important to help clients remember that *the two-chair process is not about realism.* There is no effort to figure out what the other person, the absent or vacant chair, might say in real life. Instead, it is about speaking whatever feels natural in the other chair, whatever spontaneously arises. The emphasis is on the experience. Most sessions include me saying some form of the following general statement, "Just be the person, in the moment. Whatever arises is of interest, regardless of whether it would ever be felt or spoken." Another common phrasing for the same purpose is, "This is just an experiment."

Obviously, the other person or condition is not really present. The client may need to be reminded of this repeatedly during the session because the sensations, gestures, postures, movements and emotions that arise can be so strong and compelling to be mistaken for an actual presence. Again, nothing that is spoken in the two chairs needs to be spoken in real life, and clients are free to experiment with options such as trying a particular phrase, exploring its effects, then coming back to the first chair and trying a different phrase.

• The practitioner must remain composed and neutral throughout the session. This can be hard when difficult feelings and sensations arise. Insecure practitioners might naturally fear strong emotions, since a theme of the whole therapy is gentleness instead of catharsis. But the two-chair method is inherently safer than most expressive therapies, because, again, there is always a quick solution to overwhelming dramatic situations, simply saying "switch." Whatever is happening in one chair will be transformed by moving to the other chair, thereby enabling a slow, gentle charge release. For beginning facilitators, a guiding principle is, "When in doubt, just say switch."

• As much as possible, part of our job is to see that no one, or no thing, is characterized as pathological. For all the reasons discussed in Chapter 1, the healing process is enhanced by reversing the tendency to cast events and people in negative lights. Of course, there are abusers whose behavior is entirely hurtful, and there are conditions that could be fatal. However, part of the art of the two-chair process is to find the intelligence in everything; every evil event had preceding conditions leading to adaptations that served a purpose. By switching to the other chair, the victim can reach compassion and a release from the long-term fixation or static pattern of victimhood. The two-chair process makes such a transformation easier than it might first appear.

• Working in the client's native language has many benefits. If a person grew up speaking a different language, we can help by suggesting that the communication be in the first language. This works better for clients working with child states, before a new language was learned. Even though I no longer understand what is being said, I can often still read the body states. Entire weekend workshops have been led in a foreign language, with a translator; the subliminal ANS value of the original tongue can supersede the value of

---

*In their own words...*
### *Clients describe their two-chair experiences*

*Two-Chair is a subtle yet deeply rich and insightful technique. I find it to be very helpful for understanding my own patterning.*

*For me specifically, it shed light on the method to some of the chaotic madness that seemed random in my life; a simple understanding of what I had been choosing to do for years (sort of auto-pilot). Never before this had I grasped my own behavior in such light! It helped me understand what it is I am doing, the motivation behind it and most importantly where my intentions are. I am still a work in progress grasping all of this.*

*What a gift to be able to see! The Two-Chair process illuminated this path for me.*

*In my past experiences with conventional talk therapy, reaching this level of depth and understanding did not really come up. In traditional talk therapy, I never felt productive and not buried by self-doubt, guilt and inner anger. Two-chair made me feel light hearted with fuzzy warmth all over my body. I actually felt good! That "Ah Ha" moment was priceless. I needed to rest afterwards as it was very deep and intense.*

*By embracing Two-Chair and going "there," which also means into these "characters," I was able to unlock long-buried feelings deep in the recesses of my body and being, as well as understanding my loved ones. It's a wonderful and productive feeling. I needed to rest as the insight was so vast.*

*So simple and yet completely moving as it changed the way I view my life just by providing me with some answers and understanding. Like, finally opening a locked window that was forgotten but always there, just never utilized or enjoyed due to the years of accumulated dust, dirt and decay. The new view is remarkable.*

---

our knowing the content of what is said. After all, it is the client primarily doing the work, not the facilitator.

• Utilizing "traffic light" terminology, such as "Red light, Yellow light, or Green light," simplifies interpersonal binds. This traffic light analogy reduces the complexity of situations to just three options: "go, stop, wait," or "yes, no, maybe." Typically this is used when the client is working on the two sides of a relationship, and it is unclear whether one approves or disapproves of the other. We can simply ask for a summary: "Does what you just said mean red light, yellow light or green light?"

People depend on clarity when driving across town; if the traffic lights are not working, or if they are all stuck on blinking yellow, chaos is sure to follow. The same is true for relationships; if one person is all green and the other is yellow or red, problems will arise. Even at a cellular level, life's choices can be reduced to these three: approach, wait and see, or turn away.[242] Is the other person sending a clear signal? How is that signal received? Prolonged ambiguity is exhausting and needs to be resolved for the relationship to prosper, at any stage. The key phrase is, "If it's not a green light, don't proceed." The alternative is that the uncertainty may drag on and deplete the relational vitality. The two-chair method quickly cuts to the core of such situations and reveals mismatched intentions.

The "traffic lights" inquiry has been very effective at penetrating complex relationship problems and finding effective solutions. Using the two-chair process, green light/red light will be obvious on multiple levels for the practitioner, but often invisible to the client. If the light is green for both sides, the relationship can progress. If one is

---

[242] For an excellent discussion of this cellular simplicity: Bruce Lipton, *The Biology of Belief.* Hay House, 2008.

green and the other is yellow, the green risks over-stepping boundaries and missing important cues, leading to problems in the future. The focus is on clarification so the relationship can evolve to its next stage.

• Journaling is used to involve additional brain resources, which seems to boost processing and help changes become more long-lasting. The language function in the brain is strongly organized around a witness consciousness; the very act of naming something objectifies it. Usually I offer to help fill in the script with additional details as needed later in the week because clients are often unable to remember the dialogue. The offer for support can be much appreciated. In addition to creating a more accurate script, the awareness of my support adds to the witness consciousness of the client, knowing that someone else is participating as a supportive ally. Clients are much more likely to "do their homework" when they know they are being observed by a friend.

• A numbered scale can be very helpful, and further supports the traffic lights analogy. I often ask clients to give a number to quantify the range of feelings, using a scale from one to ten. Quantifying a subjective experience increases the capacity for objectivity and cuts through mixed messages and other confusions.

For example, a couple came for sessions to get help with their relationship, but it soon became evident that he was more eager to move forward than she was. When he was seated in a chair, with his partner watching from a comfortable distance, I asked, "What number would you rate yourself, on a scale of ten, for making this relationship into a life partnership?" He quickly answered, "Ten" implying a total green light perspective and attitude. When he switched to the empty chair as his "partner," the felt sense and body language was one of caution and defensiveness, more appropriate for a yellow light, and "her" self-assessment, numerically, was six. This was a revelation for him, as he had basically been ignoring the signals (excess Yang, leading to frustration) in his eagerness to move forward. As a result, he had been putting subtle pressure on her to go along with his momentum rather than listen to herself (excess Yin, leading to resentment). Their relationship problems stemmed from ambiguity of the situation as much as it did from character traits. Once this was revealed, they could move forward to either resolve the resistance, quit the relationship or any number of now better-informed options that they could explore together.

The numeric scale approach can be used in many different situations, not just with couples. Quantifying a feeling reduces some of its potential for being overwhelming. Quantifying situations as numbers also helps us because, in a subsequent session, there can be a quick resumption of the process by just recalling the number, which sums up a complex situation in a simple way. In the example above, all I had to do was cite the number, such as, "Are you still a 10 and is she still a 6?" and he knew exactly what I meant.

• The use of "anchors," discussed above, can help a person solidify the newly achieved balance between the two sides of the self. When one side of a dipole has a resource for the other side (for example, when the higher mind wants to uplift the lower mind, or a departed parent wants to support the surviving child) the client can be asked to imagine some "gift" that would represent the resource and the intention or message. The giving and receiving of the imaginary token can be acted out with full attention to experiential processing, so that it really becomes firmly absorbed. Later, clients will sometimes create or purchase something similar to what was described in the session and place the item in a prominent place for a daily, tangible reminder of the resource. Anchors can vary widely: gemstones, works of art, articles of clothing and memorabilia are some of the many possibilities that can be very meaningful in this way.

For example, a client felt out of touch with his power, feeling weak in his current fields of action. Switching between chairs a few times, the non-dominant consciousness gradually manifested with a much stronger sense of will power and determination. I asked the client to imagine something in his hand that would symbolize this previously unavailable sense of being, and he came up with a particular gemstone, a smooth, pink quartz oval. I guided him in imagining every detail including color, density, weight, texture, size and shape. When this process was complete, I invited the stronger self to offer the imaginary gemstone to his other, previously dominant self, including physically extending his hand toward the empty chair as a reminder of the strength that had appeared in the session.

Switching to the other chair, the dominant, but originally weaker self, accepted the "gift," using the physical motion of reaching out with an upturned palm. Later, the client reported that the overall sense of inertia in his life had faded, and that he had actually bought a gemstone approximating the one he had visualized. He carried the small stone in his pocket and touched it occasionally during the day, reminding himself of the empowered state he had experienced in the second chair. Through repetition, the new state of being became well-established, as if the brain was re-wiring itself.

• Some clients have a hard time switching between chairs. They will make a statement in one chair, then continue to be in the same perspective, or tell the same narrative, in the other. The benefits of the method are not available unless there is a real switch in perspective. In this situation, we can guide the client to slow down and simplify the message, or use another "person" in the second chair with whom there is a clearer polarity. I can even suggest that I, as the practitioner, be imagined in the other chair, to heighten a felt sense of stepping outside the habitual mind. Another possibility is to take the client out of the equation entirely, having one chair be the client's mother and the other chair be the client's father. With creativity, trying different candidates, most clients who are initially unable to switch between chairs can find their way to an effective use of the two-chair process.

In a similar vein, some clients will be averse to being in the chair of an antagonist. For example, if the mother was experienced as toxic, then sitting in the "mom" chair will naturally be avoided. The approach is to avoid forcing anything, whether dialogue, movement or feelings. There are innumerable possibilities for the other chair, and there is always some alternative if the process is not working. Also, when the other chair seems toxic, the time spent can be abbreviated instead of the usual equal time being spent in each chair.

One client had parents who were extremely damaging throughout her childhood. The last thing she would ever want to do is "be" either one of them. In this case, the first session was with her youthful self in the other chair at a time of maximum happiness. She remembered a favorite spot in the woods behind her house where she liked to go to be in nature and escape the domestic chaos of her childhood home. When she sat in this chair she instantly felt better than she would in her normal, predominant state. Switching back and forth, her whole state of being could be observed to change, and the more she had these experiences, the less fixation she experienced about her parents. A few sessions later she was able to do a two-chair process with her parents, and began to feel better in her life because some of the charge had been reduced. In this situation, it was important to offer reassurances and keep emphasizing that in the second chair she was not actually her mother or father, that this was all just an experiment about ANS states.

• Compulsive behaviors and addictions are excellent candidates for this kind of therapy. One chair can be us at our best and healthiest, and the other, at our worst or most addiction-prone. This is similar to how "higher mind" and "lower mind" can make an interesting duality. The conversation that ensues can be very helpful, and often the troubled part of the polarity relationship will often identify what it needs that is driving the behavioral disturbance. Most addictive substances are playing a role in supporting the client's management of life experience, so I like to de-pathologize the usage so that the conversation can progress. A person wanting to quit smoking could put cigarettes in the other chair, make a statement, then switch and see what emerges from the other point of view. This approach can be used for any substance, including alcohol, drugs of any kind, sugar, caffeine or any other habitual support dependency.

A male client in his forties had a vague desire to quit smoking before his young son was old enough to become consciously aware of his habit, but there were always excuses and distractions, not least because smoking was really helping him manage his inner state. In the two chairs he had a conversation with tobacco as an old and valued ally in managing his anxiety, and they ended up bidding each other a respectful farewell. Then the second chair became his son, and the sense of determination increased enormously when he experienced how much his son looked up to him as a hero. He re-framed quitting smoking as a heroic act for the benefit of his son, a real-world field of action for his fatherly instincts.

He was able to quit smoking after that session, and later reported that his relationship with his wife had also improved as a side-effect, not only because she appreciated the change in odor but also because he felt less ashamed and generally better about himself as a result of being more in command (balanced Yang) of his life.

• The two-chair method is excellent for practicing or "pre-exercising" a conversation or encounter that is expected to be difficult. A client might be facing a tough job interview, legal challenge, domestic quarrel, parenting stress or any other complex situation. By putting the other person in the second chair and having the conversation in advance, without the other person being physically present, the real issues will be identified, the pent-up emotions will be reduced and new solutions may become available. In particular, a message or style of communication that may have been used in the conversation may be revealed as ineffective by giving it a test drive. When it becomes obvious that the approach does not work, a new strategy can then be developed. Clients have often reported that the tension in the situation was reduced, and the actual conversation went much more smoothly than expected.

One client was in the process of separating from her husband and was very concerned about an impending negotiation regarding terms. Using a two-chair process, with her imagined ex-partner in the other chair, old emotions were discharged and new insights were revealed. She had a refreshed and more accurate understanding about his longstanding frustration, a key factor in the separation. Before the two-chair process, she had a mental idea of the problem, but by sitting in "his" chair, she found that her awareness became more embodied and compassionate. Through the process, the emotional charge was reduced and she experimented with different language. Later, in the real conversation, she found herself with better access to empathic equanimity, and he voluntarily softened his position in the negotiation as a result. I think this was another marriage that actually could have been saved, but by then it was too late.

• There can be more than two chairs. After an initial phase, orienting to the process, an additional chair can be placed to hold the representation of another significant presence. For example, a client was exploring stress with her mother, who had always been critical of her. After some time the "father," who was much more supportive, was brought into the process and placed in an additional chair. With both imaginary parents present, the client could get a much stronger sense of how she had been placed in a very difficult bind by the enormous difference in her experience of the two parents. Her sympathy for her father's situation also caused her to have a special bond (see "surrogate spouse" in Chapter 11) relationship that undermined her ability to have a real relationship of her own. Experientially understanding all this enabled her to get some distance from the interpersonal complexities. She felt less impacted, calmer and more integrated within her own self.

• An area of the body that is experiencing problems can occupy the second chair. A person with breathing issues could be asked to put the imaginary lungs in the other chair, or a chronic health problem could be projected to be separate from the rest and sitting in the other chair. Many times, the second chair will come up with remarkable insights about the context of the disease, and the client subsequently may experience relief of symptoms. A liver cancer client put her liver in the other chair, switched chairs, and the "liver" spontaneously blurted out, "Stop being so angry!"

• Close attention to language is an important skill. The field of "psychosemantic parenthetics" describes how word choices contain subliminal messages.[243] Detecting these

---

[243] James Russell, *Psychosemantic Parenthetics*. IHTR, 1988.

hidden meanings is a highly developed art in hypnotherapy. By re-phrasing the client's statements to the fewest syllables and words, and being blunt and concrete instead of abstract, the process can move along much more efficiently. A client in conflict with her spouse started with a lengthy monologue of complex meanings. When that wave seemed finished, I tried an abbreviation, "Would it be accurate to say that you were disappointed with what happened?" It is important to have any re-phrasing confirmed by clients, because the statements must authentically represent their experience of reality. Simplified, direct language can cut through the fog of interpersonal confusion. Once language has been used that really fits for the client, I try to use the same exact words and phrases repeatedly in the session, and later in future sessions, so that the process continues in the client's own terms.

• An advanced facilitation skill is to experiment with providing beginnings of sentences and asking the client to fill in the blank. These can be oriented to the Five Elements for efficiency and precision. A client exhibiting signs of grief (typically managed by the Ether Element, located at the throat) or symptoms related to the throat, such as thyroid problems, could be offered "I feel_____ [the client is asked to fill in the blank with whatever seems appropriate]_____" as a means to initiate the conversation. Using these fill-in-the-blank phrases is a way to prime the pump of the process, and move quickly to core issues.

The elements, their associated body areas, and leading phrases are:

| Element | Body area | Leading Phrase |
|---------|-----------|----------------|
| Ether | Throat | "I *feel*..." |
| Air Element | Chest | "I *want*..." |
| Fire Element | Solar Plexus | "I *will*..." |
| Water Element | Abdomen | "I *need*..." |
| Earth Element | Seat | "I *fear*..." |

Using leading phrases, and getting the client to fill in the blank, is an advanced skill because it requires knowledge of subtle anatomy (Chapter 13). Clients exhibit Three Principle and Five Element signals very frequently, but these are likely to be missed by the untrained practitioner. The method still works without these more advanced aspects.

• Repetition is useful in the two-chair process. Statements can be embellished by the facilitator and the client can be asked to repeat as the process unfolds. Often a brief synopsis can be offered and when the client switches chairs we can repeat what was just said in the other chair, to maximize the pendulation action. This repetition is especially useful when emotions are high. Repeating what was spoken by the client amplifies the effect of the communication and helps when there has been long-term denial about a particular topic or antagonism with a certain person.

• Humor can be very helpful when facilitating a two-chair process. Amusing comments loosen up fixation and support the "witness" consciousness more securely. Some humor has an autonomic dimension, as the Moshe Feldenkrais quotation illustrated earlier. Humor is an art in itself, however, and if it does not come naturally, it is probably left excluded.

Humor should never be negative: no sarcasm, criticism or ridicule. Also it should never be at the expense of anyone neither the client nor the "person" in the other chair. A constructive and funny possibility is the "Exaggerated Yin and Yang Practice" (Chapter 9), which can be very effective for couples who have become de-polarized.

• The person in the chairs can also be guided to experiment with alternative language in the form of phrasing, body posture or gestures. A person showing an imbalanced Yang archetype could be coached to try out a balanced Yang statement, in order to experience the effects on whoever is imagined to be in the other chair.

A couple was drifting apart, the woman becoming increasingly discontent and the man feeling less certain about his direction in life. This appeared to be a critic-wimp (Yin-deficient, Yang-deficient) scenario. They came in together for counseling and each one took turns in the chairs, for about 25 minutes each. She started and expressed her discontent, and when she switched to the other chair, as her husband, she immediately began to shrink and lean rearward and to the left side. This caught her attention; she had not previously had any sense of what it felt like to be him in the presence of her criticism. After two more shifts, discussing issues and softening the entrenched positioning of their familiar quarrels, I suggested that she try something new, as an experiment. For the next chair-switch she was asked to lean slightly rearward (more Yin) in her chair, relaxing her hips, and lean slightly forward (more Yang) in his, with more weight on his feet. The effect was very different and she reported that she definitely felt more at ease when "he" was leaning slightly forward.

Then it was his turn to be in the chairs. The same conversation was continued, and the now-familiar posture was again spontaneously expressed. In the man's chair, the leaning forward posture was repeated. This time it was subtly amplified with gesture (moving the right hand while talking), tone (slightly more firm sounding) and intention (stating his direction for life and the relationship). Switching chairs, the effect was immediate as "she" relaxed and felt a lower center of gravity (less Yin-deficient). A reconciliation process began because their Yin and Yang equilibrium had been moved into a more functional range.

Similarly, a problematic autonomic state can be experimentally shifted. A person in a dissociated parasympathetic ANS state (flat affect, withdrawn, spacey) can be asked to lean forward (more Yang, and more sympathetic ANS) while continuing the conversation, just to stimulate movement within the conversation. Similarly, a wimp archetype can be asked to lean forward, speak more loudly, and perhaps emphasize the statement with a firm gesture, such as pointing the finger, pounding on the thigh or other indications of strong conviction, commitment and responsibility. The effect can be quite profound for the ANS state experienced by the person in other chair.

• Occasionally, sequences unfold in the chairs that defy explanation, and the process can even take on a life of its own with clients basically doing their own facilitation. In one case, a female client troubled by chronic fear conjured up (on her own, I had no direct part in the choice) the imagined presence of her grandmother in the other chair. Her grandmother wanted to give her an important message about non-violence. Switching back and forth on her own, a story unfolded that the grandmother was pregnant with the client's mother when she participated in a depression-era gangland murder. The grandmother described how the egg that later became the client was in her fetal daughter's body during the violence, so her granddaughter also carried an echo of the experience. In effect the granddaughter was somehow shell-shocked by an event that happened long before she was even conceived.

The "grandmother" sincerely wanted to release the wounding that her behavior had caused. Several more switches ensued, with detailed descriptions of the crime and release of old emotions; in time a great peace came over the

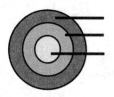

• *Grandmother (dark shading) was pregnant*
• *Mother (lighter shading) was a fetus inside Grandmother*
• *The fetus contained the egg (lightest shading) that created the Daughter*

client. This all happened without much prompting from me; the mechanism is unknown, but the effectiveness was clear.

Later the client reported that she did not need further support; the effect of the session had been long-lasting, and she had been able to move on with her life, including making long-postponed career decisions.

• The session does not have to end in resolution. There may be a dynamic tension between two chairs, such as between a husband and wife in conflict. Switching back and forth between chairs and roles, the issues are likely to be identified, but one or the other may not be ready to take the next step. The session can end in this unresolved state, because the unfolding of the process will continue after the client goes home. The process needs time to mature, just as homemade soup tastes better if we give it a chance to sit for a while. When I get a sense of dynamic tension not ready for completion, I simply say, "I think that's a good place to stop." In such a situation, I make it clear that this is not the end of the process and that I am fully available for the follow-up, when the time feels right. Usually I will hear from the client later saying the process continued over the course of hours or days, and in a return visit the resolution will arrive at the client's own pace.

• Switches between chairs and roles can be prolonged or abbreviated, whatever is most appropriate for the therapeutic moment. Sometimes "less is more," and switching back and forth a few times only takes a few minutes, with a key message being sent and received. This can be useful when trying to combine several processes in just one session. In other situations, staying in one chair, such as a relaxed state for a person who is chronically tense, can go on for five or ten minutes so that the unfamiliar state has adequate time to take hold and become normal.

## *Relationships and Couples Counseling*

As introduced above, the two-chair method is quite effective and efficient in relationship situations and couples counseling. Instead of having the couple talk to each other, the conversation happens in the chairs, with one person talking to an imagined other, in the other chair. Switching back and forth engenders a wide range of responses. Attachment styles become quickly evident, but instead of becoming even more fixated, as can happen in direct communication, the two-chair conversation is much more dynamic. Often an avoidant (Yang, distancing, self-regulating) style is in conflict with an ambivalent (Yin, merging or pulling back, other-regulating) style, or a disorganized style is self-defeating by sending complex, confusing messages.

As is the case with individuals, all states and expressions within couples are seen as the inner intelligence trying to survive, especially under threatening conditions in early childhood. Being in a state of too little Yin (the critic archetype) is not a "life sentence" or a lifelong disability. Similarly, an avoidant attachment style can be appreciated for the wisdom that it represents when considering the parental dynamics that preceded it. ANS states can be fully experienced and appreciated as a form of wisdom, then they can be transformed by switching to the other chair. When this is experienced in the chairs, the hypnotic spell of habitual behavior begins to loosen and real transformation can begin. Issues are experienced and positions are made more flexible. The actual chemistry and neurology of secure attachment can be induced and made memorable and the social branch of the ANS is often elevated.

Practitioners who counsel couples are well advised to study the Yin and Yang archetypes, autonomic nervous system states, attachment styles and life situations (Chapter

11) in depth. Many clients do not know what to do in certain situations such as becoming new parents or being in new relationships, so opportunities for education often arise. After both partners have had a turn in the chairs, I often provide an educational interlude, summarizing what I observed so that we can recognize and understand the therapeutic process that was just completed.

Guidance for couples is often particularly lacking. There are many excellent lists of recommended conduct, such as "don't argue at night," "always give appreciation," "take time for each other," and so on, but these often lack a larger and more complete context.[244] A Yin and Yang approach starts with the big picture and proceeds to details. An educational phase of the session is often fascinating for two-chair clients who have been emotional and uncertain about what was happening and are ready to improve their situation.

Yin and Yang polarities, ANS responses and attachment styles can all be explored thoroughly through two-chair switches. Once the system is flowing, clients can be gently guided in a series of two-chair experiments to provide an experience of alternatives, in basically any context. Switching to the other chair gives a body-centered experience of the new experimental state on the imagined other person.

One couple had a habitual tyrant/doormat dynamic. After this dysfunction had been experienced on both sides by taking turns in the chairs and feeling the experience of the other person, and also watching each other do the same, the session progressed to trying something different.

---

244 Michele Weiner Davis, *The Divorce Remedy: The Proven 7-Step Program for Saving Your Marriage*. Simon and Schuster, 2002. This is a great book with a terrible title, because the family may misunderstand the intention. I advise clients working on upgrading a relationship to cover up the title if they are going to leave it lying around the house, so that the spouse or children do not get the wrong idea.

The tyrant represents too much Yang, so I suggested leaning rearward by one or two degrees, thereby making the presence a bit less Yang. Attentive sensation tracking was used to explore this, and then the client was advised to switch chairs and be the other person. The previously habitual "doormat" immediately got a sense of a different possible state, because the two were naturally wired to constantly adapt to changes in one another.

ANS states can also benefit from experimentation. One may be more parasympathetic (withdrawn) and the other more sympathetic (combative or fleeing) by habit. Experimenting with muscular embodiment, such as flexing all the muscles, then releasing and tracking the ensuing sensation, then switching to the other chair and experiencing the effect, can be informative and supportive.

Couples often have one partner who is interested in improving the relationship while the other is less active or less interested in having sessions. One may make the appointment and have a hard time persuading the other person to attend counseling in any form. Often, the more actively healing role also has the more Yin position in the relationship, because Yin naturally seeks a "return to source" and holds a bigger picture, while Yang is absorbed in its materialistic interests. Progress can be made even if only one of the two is willing to participate. Again, this is because the two are energetically connected, especially if there has been sexual intimacy. If one starts to move, the other will feel a subtle effect, and be gently nudged to participation.

## Using the Two-Chair Method with Babies and Mothers

Yin and Yang counseling is exceptionally effective with prenatal, birthing and post-natal situations. I have shown this method to midwives, doulas, nurses and other baby specialists, and it has never failed to amaze and strike a chord.

The most frequent issues are about the baby's sleep, nursing and agitation (the condition known as "colic"). Obviously babies cannot directly express their needs in ways that most people can readily understand, but putting the "baby" in the other chair can often illuminate the dynamics of the situation. The mother is basically being a surrogate for the baby in order to discover the subtle energy dynamics that are in play with whatever problem may be present.

The birthing environment is unique in human experience and in Yin and Yang archetypes. Being a mother is the most Yin condition of all possibilities, and out of that extreme arises the extreme Yang of muscular force and powerful determination that appears with the delivery process, followed by the intense protective instincts of the "mother bear" experience.

Having a mother talk to her "baby," at any stage of development, is an extremely productive pairing. Babies in the other chair are often fountains of wisdom and innocence and often provide relief for their often anxious, overwhelmed mothers.

With prenate or baby sessions, we do not really know who is actually talking in the "baby" chair. In theory it is the unseen inner knowing of the mom, which has been sublimated in the stressful fixations of the moment, possibly compounded by her life circumstances. But there is also an uncertainty factor: babies, like departed loved ones as we've seen above, often come up with surprising and remarkably wise statements, beyond what seemed to be possible for the client. When the pole-to-pole movement is restored, transcendent information often appears, seemingly out of nowhere.

Similarly, the interpersonal relationship between the parents may come to the foreground and have a big effect on the baby. If there is Three Principle archetype trouble between the parents, appearing as tyrant/doormat or wimp/critic, the baby will detect a disturbance and try to compensate. When the imbalance of the parents is resolved, it can have a calming result for the baby. Babies respond naturally and predictably to balanced Yin and Yang in the surrounding field, almost as if they have more access to wisdom than the adults.

Effects of birth interventions are very significant, but often go unrecognized. "Interventions" here means anything that is done to support birthing that would not happen in nature; these are typically medical procedures deployed to protect life and safety. A two-chair process can be very helpful in resolving problems before or after interventions. A *before* application would be to anticipate an intervention and explain it to the "baby" in the chair, to persuade the baby on the benefits; babies are less affected if pre-warned. An *after* application would be to review what happened in the intervention, resolving residual feelings that may be present.

As described earlier, babies are actually super-sentient. Using two chairs, a voice can be given to that sentience. The voices coming from the second chair, the "baby" chair, are consistently clear about how interventions should be handled in order to minimize the ANS damage.

For a two-chair process with a baby, the mother or father can start in one chair and, when the time is right, imagine that the baby is in the other chair. A discussion can ensue, often leading to new insights about the procedure. Babies are very resilient and when held in a secure supportive field of sufficient maternal bonding, they can recover readily from most treatments. The two-chair process can efficiently re-balance the field so that the whole family system can move on from the traumatic sequence of events.

The method is recommended early in the pregnancy and again periodically as the baby develops, and particularly in the adjustment period just prior to, during or right after the birth. It is most useful for first-time mothers and their babies, because the novelty factor is higher and more anxiety is likely to be present. Babies are hitchhikers on their mothers' ANS states for the first few years. If mom is upset, the baby will often reflect the disturbance with difficulty eating, sleeping or relaxing. In Yin and Yang theory language, fixation has arisen in the nervous system under the stress of the circumstances, and the remedy will have to do with restoring pole-to-pole flow in the dyad, by switching back and forth between the two chairs. The parents are Yang relative to the baby's Yin in all cases.

A new mother scheduled a session because her baby of two weeks was not nursing well. After twenty minutes of craniosacral work to release the occiput/temporal suture, which is often compressed during birth, I held the baby while the mother did a two-chair process. In the first chair, as herself, the mother expressed a wave of emotion, with pent-up feelings about the whole experience of birthing, her desire for perfection, and the adjustments of being a first-time mom including postponement of her professional aspirations. Body-Low-Slow-Loop was used to help her system stabilize.

Then the baby was imagined to be sitting in the other chair. Immediately more emotions came to the surface and were digested, again using BLSL. Then she posed the question, "Baby, what is happening with the nursing?" When she switched to the other chair, the imagined baby immediately observed that the mom was so nervous and stressed that nursing was ambivalent at best. There was a need for nourishment coinciding with a fear about mom's well-being and a strong desire not to add to her already overwhelming stress. Switching back and forth between the two chairs helped clear the air: the mom had a fresh perspective about her own inner anxiety, which had been so all-consuming that it had become invisible to her. Meanwhile the "baby" was reassured that mom was all right, ready for nursing. There was a repeated observation that the mother's anxiety was not about the baby, it was her own process and had been present long before the baby's arrival. Emotions were released on both sides, with anxiety yielding to joy. Gradually the mother found a new ANS state for herself. After the session the baby nursed fully and easily, and after ten days the mom emailed to say the problem was entirely gone from the time of the session and had not returned. She said, "I have a whole new baby!"

In another instance, a client called from the hospital delivery room saying that the labor seemed to have stopped and major interventions were being discussed. She was familiar with the two-chair process, having done it as part of her pre-natal self-care, so I asked her, "Have you talked to the baby?" In the strenuous excitement of labor she had forgotten about the method. "Imagine that the baby is in the other chair (in this situation, she was in a hospital bed and there was not an actual chair), what would you like to say or ask?" The answer was immediate, "Baby, why are you not coming out?" I said, "Good. Now switch and be the baby." Immediately the "baby" said, "What is happening out there? Why is everyone rushing around with sharp instruments?" Switching back, mom said, "Oh, everything is fine, these people are just here for our safety, pay them no mind." Switching back to the baby, the spontaneous response was just, "Oh." Abruptly she said, "Ooops, gotta go!" and she hung up the phone. The baby was born with no interventions or complications.

Another baby story with the two-chair method shows additional possibilities. The mother was close to delivery but the baby was turned the wrong way. The mom was very well-educated and knew that this could be a great complication, involving significant pain for her and possible risk for her child. Putting the baby in the other chair, the two had a conversation and I encouraged the mom, "Sell the idea of turning to the baby!" She imagined the baby in the other chair and switched back and forth once, to get some flow going between the two in dialogue, then she talked to the baby about the advantages of turning.

When she switched to the other chair and role-played as the "baby," the posture and gestures suggested that the baby was not actually paying attention; instead the baby seemed to be obliviously enjoying just floating in the womb space. Switching back and forth he became much more engaged, and the advantages of turning were repeated again, and this time the "baby" was much more available for interaction. There were some poignant sentiments expressed back and forth, including the mom being able to express some of her fears, and the baby gradually becoming more cooperative. That night the baby turned, with the help of massage, and the next week the birth happened without complications.

Another client came in with a week-old baby saying that the little boy was not nursing. The situation was becoming serious due to numerous side effects. There was a major concern that breastfeeding would have to be abandoned altogether. After some biodynamic craniosacral therapy for the baby, two chairs were set up for the mom and a "conversation" with the baby was initiated. In the first chair the mom expressed a wave of emotion, including the whole intense drama of birthing as a first-time mother. Body-Low-Slow-Loop was very helpful to reduce the feeling of being overwhelmed in the presence of strong feelings.

Then the question was asked, "Baby, why are you not nursing?" Upon switching chairs, the "baby" said, "Mom, I am so worried about you, you are so anxious!" Switching back and forth between chairs a few times, the mom experienced an unacknowledged, intensely stressed side of herself. Gradually she came into a state of equilibrium and understood that she could trust and yield (embracing and celebrating archetypal Yin) to the larger forces that were at work. The next day her husband emailed to say the baby had nursed and slept, then nursed some more during the night, and that the whole problem seemed to be resolved. No further sessions were requested and the boy flourished.

In an advanced application, two-chair processing can be used with babies without the parents' actual participation. An emergency call came in from a client at night, saying that the birth of her first child had complications and that she was recovering but that the baby was away in the nursery. I went to the hospital nursery (this was an adventure in itself), found the baby and picked her up. Palpating the system, I found that she seemed to be totally dissociated, as if she was hovering on the ceiling of the room instead of being in her body. This would be a case of parasympathetic ANS shock, often misinterpreted because the flat affect seems like just a "good" baby that is super-quiet.

Holding the newborn girl, I used a two-chair process, without chairs. I commended her for dissociating because it showed a great intelligence being deployed after a complex birthing sequence: "That's great, you are coping in the best way possible under the circumstances." This was a form of de-pathologizing the parasympathetic stress response, even though it is a serious condition.

Once the appreciation felt complete, I non-verbally "invited" the baby into her body, "And you could come in now, it's safe and I am holding you." Gently there was a palpable warming and animation in the baby's body, including an appearance of a craniosacral tidal movement for the first time, then she "vacated" again. After two or three switches between embodiment and dissociation, she seemed to settle and went to sleep. She slept peacefully until mom was available, then nursed and seemed to flourish thereafter.

These kinds of outcomes are common and the practice is most gratifying and fulfilling. Working with babies and their families presents the greatest leverage of any time in life. This is when "a stitch in time saves nine" is literally true. In Yin and Yang jargon, the phrase might be amended to "a switch in time..."

### *Verbal Work on the Table*

For touch therapists with an appropriate scope of practice, verbal processing can be effective during a table session, though obviously without the chairs. For example, while holding supportive contacts, I might facilitate a process by suggesting that the client imagine that a key person, or condition or body area, is present in the room. The client's physical response is often palpable to the touch, such as a congestion pattern appearing in the presence of a person with whom there has been incomplete communication, or a defensive response pattern arising in the case of a person who has been threatening.

When suggesting the presence of another person in the room, it is helpful to ask the client on the table about the location of the imaginary person. This can help the client orient to the process; otherwise lying on a table can feel confusing and stimulating. Directionality is established by asking, "If _____ is imagined to be in the room, where would you locate him (or her)?" Most clients will have an instant opinion about the location, for example, front, side or rear, above or below. Establishing location makes the dualistic arrangement a bit more real, which can be helpful because the physical chairs, which are the normal way to make the process tangible, are not being used.

If the client is very distressed, or distress arises during the session, guidance in Body-Low-Slow-Loop can help create a basis for energy balancing. In biodynamic craniosacral therapy, it can be used if the client does not seem to express palpable tidal movement, as a way to support initial movement. Other practices from the Self-Help section that are often useful on the table include Left/Right, Belly Breathing and Boundaries.

As a final piece for this chapter, and to illustrate all this in a different format, the following sample gives a "tabular" version of a two chair process. To read this script, the horizontal rows are progressing through time, while the vertical columns are the occupants of the three chairs and what they say. At the far right, in italics, are comments about what is happening. These comments are unspoken in the session. When I am training people in the method and we review recorded demonstration sessions, these are the kinds of comments that I often make.

The client, "Mary," is 32, married, with one very young child, and feeling "out of love" with her husband, "Joe." In the initial interview she complains that he is not attentive like he used to be, and she does not know why. She fears that he is losing interest in her and that he is avoiding meaningful dialogue. Meanwhile the baby is quite demanding. She is feeling stressed.

| Facilitator | Mary | Joe | Comments |
|---|---|---|---|
| Let's begin with a scan of the body. Bring your attention in to the body and notice what is present, as sensation. Naturally there are also thoughts and feelings, but just now let's focus on physical sensation. Notice your contact with the chair, your feet on the floor. Notice the movement caused by breathing. If neither of these is present, we have a problem! | | | *The session begins with a few minutes of "Body-Low-Slow-Loop" especially if the preceding discussion has been about stressful topics, if there is agitation, or if there is significant pain such as a headache or stomachache.* |
| | I can feel my seat on the chair and my feet on the floor, and a there is pressure in my upper chest. | | *It is common to have some trace or major expression of body activity, within the overall sensory scan; hypothetically this is how the body is managing experience in the present moment, given all the factors that are present going all the way back to infancy and even before.* |
| OK, in the upper chest, notice the boundary of the sensation group, the depth and the temperature. Is it more on the left or right, moving or still, shallow or deep? | | | *It is helpful to give specific guidance, especially for those who are new to the process* |
| | It is slightly more on the left, and sort of swirling; it feels a little warm as if there is weight pressing down on me. | | *At the start, warmth often indicates agitation; later it can be a form of release. "Swirling" is a better state than dense or "Block-like" because at least there is movement already. Weight means constriction.* |

| Facilitator | Mary | Joe | Comments |
|---|---|---|---|
| (After a short continuation of tracking what is happening in the chest) Now let's shift and bring your attention to the feet. Please wiggle your toes inside your shoes and focus on every detail of sensation: the texture of your socks, the contact with the floor, the temperature... (two minutes)... now shift to just one foot and continue with even more detailed focus, and shift to micro-movement in super-slow motion. | | | *This is the "Loop" part of the BLSL practice, the great innovation perfected by Peter Levine. Where earlier body-focusing therapies often stayed in one place, and perhaps found a word for that place, Levine discovered that shifting somewhere else and coming back had profound benefits.* |
| | (Follows guidance; a deeper breath is taken spontaneously) | | *A spontaneous shift of breathing means the ANS is becoming engaged and reducing fixation.* |
| Now let's have another shift of attention, back to the body, including the chest. What do you notice now? | | | |
| | My chest feels lighter, and I can breathe a little easier. | | *This is the common result of BLSL, and sets the stage for the next steps.* |
| That's great! That means your system is loosening up a little. Now let's progress this one step. Imagine that your husband Joe is in the other chair.... (pause for 20 seconds)... now, again, what do you notice in your body, in the imaginary presence of Joe? | | | *The client is reminded that this is the imaginary presence of her husband; the experience of the other person could be quite realistic, but it is also still just the client and her "secondary, non-habitual" perspective.* |

| Facilitator | Mary | Joe | Comments |
|---|---|---|---|
| | There is a rush of sensation from my chest to my throat, and it feels tight there now. | | *Sensation in the throat often means emotions are coming to the surface; this relates to the ether element. I am using "body reading" to make the process more efficient by recognizing core issues based on physical gestures and sensation location.* |
| Can you just let that happen for a few seconds?...(20 seconds)... and what happens next? I see there is a tear in your eye and your face is getting a bit flushed.... (20 seconds)... Now let's take another step: What arises that might be spoken to Joe right now. Please understand that we have no obligations to reality; this does not have to be anything that was ever said or will ever be said, it is just an experiment. | | | *I am noticing and verbalizing phenomena that are happening because sometimes clients are not aware of them. The comments about reality are very important and used with almost every new client. The emphasis is on the imaginary presence. This is true even if the spouse is actually in the room, during a couple counseling session.* |
| | (Emotions increasing, no words); (Pause) | | *Here we give time for her to experience her feelings* |
| Let the wave of feelings be present, it is good to cry. It is just a wave and it will pass if we give it some time... (pause)... Now again, what arises that might be spoken to imaginary Joe just now? | | | *Many clients are afraid of feelings, that if they let them run, they will become overwhelming. Reassurance about the wave nature of feelings can be helpful here.* |

| Facilitator | Mary | Joe | Comments |
|---|---|---|---|
| | I really want to have a warmer, closer relationship with you, but you seem distant and you're always at work... | | *In the Sun and Moon archetype, this statement shows that the dynamic is starting to shift to a more functional state, for any of several reasons. The game plan is to restore flow.* |
| That's great, (repeat what she said), now once again please notice what is happening in the body. | | | *At every turn, the body processing is continued again; this maximizes the ANS flow.* |
| | (Still crying)... I feel a little less tight in the throat. | | *The ether element is loosening up a little.* |
| That's good, now please **change chairs**... (pause while she switches)... now in this chair, just be Joe. We have no obligations to reality here, it is just about whatever arises naturally as you sit in the chair. What do you notice now? | | | *This is to reinforce the idea of being in the present, and not trying to replicate anything else such as a conversation that happened yesterday.* |
| | | (As "Joe" the client's body turns leftward and leans backward)... I feel a little uncomfortable being here and I sort of feel like getting away. | *This posture suggests Joe is feeling pressure, possibly an "Avoidant" or "Ambivalent" attachment style plus dissociation (parasympathetic ANS stress response). These suggest Yang-deficiency as the regular state.* |
| Would It be accurate to say that this is a really different state of being for you? | | | *A reminder that states are changeable— many clients have forgotten this.* |

| Facilitator | Mary | Joe | Comments |
|---|---|---|---|
| | | Definitely yes; my throat stuff is gone and I feel really spacey, and a little upset in my stomach. | *Ether element is looser, fire element is awakening, suggesting old frustration of some kind perhaps unrelated to Joe.* |
| (Pause)... So let's progress it another step. She said (repeat what was just spoken), how is that for you? How would you respond to what she said? | | | *Repetition of what was said before is frequently helpful.* |
| | | I don't know how to approach you any more. You are so busy with the baby, and I feel like I have no place to rest any more, there is too much pressure and you are so uncomfortable. | *As "Joe," she is having a felt sense of being him, which opens the Yin and Yang pathway. His aversion and dissociation had a basis in experience, not just old trauma or developmental wounds, though those are also factors for him.* |
| Now please bring your attention in the body, what happens now? | | | *Another body check-in.* |
| | | It is shifting a little, less leaning and a little more focus. | *Now the system is re-mobilizing.* |
| Now please **switch back** to the first chair. | | | |
| | (Pause)... Wow I feel so different. I did not realize how you felt. | | *Commonly the switch back to the first chair reveals a very different state, which can be a revelation for the client.* |

| Facilitator | Mary | Joe | Comments |
|---|---|---|---|
| How is that for you?... How do you respond to what he said?... What do you notice now?... What would you like to say?... Can you begin a sentence with the words, "Joe, what I want is..." and fill in the blank? | | | *"I want" is chosen as the prompt here because the initial sensation was in the chest (air element). Prompts are frequently used to work within the specific body response process, which saves time in the whole process.* |
| | (Sigh)... Joe, what I want is to feel close and supported. | | *The sigh is an indication of air element release, a good sign for the whole process.* |
| To feel close, he may need to feel that there is a safe space. Can you imagine a safe space right now? Where would that be in your body? | | | *The offering of guidance about "safe space" comes from knowing Yin and Yang archetypal dynamics. The selected body area is useful for ANS processing.* |
| | (Body scan)... I think it would be in the heart area... | | *The area of opportunity (heart) coincides with the first area of stress signaling.* |
| At the heart area, what do you notice? If there is a safe space for Joe, what does it feel like? | | | *More ANS support by asking a detailed question or two, thereby slowing the system down and engaging the curiosity.* |
| | It is warm and has an open feeling. | | *Now the ANS change is accelerating.* |
| This is different from the first sensation of tightness and pressure? | | | *Confirming what is happening at every opportunity.* |
| | Yes definitely... | | |
| Now **switch chairs** again... (pause)... What arises that might be spoken now? | | | *By now the Yin and Yang pendulum is swinging freely and the healing process is well underway.* |

| Facilitator | Mary | Joe | *Comments* |
|---|---|---|---|
|  |  | (Posture is now more centered and "Joe" is leaning forward a little bit)... "I love you..." | *Leaning forward means more Yang; "Joe" is coming back into himself; true original feelings can now be expressed.* |
| Now **switch chairs** again. |  |  |  |
|  | (Posture changes to slightly rearward), more tears. |  | *More rearward is slightly more Yin, tears represent release of old residue from earlier times.* |
| That's a good place to stop for now. If you can, please write down everything that you can remember from this, while it is fresh in your mind. You can email that to me if you want, and I will maybe have some additions of bits that might have been forgotten. |  |  | *Writing down what happened helps the client "digest" the process, bringing additional brain resources into play and helping the client feel like the process was "real" beyond just the session time.* |

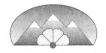

## Chapter 11

# Yin and Yang in Life Situations

This chapter offers a "User's Guide" for stress reduction in life, based on Yin and Yang principles. The term "User's Guide" means a set of recommendations for common challenges that many people face, all derived from the Yin and Yang model. While the two-chair chapter was about treatment, now prevention becomes our focus.

A User's Guide suggests that those who have traveled the path of human challenges in the past might have left us good and relevant instructions. Human challenges do not change all that much: teenagers face a particular set of problems, and new parents face another. Our parents or extended families might be a source for guidance, but they may not be very credible as role models. Our culture is another possible source for "how-to" information, but a similar problem still exists: among all the multi-cultural voices, which or who can we trust? We may end up with a patchwork approach, without a unifying foundation, or we may blindly be pulled in whatever direction by simple happenstance or sheer inertia.

We also may suffer from too many choices. As the *I Ching* says, "Unlimited possibilities are not suited to man; if they existed, his life would dissolve in the boundless." [245] In a

---

[245] W. Reich and C. Baynes, translators, *I Ching*. Princeton University, 1967. See Hexagram 60, "Limitation."

time of globalization, "anything goes" in personal and social conduct. Old constraints have fallen away and new options constantly come into view. The Yin and Yang model has the potential to cut through the noise of trial and error, supporting much-needed coherence. Instead of feeling like we are running a series of random experiments with too many variables, the Yin and Yang approach gives advice that proceeds in an orderly way from the big picture to the small details.

This chapter is another application of the "pebble in the shoe" metaphor. If we are doing something that is not working, we will begin to limp in some way. Imagine again the health care of the future, when the intake form includes the question, "Are you doing anything in your life that is not working?

Because the stages of life are fairly universal, we can benefit if we can be warned about what common errors to expect along the way, and keep our shoes relatively free of problematic debris. Ideally, we will not have to suffer the consequences of experiments that went awry, especially considering that some consequences can continue for a long time. A little prevention goes a long way!

When I have a pebble in my shoe, the top priority is to take it out. It may be interesting to figure out when I acquired it, what kind of minerals it contains and what its ramifications for my knee and hip might include. But the first order of business is to take it out so that the pain subsides before it gets worse. For our purposes here, complex psychological interpretations are secondary to just validating and then following the User's Guide to build a life for ourselves that will support our true purpose.

A User's Guide runs the risk of being politically incorrect. In an era of "anything goes," it is difficult to take a stand about anything, for fear of offending someone. No one wants to tell others what to do, or be told what to do. This chapter should be taken with a grain of salt, with the expectation that the whole approach has to make sense and be tested before it is widely applied. I feel quite free to move forward based on my life experience, but I expect my clients, students, fellow practitioners and readers to validate these theories for themselves before applying them. I do my best to be diplomatic and respectful when venturing into User's Guide territory.

To start with an example of how a User's Guide can relieve mental and emotional stress, a woman in her early thirties sought counseling for turmoil in her intimate relationships. She was experiencing turbulence repeatedly and wondered how she could get to the bottom of the problem. She had trouble sleeping and was being diagnosed with an anxiety disorder, although she had not yet actually started medication. Observing her tell her story, I thought that there were as many potential paths of inquiry as there were psychotherapy modalities.

In the two-chair process, her sublimated, untroubled self in the second chair spoke plainly to her primary perspective in the first chair and said she was having sex too soon with new boyfriends. This was leading to multiple complications due to the multi-leveled emotional intensity of sex. Because the advice was self-generated, she was receptive, and resolved to change this related behavior without trying to "figure it all out." In effect, she looked up that topic in her own inner "User's Guide" and followed the directions in order to reduce her ANS symptoms. The topics of when the behavior originated and how it was played out were left for later.

In a later session, she reported that she had applied the instructions that came through her, and her relationship issues were no longer quite so burdensome. The "pebble," so to speak, had been removed from her "shoe," and her anxiety level had receded. It was another example of how the conscious mind can give relief for the unconscious by making good choices and staying away from known pitfalls, even if the complexity of the underlying situation has not necessarily been addressed.

### Conscious and Unconscious Interactions

Stone emphasized the value of a top-down Yang approach to major life events, applying consciousness as much as possible instead of being pulled about by subconscious impulses. This is easier said than done, given the enormous power of the subconscious mind, but it can be achieved. To convey a sense of the size of the problem, biologist Bruce Lipton explains:

> The subconscious is associated with the neural activity of a much larger part of the brain (approximately 90 percent) than the conscious mind's prefrontal cortex. The subconscious mind is also a profoundly more powerful influence on our behavior than the conscious mind. The conscious mind's prefrontal cortex can process and manage a relatively measly 40 nerve impulses per second. In contrast, the 90 percent of the brain that constitutes the subconscious mind's platform can process 40 *million* nerve impulses per second.[246]

It is not possible for the conscious mind to directly tell the subconscious what to do. However, if the conscious is able to do something that supports more harmony and order, the subconscious will often respond. This is an indirect way of working; the conscious does something to address a particular life situation; subsequently the subconscious feels

---

[246] Bruce Lipton, *The Honeymoon Effect*. Hay House, 2013. p. 75. Lipton's footnoted source is T. Norretranders, *The User Illusion: Cutting Consciousness Down to Size*. Penguin, 1998, pp. 124-5.

more safe and the ANS shifts away from anxiety or depression.

## *The Stages of Relationships*

The idea of "stages of life" is well-developed, particularly by psychologist Erik Erikson, who described the challenges and successes/failures of eight developmental phases, from infant to elder. [247]  In contrast, in the Vedic system, three stages are envisioned: student, householder and retiree. In Shakespeare's *As You Like It*, a character describes seven life steps in the famous monologue, "All the world's a stage..."

For a Yin and Yang adaptation of Erikson, we can combine "stages of life" and the "hierarchy of action fields" to create "stages of relationships" as a focus for this approach to psychotherapy and healing in general. Personal integrity and self-esteem are at the very top of the hierarchy pyramid described in Chapter 5, and therefore these are the first targets in counseling.

Relationships immediately follow, so this field of action closely follows as the next priority. Even personal integrity and self-esteem are significantly derived from relationships, initially from the parents' relationship with each other. In relationships, the dualistic forces of Yin and Yang are brought into sharp, real-world intensity, in ways that an isolated, uninvolved person might not experience. Relationships, particularly intimate ones, are the great laboratory for personal growth, when self/other resistance provides an immediate mirror for maturing, refinement and the learning of life's lessons.

Intimate relationships can be observed to move through a progression of events, from casual initial contact to

---

[247] Erik Erikson, *Identity and the Life Cycle*. Norton, 1994.

deepening interest and increased mutual intention. Eventually, longer-term arrangements may arise, including the possibility of a commitment with a life partner and raising children together.

Relationships do not stay frozen in one state; they are always dynamically evolving through natural progressions. Similarly, a single individual is always moving through natural developmental stages, observed as babies inexorably raise their heads, then pull themselves up, then crawl, walk and run. Relationships also have a developmental sequence, beginning with immersion in our mothers, to partial autonomy, to full differentiation, and eventually reversing roles to become our parents' caregivers. It is unrealistic to expect for a relationship to be static, as some people seem to believe, any more than a tree can stop growing or a leaf dropped into a moving river can just stay in place.

The Yin and Yang model offers insights all along the way, providing a guiding framework to keep our lives more coherent and healthy. Effective guidance for relationships serves as a preventive measure to minimize health issues, including mental/emotional disturbances.

The following pages describing intimate relationships seem to be equally applicable for all relationships. In theory, the same Yin and Yang phenomena will be present, and harmony will be a natural side effect of using energy principles appropriately. The language used here is often about male/female relationships, but the concept applies to all relationship configurations.

The same principles can be expected to apply in all social structures, not just in the nuclear family arrangements that prevail in Western culture. Yin and Yang is about biological sequences, which underlie social differences. The nuclear family is more a cultural construct than a biological mandate; we know this because there are so many exceptions in anthropological literature. A Yin and Yang model is hypothetically applicable to other social structure models, although I have not tested the theory with different cultures.

In the Yin and Yang "Stages of Relationships," eight steps are identified along the path of creating and sustaining a life partner relationship:

- Dating
- Courtship
- Engagement
- Marriage
- Sex
- Parenting, including birthing
- Career
- Elder care and deathing care

This sequence is obviously not necessarily how events actually unfold. The sequence can be scrambled. Here I will use an order of events reflecting the steps that might be most common. Also, the terms used here do not matter so much as the concepts: the word "dating" may seem to be obsolete, but "being socially active and receptive to the possibility of forming a relationship" still happens.

## Dating

Dating, the first step in creating an intimate relationship, means meeting new people and having fun. A sense of caution is appropriate, in order to protect against unexpected problems. A respectful distance helps us determine if the person is a real candidate for a more substantial relationship.

The ability to engage in the dating phase indicates that we have significant sympathetic ANS resources. Sexual magnetism is a positive indicator of overall vitality, but it needs to be managed. Dating is hugely preferable to self-isolation, resignation or avoidance of any social risk because these indicate a parasympathetic ANS state that is much more restrictive and difficult to manage. The situation is an echo of how anxiety is preferable to depression, as discussed in Chapter 6, because the sympathetic ANS is a higher order of response compared to the parasympathetic ANS. Lord Tennyson's statement, "It is better to have loved and lost, than never to have loved at all," is justified from an ANS perspective.

In the beginning phase of a new relationship, some inquiry about intention is very helpful. The ability to discuss this openly is a good indicator of whether the relationship will work. Often people will mill around in a social setting, perhaps with the inhibition-bypassing support of intoxicants, and end up randomly "hooking up" with someone, with no clue as to underlying intention. This is a recipe for future problems.

Even in a chaotic environment, such as a college campus with hormones at a peak and new freedoms available, the Yin and Yang emphasis on intention can help give a frame of reference. The best approach is to have the conversation early in the relationship. This may go against the grain of youthful exuberance and popular culture, but will serve both people in the long run and help to avoid hurt feelings and other problems. It sounds preposterous in today's climate, but I have seen far too many casualties as people try to fit in with the stereotypical, media-driven illusion of carefree singles action.

Yin and Yang understanding informs the dating process profoundly. The Yang person will be more oriented toward sense pleasure and materialism, and the Yin person will be more oriented to companionship, communication and awareness of the big picture of life. If these are well-understood, the new pair can recognize what is going on and have more fun, with more security because each is guided by a level of self-awareness about the underlying nature of phenomena. Otherwise each might try to bend to meet the other; this might feel good initially, but it leads to confusion later.

The get-acquainted phase is being revolutionized by online dating. Statements of intention are becoming more common, however the potential for deception is also increasing. Meanwhile, the online popularization of pornography can confuse the mental/emotional program for a young person, because expectations and pressure to fit in with extreme behaviors arrives before the brain's capacity for risk-assessment and self-individualization has actually matured. With so much freedom and examples of every kind of behavior all around, it is difficult for young people to get to a brain-mature age (approximately 22-25 years old) without wounds from problematic first explorations of intimacy. These wounds can take years to be resolved; the occurrence of thirty-somethings who suffer lingering problems from bad first experiences in their teens and early twenties is very frequent in my counseling practice.

The dating phase is also changing due to modern career pressure. If a person has a clear career plan that means total dedication and few choices about location for many years, such as an intention to go to law school or medical school, dating may seem to be pointless because there is no clear pathway for the relationship to deepen. The hierarchy of action fields has already been rearranged, in this example career has been placed above relationship. Extra care will be needed to end up in the desired location, whatever it may be. The number of clients with career success but relationship problems seems to be increasing. If my perception is correct, this trend does not bode well for the future, either personally or societally.

## Courtship

Courtship is an archetypal phase when people muster up their best behavior in order to endear themselves to the other person. Courtship overlaps with dating; it is just a matter of degree of intention and increased exclusivity; it was known in an earlier age as "going steady." Courting is not necessarily realistic in that people are performing to some degree, trying to impress each other. Courtship can provide a basic qualifying process to determine if the prospective partner is actually a candidate for real intimacy.

Courtship is very often the entry phase into sexual activity, if it has even been postponed past the dating phase. Sex engenders intimacy, but it can also cloud and confuse all aspects of the progression of an intimate relationship. The earlier the sex, the more confused the process may become. As discussed above in Chapter 4, the relatively modern idea of "free love," in which sex happens without much development of relationship, and usually without clear mutual intention, rarely leads to energetic coherence. Again, the problem is that sexual activity invokes super-intense emotional responses, often subconscious, that may not be fully appreciated at the time. These intense feelings are rarely equal on both sides; one person is often hoping for a different outcome, such as a more substantial relationship, while the other just wants to have fun. It is common to believe erroneously that pleasure comes without any price. Often one or both people involved are in denial about their real feelings.

If two people are truly in agreement about most of their attitudes and expectations about having sex together, problems are minimized, but realistically this is rarely the case. Ever since the "sexual revolution," experiments have been underway, and the exploration of possibilities continues today.[248] Because of the intensity of the experience and the frequent mismatching of attitudes and expectations, I am skeptical when I hear about casual sex being promoted as a way to just experience free pleasure.

Emotional turbulence after premature sex leads to a host of psycho-emotional complexities; sex without attunement between the two people's attitudes and expectations could even be considered a form of emotional violence, as described in Chapter 8. The intensity of sex usually activates subconscious attachment style issues and developmental wounds.

Furthermore, the effects can be long lasting, as the intensity creates an imprint that is hard to clear. A person will tend to compare a new lover to previous experiences and therefore be less present in the actual moment. In *Hands of Light*, author Barbara Brennan describes echoes remaining from past lovers that subtly disrupt a person's capacity for intimacy in the present and for many years after.[249]

Unconscious deception is very common in the courtship phase. Conscious deception is less likely. Usually the deceiver wants something and will do whatever it takes to achieve the goal. For example a person may make implied promises that have not been actually thought through, or exhibit behaviors that are not actually representative of the inner reality. By proceeding more slowly in the dating phase and being alert to the likelihood of confusion, some of these effects can be softened.

---

[248] Kate Taylor, "She Can Play That Game Too." *New York Times*, July 14, 2013. This feature article describes a campus scene in which casual sex is supposedly a clear mutual intention. However some of the interview comments seem a bit suspicious from a Yin and Yang perspective. Some of these students may show up for sessions ten years later with turbulence about intimacy.

[249] Barbara Brennan, *Hands of Light*. Bantam, 1987, p. 259.

Relationships tend to progress in a steady march, with cycles of expansion and contraction. This is confounding for some people. I often encounter couples for whom the progression is not mutually shared. One person may want the courtship phase to last forever, while the other is feeling the inevitable progression to something more. One is getting what is wanted but the other is not, an obviously unfair arrangement.

I try to explain that relationships do not stand still, any more than the seasons can last forever. The plots of movies such as *Friends with Benefits* (2011) and *No Strings Attached* (2011) have some validity, showing one partner feeling pressure to deepen to something more, while the other was feeling satisfied. Basically, the situation gets awkward when the natural progression is denied, unrecognized or pathologized.

## Engagement

Engagement is an archetypal phase in which people reveal more realistic behaviors and attempt to fully describe true attitudes and expectations about all aspects of life. At a subconscious level, they may act out behaviors that actually do represent their inner world and family patterns. Counseling support is highly recommended but rarely used during this phase.

Topics to be addressed that are of particular importance during engagement include:

- Sex
- Money
- Politics
- Intoxicants
- Children and parenting
- Division of labor
- Values
- Communication beliefs
- Religious and spiritual beliefs and practices

These are the fields that may later become issues; it will be easier to manage if both people can understand and agree (or agree to disagree) on their attitudes and expectations during the engagement phase, instead of later. I highly recommend that engagement include a clearly-established time and space for both people to describe their thoughts and feelings about each of these topics, basically creating an unwritten, non-legal, "pre-nuptial agreement of intention" for each other.

One of these topics can be selected, and the couple can spend fifteen minutes each in a monologue about all aspects of what is important in that particular subject, repeating as needed until both feel complete and there is nothing left to say.[250]  Later what was expressed in the engagement monologues may serve as a reference point for negotiation when these issues arise, as they often will.

If people feel trapped already during engagement, the Body–Low–Slow–Loop practice can be effective first aid. Outside support may be helpful. If there is ambivalence during this phase it should be taken seriously and resolved without long periods of elapsed time, because sustained ambiguity can be exhausting. Each person should feel "green light" to a high and matching degree (recognizing that 100 percent probably does not exist), otherwise it will be hard to sustain the relationship under strain.

Concern for the other person's feelings (such as staying together because the other person is so intent, dependent or emotionally invested), while noble on one level, is not auspicious for long-term stability. The two-chair process can be very efficient in clarifying these situations.

The word "Love" has too many meanings (love of partner, child, parent job, recreation, country, etc.) to be helpful. The same verb is used for describing good food,

---

[250] A.H. Almaas, *The Unfolding Now: Realizing Your True Nature through the Practice of Presence.* Shambhala, 2012. The Diamond Heart approach, also known as the Ridwhan School, uses repetitive monologues as a method of safe self-inquiry.

beautiful weather and long-term loyalty, and can have many meanings in the context of relationship intimacy. "Love" changes in meaning over time, from fickle passion to time-tested interdependence. Love means something, but what?

When a couple is struggling, it is not uncommon for one to say, "I don't love him/her any more." When I hear this kind of language, I usually request alternative wording, avoiding the term "love," to get more specific insight into the exact nature of the disturbance. It is likely that the person is applying unworkable attitudes or unrealistic expectations, not taking responsibility for some aspect of the partnership, lacking mutual intentions in an important field of action, or the partnership has become de-polarized.

Stone described "Love" as one half of the cycle of energetic flow, when particles are pulled by centripetal Yin force to merge ecstatically in the restful center. Interestingly the popular descriptive phrase is to "*fall* in love," as if two lovers collapse into union. The inverse phrase would be to "*rise* in love," but that just doesn't have the same subliminal feeling because the energetic reality is not represented.

The attraction phase is compellingly irresistible in its power, as we experience in sexual magnetism and see displayed in movies. Over and over, "moth meets flame, flame wins." What the movies don't tell us is that this is inevitably followed by an expansive Yang phase, in which particles fly out again from the center, differentiating into their more individual arcs and adventures. Stone did not assign an emotion to this centrifugal phase but I am sure it feels different from the magnetic attraction of the "Love" experience. In his words,

> Opposites attract on the ingoing waves and repel on
> the outgoing currents, such as the top and the
> bottom, the center and the circumference, the within

and the without, the "I" and the "you." Love itself is an attraction in one direction– toward its center.[251]

The last sentence is another true gem from Stone's writing, with profound implications. The basic nature of all phenomena includes cycles of Yin and Yang, attraction and repulsion, expansion and contraction, night and day. There are no exceptions to this pervasive pattern throughout the natural world, even scaled down to the atomic level or scaled up to the size of galaxies. Why would we expect the relational field to be different?

After a centripetal phase, a centrifugal phase will surely follow. Many passionate love relationships end in tragedy including the surprisingly large incidence of domestic violence, and "hell hath no fury" like what happens when "love" attraction turns to its natural repulsion complement in a relationship that is unaware of the principles of nature. The primary mainstream culture offers little understanding to help the couple to recognize and buffer against what is happening. They may feel blindsided by what is actually just a natural phenomenon. An ounce of realistic expectation provides a pound of relief for the inevitable effects of this cyclic process.

The popular idea of there being a perfect "soul mate" partner, who will bring permanent, unchanging happiness and fulfillment, is for the most part just another fantasy. This unrealistic attitude makes people reluctant to ever make a commitment, or if they are in a relationship it will make an easy escape route when the situation becomes difficult. In addition, this flawed attitude creates enormous pressure on the other person in the relationship.

When I have clients in the engagement phase, I like to ask if they have a vision for their relationship future. Do they

---

[251] R. Stone, *Polarity Therapy, Vol. 1.* CRCS, 1986. Book 3, p. 14.

actually want to have a life partner? Is there a clear intention about commitment? If there is not a "green light" for these kinds of basic questions, going slower in the engagement phase is probably going to make sense.

## Marriage

Discord and turbulence in long-term relationships, including marriage, is widespread and a root cause of great suffering including health issues. From a Yin and Yang perspective, one huge factor is a cultural misunderstanding about the meaning and purpose of marriage. Western cultures mainly subscribe to the "Hollywood" idea of marriage, in which people meet their perfect match and supposedly "live happily ever after," fulfilling each other's needs all along the way. This concept is rarely articulated clearly but is predominant and assumed to be true in the culture. It is constantly reinforced through popular mythology and entertainment, as the movie stars ride off into the sunset and the credits start to roll. We don't get to see what happens after that.

In a Hollywood scenario, the pressure is high for the individuals to meet the needs of their partners and also have their own needs met. Realistically this one-on-one setup makes a risky basis for a marriage because it is based on a projection of early attachment experience. What are the realistic chances that one person can fulfill the unmet needs created by a long-gone phantom mother or father?

Another reason one-on-one is not a stable foundation for marriage is that people change, pressures build and new challenges arise. Because the focus or foundation of the relationship is just the other person, who is constantly changing, the base of the relationship is constantly in flux. This often leads one or both individuals to say, "This is not what I signed up for" and the separation process begins. An analogy for one-on-one from geometry is a single line, pole-to-pole. It is hard to build a lasting structure with just a stick, without somehow triangulating the pieces into a stable structure.

Meanwhile, another model exists and deserves consideration. Over half of the world's population does not use "romantic marriage" and presumably some of these relationships are also successful. The very existence of "arranged marriages," so totally implausible for our western sensibilities, leads to the curiosity, how is this possible? From a Hollywood perspective, a marriage between two people who have maybe never even met is entirely preposterous.[252]

My guess is that in an arranged marriage, the couple is brought together with a Third Presence, the *idea* of being married. Throughout life they are constantly, sincerely playing the role of a marriage partner (lover, companion, supporter, co-parent) as their primary intention. The pressure is not so focused on the individuals; the commitment to the third entity, the state of marriage, is primary. A different part of the brain, the orbitofrontal cortex, is possibly more active.[253] Experiences of the past, such as each partner's maternal bonding history, attachment style or object relations history, have a reduced impact.

Mutual acceptance of a third presence in the relationship, the "idea of marriage," can have a profound effect on coherence. Instead of a dualistic back-and-forth focus, each partner aspires to the standards of the ideal, and the other partner's performance becomes less critical. In this way the partners can have a much stronger basis for studying the art of relationship including sexuality, parenting, financial

---

[252] This discussion is not a promotion for arranged marriages, it is an inquiry into the psychodynamics at work. Again, we seek theories that can accommodate the evidence.

[253] Joshua Jones *et al.*, "Behavior and Learning Using Inferred But Not Cached Values." *Science*, Vol. 338, p. 953. Nov. 16, 2012.

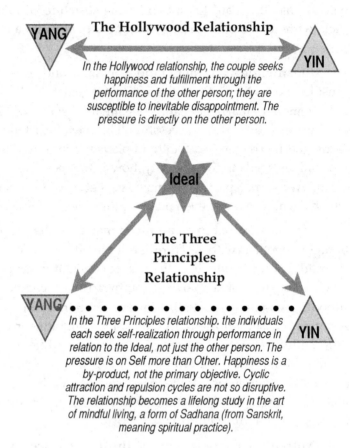

**The Hollywood Relationship**

*In the Hollywood relationship, the couple seeks happiness and fulfillment through the performance of the other person; they are susceptible to inevitable disappointment. The pressure is directly on the other person.*

**Ideal**

**The Three Principles Relationship**

*In the Three Principles relationship. the individuals each seek self-realization through performance in relation to the Ideal, not just the other person. The pressure is on Self more than Other. Happiness is a by-product, not the primary objective. Cyclic attraction and repulsion cycles are not so disruptive. The relationship becomes a lifelong study in the art of mindful living, a form of Sadhana (from Sanskrit, meaning spiritual practice).*

security and similar hot-topic areas. This approach could be called "The Marriage Triangle" (two spouses and one ideal) as a reflection of the Three Principles, providing much great stability for building than a simple dualistic configuration.

Yin and Yang understanding supports the triangular approach to marriage. If both partners have a clear understanding of the other's inherent nature and challenges, they will be less likely to look to the other for self-fulfillment. As author Michael Brown says, "Let go of the messenger and get the message."[254] In a Hollywood marriage, they may be drawn into wishing the other could be more like themselves, which is not possible. In the Three Principles Marriage there is much more room for appreciation of the differences between Yin and Yang. There is likely to be more flexibility and adaptation.

This idea of marriage agreement and commitment is recognized in many cultures, with "God" being invoked at the ceremony. The "Third Presence" is also found in other sources.[255] Focusing on the state of being married more than the other person means that the experience is about oneself in relation to an ideal, which implies much more personal responsibility.

### Using Marriage to Increase Consciousness

A second pillar of marriage is mutual understanding and agreement that the purpose of marriage is personal growth, facilitated by intentionally entering the process of intimacy for the long term. The primary purpose of marriage is not romantic love, personal happiness or gratification; these are highly valued, super-rewarding, enduring by-products of personal growth, rather than the first objective of the marriage. As Reichian psychologist Alexander Lowen put it, "Happiness is consciousness of growth."[256] A long-term intimate relationship can be very effective as a field of action for personal growth, with constantly-changing conditions

---

[254] Michael Brown, *The Presence Process: A Journey into Present Moment Awareness*. Namaste, 2010.

[255] Robert Bly, "The Third Body." From the collection, *Ten Poems to Open your Heart* by Robert Housden. Harmony, 2003. Also, Morag Campbell, *Sink the Relation Ship: Transform the Way You Relate*. Masterworks, 2010.

[256] Alexander Lowen, *Bioenergetics: The Revolutionary Therapy That Uses the Language of the Body to Heal the Problems of the Mind*. Penguin, 1994.

inspiring constant adaptations. Long-term intimacy can be a crucible in which distortions such as ancestral patterns can be pulverized and transformed in the heat of daily interaction within life's ever-changing real-world challenges.

Buddhist author Sandy Boucher put it this way:

> Many Buddhists look to their sexual relationship as a fertile ground in which to practice loving kindness and compassion, to learn patience and large-heartedness. They recognize that our primary, committed relationships challenge us to confront our most troublesome tendencies and to act decently and supportively with our partners. [257]

The resulting dynamic is similar to a yoga or mindfulness practice. Many wisdom traditions have described the process of living each day, even each minute, in maximum mindfulness, intentionality or awareness. Even the most trivial or burdensome aspects of daily life can be experienced as opportunities for awareness or personal growth. [258]

In a triangular approach, both partners agree to keep referencing their reactions back to themselves as an inquiry into their own personal processes. From such a conscious base, the partners can even begin to recognize the attachment style responses of their partners and compassionately, sensitively attempt to meet each other's needs. If they are able to do this, the partners become mutually co-regulating.

The result of such a practice could be called a *sadhana*, (from Sanskrit, meaning personal or spiritual practices that enhance connection with deeper forces). The partnership can

---

[257] Sandy Boucher, *Opening the Lotus: A Woman's Guide to Buddhism.* Beacon, 1997. p. 120.

[258] Rick Fields, *Chop Wood, Carry Water: A Guide to Finding Spiritual Fulfillment in Everyday Life.* Tarcher, 1984.

increase our capacity for understanding, compassion and service. Being in a long-term intimate relationship can be a supreme yogic enterprise, if the triangle approach is used. If the Hollywood approach is used, the relationship is vulnerable to shifting emotions that often lead to decreasing consciousness, not increasing.

The experiment has to be sustained long enough to fully harvest the fruits of the process. Using a triangle approach, a couple shares a clear intention that can withstand the trials of life's setbacks and confusions. Then the long-term harvest will be more likely to be sweet, as the elderly couple enjoys the coherence, satisfaction and security of each other's growth, support and clarity together.

Using a Hollywood approach, when people grow tired of the relationship, they often believe that they can just start over. But each start-over does not necessarily begin with a clean slate; it picks up pieces and impressions made in earlier attempts. The phenomenon is true in all intimate relationships, but it is perhaps compounded in multiple marriages. Comparisons remain after the former lover has gone. The next partner has to navigate through the incrementally increasing fog including remnant feelings such as betrayal, distrust, disappointment, frustration and fear.

This is not to say that second or later marriages cannot be successful. Later marriages benefit from lessons learned earlier, including re-doing the preliminary steps with much more consciousness, and having a more clear idea of what to expect and how to manage challenges. However, in many cases, perseverance in the first marriage can also be effective, without some of the costs and disappointments. When children are involved, the value of perseverance is greatly magnified.

Having a primary relationship with the third presence, and a secondary relationship with the significant other changes the whole game. An analogy is found in the fable from India of a teacher who sends a student to a carnival, to sample the stimulating pleasures to be experienced there.[259] However the teacher makes one stipulation: the student has to go through the whole day carrying a cup of milk filled to the brim, and not spill a drop the whole time. At the end of the day the teacher asked, "How did you enjoy the carnival?" and the student responded, "It was nice but I was so focused on the milk that the carnival's peaks and valleys of experience were hardly noticeable."

Having a mutual agreement to focus on the third presence lends a stability and durability to the long-term relationship. The marriage becomes less vulnerable to the ebb and flow of normal, universal, attraction-repulsion cycles of movement from the periphery to the core and back.

### Other Yin and Yang Marriage Ideas

• Pre-marital counseling is highly recommended. It is an insightful commentary on modern culture that young people learn historical trivia but not how to be in a functional relationship. Study of effective relationships should be a primary objective of teenage learning, because this is the field of action with the next-to-highest impact on lifelong wellness. In Yin and Yang-based premarital counseling, high emphasis is placed on educating the couple about how to triangulate the experience, and on helping them arrive at a clear mutual intention. Clear common agreement on this one major point will have a stabilizing effect throughout life, and the relationship experience can become more of a mindfulness practice.

• Sun and moon archetypes serve as a key reference point. The first object of the game is to fulfill one's archetypal

---

[259] Huzur Maharaj Sawan Singh Ji, *Tales of the Mystic East*. RSSB, 1961. p. 51.

tasks. As a female respondent in a survey of long term baby boomer marriages put it, "He keeps me grounded and I give him wings."[260] The art of relationships is to fulfill the primary job description while not losing flexibility, and not becoming too much or too little Yin or Yang.

• Division of labor needs to be mutually agreed. Yin and Yang should not be confused with old-fashioned male chauvinism. A balanced and functional life is much more nuanced and sophisticated. Both partners need to articulate their assumptions clearly and negotiate in good faith, to make sure that both people authentically feel that the workload is fair.

• It may be helpful to "re-polarize" in some situations such as interpersonal stress. Re-polarizing means that in the heat of conflict, each person pauses to reflect on what would be the archetypal Yin and Yang characteristics, and experiment with those. David Deida's book *Intimate Communion* is highly recommended for this purpose.[261]

• If one person is moving into a dysfunctional role, there will be a natural pressure for the other person to begin to manifest the complementary dysfunction. Focusing on the marriage triangle, and remembering the intention for personal growth, can help ward off dysfunctional archetypal tendencies and keep the relationship process on track. If our partner is having a bad day, we do not have to take it so personally or react so dramatically.

• It can be helpful to consider the other person as an expression of the invisible part of oneself, in sickness and in health. In this way the marriage partner is constantly in more sympathy and compassion for the suffering of the other when

---

[260] Erika Allen, "Booming: Making It Last." *New York Times*, Sep. 20, 2013.

[261] David Deida, *Intimate Communion.* HCI,1995.

challenges arise. The two-chair method is excellent for making this obvious, quickly and painlessly.

• In marriage there should be no violence, and no leaving or threatening to leave. Threatening is similar energetically to actually leaving, just not manifested. Talking about leaving is a subtle form of violence and serves little positive purpose. One person constantly talking about leaving is a valid indicator of archetypal disturbance: one person has become tyrant or wimp, or critic or doormat, and pressure is building as a result. Talking about leaving is often one of the "games people play," a way to manipulate the relationship.[262] Complementarily, one should not stay if violence threatens self, spouse or children.

• Sexual frustration should be minimized and discussed openly. Sexual problems are likely to be symptoms of deeper issues, including autonomic or archetypal imbalances, or a Hollywood scenario. Sexual frustration deserves close attention, so that unwanted side effects do not take root and proliferate. Both people can negotiate to reduce sexual frustration if it starts to arise, hopefully arriving at a mutually acceptable solution. Counseling and autonomic exercises to deal with the subconscious factors can be very helpful. This is another area where the two-chair process really shines and gets to the central issues quite efficiently, because each partner has a chance to experience the other's perspective.

• Children or parents should never be used to gain advantage in arguments. If there is disagreement, the children will not flourish if placed in the middle in any way.

• Generally children should not even be exposed to arguments or harsh interpersonal sounds. Children are in a

---

[262] Eric Berne, *Games People Play*. Vintage, 1969. This early pop psychology classic has enduring value with many useful insights.

state of high hypnotic suggestibility; they do not have a context and they respond autonomically, with potentially serious after-effects. The common justification, from the partner with a predisposition toward volatility, is about supposed authenticity, saying the children "should know how things really are." However this ignores the findings of child psychology and makes space for very damaging behaviors. Loudness or shocking phenomena should be shielded from the child as long as possible; the later the disturbance appears, the more solid the child's base to withstand the inevitable ANS stresses of life.

In particular, when one parent complains about the other to a child as if to an adult confidante, larger problems are probably in play. Years later the child will be susceptible to intimacy issues because their early experience of sharing was in an inappropriate context, such as being expected to converse about adult emotions and concerns, but from their position of immaturity.

• Separate money or separate accounts can be a form of energetic non-commitment and a prelude to possible separation. With separate accounts, there is less need to really develop the relationship and deal with its issues, and at least one of the partners (the one making or holding more money) has an easier out, if problems arise. This often can mean a power differential, subtly undermining the relationship triangle. The strongest bond occurs when both people are truly "all in" with the yogic commitment and both share the relationship's risks and rewards equally. One person having extreme wealth can actually be a liability for lasting intimate relationships, due to the seeds of distrust that may be present. The two-chair process can also address this issue efficiently.

Money is a taboo subject in our modern world. Prospective partners would be well advised to dig a little deeper with expectations and intentions if financial resources are very different. These relationships can definitely work, they just need extra support and clarity at the start.

• Getting help early in the form of counseling can be a great resource in marriage, as stated repeatedly above. Getting help means finding a counselor that both people trust and checking in periodically if problems are beginning to surface for either person. Ongoing support creates a sense of "emotional hygiene" to protect against inevitable disturbances igniting out of control. The use of a counselor is often resisted, and it is a relatively recent cultural phenomenon. In past generations, marriage issues were often held in tight family secrecy. Modern attitudes have softened, allowing marriage counseling to be used more freely without people feeling stigmatized by family or society. Among other benefits, a trusted counselor provides another element of triangulation to stabilize the energy system.

• Equal sharing of responsibilities based on negotiation, compromise, mutual agreement and true reciprocity can be very helpful for overall relationship health. Unequal valuation or weighting of contributions to the common good, such as an attitude that the wage-earner is more important than the primary parenting activity, is likely to lead to disturbances. If both people are really doing their best to support the whole family system, working as a team to solve problems and deal with conditions, comparative valuations are not valid or useful. The dangers of comparative thinking were discussed in Chapter 7.

• Self-Other awareness can be a tremendous resource, helpful if practiced in some form every day. The Self-Other practice means to fully experience our own sensations and feelings, and then reverse our perceptual focus and attempt to fully experience our partner's sensations and feelings. The "Resonance Practice" (Chapter 9) can be helpful as a prelude to negotiation on difficult issues or intimacy.

• Stress often arises from attitudes and expectations, more than from actual experience. When there is stress, we can examine our own attitudes and expectations and be ready to adapt, to make them more realistic. In the Yin and Yang model described in Chapter 2, attitudes and expectations are at the headwaters of the whole system, just as a blueprint shapes the eventual house. It can be very helpful for partners to take turns describing their attitudes and expectations about a particular subject (Chapter 9), then reverse roles and let the other person do the same. Comparing what arises in such a monologue exchange can be enlightening and lead to compromise or creative problem-solving.

• When partners feel frustrated or angry, they should seek something to appreciate as soon as possible, for the benefit of self, partner and the whole family.

• The words *always* and *never* are "psychosemantic" symptoms of problems. It is unlikely that they can be used accurately although they are frequently heard. Saying "I always..." or "You never..." is a reliable sign of Yin and Yang disturbance and the alert couple will pause for reflection and communication when these arise.

• Partners should be wary of counselors or friends who suggest or condone divorce, especially when children are involved. Advising divorce is fashionable, not least because so many have done it, including counselors. Instead, the partners should seek support from people who believe in the marriage triangle and the spiritual/personal growth value of marriage, and who will help defend it.

• In partnerships, the Yang role may have a natural orientation to time, while the Yin role may be more oriented to space. Understanding this division of interests can help avoid conflict, with each person expecting to yield in the other's area. Having a division of tasks can simplify topics such as calendars and appointments (more Yang) and home arrangement (more Yin).

• Non-Violent Communication (also known as NVC, developed by Marshall Rosenberg) provides an excellent communications model.[263] NVC offers a simple four-step formula for communications that is effective in defusing stress, beginning with recognition and validation of what the other person needs.

In a simplified version, relationship partners can use this particular response when tension is high (adapting the exact words to the situation): "Just now I observe [whatever is obviously happening, such as loud voices or upset expressions]; I am guessing that you have a need for [some valid need]; is that correct? Then the NVC-informed conversationalist stops talking and really listens. By making a sincere guess about the other person's needs, the tone of the conversation is steered into more mutuality and cooperation.

## Sexuality

As stated repeatedly, sex is perhaps the strongest force in nature. Yin and Yang are drawn to each other with enormous power, and temporarily resolved into a Neutral that has exceptional psycho-emotional richness and potential for nourishment.

The polarized agendas can be quite different. Yang sex is more about sensual pleasure and physicalization. Yin sex is more about bonding, companionship, communication and feeling valued. These polarities are both present for both people, but one may be more in the foreground, depending on the circumstances. By recognizing and accepting the differences, the partners can be more relaxed and generous about meeting the needs of the other person, and more flexible to be able to fully enjoy both dimensions. Again, the

---

[263] See http://www.cnvc.org

Self-Other awareness practice (Chapter 9) can be very helpful, as each side takes time to fully recognize and acknowledge the validity of the other.

Polarization is a key aspect of sexuality. Loss of polarization leads to sexual dysfunction; in many dysfunctional sexual states, identifying basic imbalances such as tyrant/wimp and critic/doormat can be very helpful in getting to the core of the problem.

The sexual physiological process is largely an autonomic function, and autonomic stress responses are significantly about the body-mind coping with threat. When a couple is having sexual problems, psycho-emotional safety may be an issue in some part of their intimate relationship. The two-chair method can reveal these problems, with the client imagining the intimate partner in the other chair and saying something about their sex life together, closely observing ANS body responses and other sensations all along, then switching chairs.

---

### Sexuality in Psychoanalysis...

Psychoanalysis places great emphasize on instinctual drives that manifest in sexuality, such as the Oedipus complex and ideas derived from similar archetypal myths. In early psychology, "hysteria" was a common diagnosis, and thought to be the result of an over-active uterus. These ideas reflected the culture of the Victorian era, when sexual frustration was high, abuse was common but consistently denied and there was insufficient understanding to deal with the real forces of the magnetic effect.

In retrospect, a simpler explanation would have served the early psychology pioneers very well: sexuality and its enormous power is not abnormal or taboo, it is a biological arrangement of essential Yin and Yang forces that can be managed to some degree with education and consciousness.

---

The ANS is "reset" in mutually-coherent sex in that all three branches of the ANS are potentially invoked, exercised and fulfilled.[264]    Arousal reflects the functioning of the parasympathetic branch, orgasm reflects the functioning of the sympathetic, and flirting/foreplay (as well as afterglow/bonding) reflects the function of the social branch of the ANS. The ANS effect makes sense of the turn-of-the-century ideas of orgasm being a remedy for mental illness, as described in movies such as *The Road to Wellville* (1995) and *Hysteria* (2012). Wilhelm Reich proposed the then-revolutionary idea that healthy full-surrender orgasm between loving partners reduces neuroticism; this seems to fit the model and deserves more recognition.[265]

As a counterpoint, some yogic and Taoist systems advise *reduced* sexual activity or even celibacy except for procreation. The theory of these pertains to conservation of inner resources; possibly marital celibacy was more viable in cultures where it was firmly established philosophically. If reduced activity was promoted in popular culture and the baseline ANS was in a more stable condition due to more coherence in society, maybe it could work.

With thoughtful arguments for either more or less sex in the discussion, each couple needs to find its own way. Openly discussing attitudes and expectations about the frequency of sex, and negotiating a mutual agreement is a high priority, as early in the relationship as possible because the topic is so highly charged and centered on the all-important ANS.

---

[264] A. H. Almaas and Karen Johnson, *The Power of Divine Eros: The Illuminating Force of Love in Everyday Life.* Diamond Heart, 2013.

[265] Richard Blasband, Book review refuting *Adventures in the Orgasmatron* by Christopher Turner, published in the *Journal of Scientific Exploration.* Winter 2012, Vol. 26, No. 4, p. 895. Blasband is a leading Reich scholar/historian. Key titles by Reich in the subject are *The Function of the Orgasm* (1942) and *The Sexual Revolution* (1945).

Another peripheral topic relating to sexuality involves the ideas of monogamy, compared to other possible systems such as polyamory and polygamy. It is clear that monogamy is not biologically mandated.[266]

From a Yin and Yang perspective, the first problem is with the archetypal nature of sun and moon, and how they have different underlying agendas; polyamorous Yang may feel fulfilled by casual sex while Yin may want more feeling of deep connection. With a "free love" philosophy, one of the partners may be at a disadvantage, especially if pregnancy happens, or later if one feels discarded for a younger playmate.

Commitment to monogamy puts pressure on the couple to deal with issues, instead of being able to bypass them. The

---

## ...and Sexuality in Five Element Theory

In the Five Elements, sexuality is in the domain of Water, and its archetype is Scorpio, ruled by Mars. The ancients saw how water could heal or destroy. Mars is the astrological planet of both the healing arts and war.

Water has the attribute of clinging to whatever it touches, attaching itself as the "universal solvent" to subtly connect all life. Similarly, sexuality is the exchange of fluids and creation of our ultimate attachments, our children.

An analogy is the water system of a prosperous town. Well-managed, water provides hydroelectric power, irrigates the crops, provides clean drinking water, supports manufacturing and carries away waste, all through designed channels. In contrast, if too much rain falls and the channels fail, flooding water causes immense destruction. Similarly, sexuality can sustain or ruin our lives, and conscious attention to clear channels is the key.

---

[266] David Barash and Judith Eve Lipton, *The Myth of Monogamy: Fidelity and Infidelity in Animals and People*. Holt, 2002.

relationship gives a direct mirror which, if seen as a practice, can motivate each person to look more, and feel more, deeply into themselves. Monogamy takes away the escape hatch of release with someone else and the ensuing emotional turbulence that often follows. It applies a form of heat to clear away issues that are being avoided. The pressure may feel uncomfortable, but if the whole relationship is seen as a consciousness practice, monogamy pushes the partners into further personal growth.

The second problem is that the chances for true mutuality of intention, and particularly avoiding the all-too-common tyrant/doormat scenario, are not good for polyamorists in a culture that is predominantly monogamous; there are too many counter-forces at work.

Thirdly, the raising of children in modern culture is already a major challenge without this added complication. Single parenting can be effective, but, based on my experience, I am skeptical of some trends and comments promoting fatherless child-raising.[267] In a Yin and Yang perspective, children need mothers *and* fathers, and not just for conception. A single parent needs to be adept at both of the main functions: protection/respect for Yang and nurturance/support for Yin. Obviously, single parents can raise healthy children; the idea here is just that the mother-father dyad has significant advantages. Unless the culture is able to provide and truly normalize an alternative (such as in some indigenous examples when parenting duties are spread more widely), the problems can be severe. In addition, kids and teenagers have a developmental need to be "normal;" parents trying a different relationship model can be stressful for their children.

---

[267] Peggy Drexler, *Raising Boys Without Men: How Maverick Moms are Creating the Next Generation of Exceptional Men*. Rodale Books, 2006.

## *Autonomic States in Sexual Dysfunction*

Autonomic states can be identified within sexual dysfunctions, as follows:

**Parasympathetic** (hypo- state) symptoms of dysfunction in sex include no interest or arousal, erectile dysfunction; a feeling of interpersonal safety may be lacking. When questioned, one person may feel that he or she is "on thin ice" or "walking on eggshells" in some way, with mixed red-yellow-green traffic signals flashing from the partner. Over time, ambivalence is exhausting and leads to parasympathetic resignation. The source of the dysfunction is likely to involve both partners, not just the one with the problem. Therapeutic support can be focused on the felt-sense of safety, using Body-Low-Slow-Loop to gently soften the extreme immobilization of the hypo- autonomic state.

**Sympathetic** (hyper- state) symptoms of dysfunction in sex include no climax or premature climax, sexual addiction, coupling of sex with aggression or violence (a fight response) or strong impulses to get away (a flight response). The sympathetic range of response may be disturbed, as in a feeling of disorientation (such as, "I don't know where I stand with you"), or unresolved anger or fear that does not find resolution. Old frustrations, set in place long before the current relationship, can be acted out in ways that initially don't make sense. The reason is that the high sympathetic ANS arousal of orgasm can easily be coupled with other high-arousal states from recent or unresolved past experience. Victims of earlier sexual abuse may have a very hard time in this phase because their sympathetic stress responses are naturally linked.

The coupling effect is commonly depicted in movies: after a harrowing chase or escape, the leading characters often fall into sexual ecstasy, whether they are a good match or not, because it feels so normal from an ANS perspective. The end of the movie *Speed* (1994) is a prime example. The characters have nothing in common but frantically initiate highly charged sex immediately when the severe and prolonged threat is finally resolved. The plot makes sense from an ANS perspective as the ANS needs to be re-set after such extreme events.

In sympathetic ANS sexual problems, therapeutic support can include gently discharging thwarted defensive responses, resolving binds from earlier times and ensuring safety. The therapeutic process should be mindful that the sympathetic stress response is a higher order of coping strategy than parasympathetic, even though sympathetic may be more dramatic and alarming.

**Social nervous system** symptoms of dysfunction in sex include sub-optimum bonding, inability to discuss intimate issues or engage verbally, lack of eye contact and lack of affirming sounds or afterglow. Casual sex that minimizes or denies the reality of a psycho-emotional component, leading to feelings of confusion and emptiness (perhaps more so for the Yin role) indicate social nervous system disability, and can also cause ANS problems later. Social nervous system problems are also indicated when the two people are far apart in their attitudes and expectations about the encounter but are unable to detect disparities or discuss them frankly.

Therapeutic support can include self-help practices, embracing differences between Yin and Yang and honest communication about needs. Ideally the partners can come to conscious balance and mutual meeting of needs, instead of just unconsciously blundering along in the unspoken dark.

### Sexuality and Youth

Sexuality is particularly awkward in the teenage and early-twenties age groups. Sexual magnetism and biological forces are at a peak; however cultural support for lasting relationships and psychological maturity are lacking. The risk assessment functions of the brain are thought to be not mature until age 23 or more, as expert Reuben Gur explains:

> The evidence is strong that the brain does not cease to mature until the early twenties in those relevant parts that govern impulsivity, judgment, planning for the future, foresight of consequences, and other characteristics that make people morally culpable.[268]

Alcohol and recreational drugs make the situation much worse, bypassing what immature restraints may have manifested at a still-early age. How many lives have been pushed in a certain direction by the inability to get past this particular gate, when hormones are highest (age 15-18) yet brain development is unfinished (age 22-25)? Again, discussion of all this, including how to be in a relationship, should be a main topic in middle and high school education.

In the case in which there is not much consideration of a lasting relationship, a minimal approach is for two young people to at least talk about their intentions before having sex. The more the intentions are congruent with each other, the less likelihood of further complications. Naturally there is a high possibility of inauthentic conversation or changing of minds, but at least the subject has a chance of receiving increased consciousness.

The challenge is compounded by today's college mentality, that assumes real, lasting relationships will be avoided ("too early"), while inter-personal contact, biological magnetism and opportunities for promiscuity are very high.

---

[268] Ruben C. Gur, *Declaration of Ruben C. Gur. Patterson v. Texas. Petition for Writ of Certiorari to US Supreme Court.* J. Gary Hart, Counsel. (2002).

A recent development in the sexuality dimension of youthful experience is described in the excellent research summary, *The Demise of Guys* by Philip Zimbardo, which is highly recommended for therapists who work with young men.[269] The Stanford-based project studied behavioral trends among substantial users of video games and internet pornography, and found that these entertainments could have the effect of de-mobilizing the users for real activity. As the authors describe:

> The excessive use of video games and online porn in pursuit of the next thing is creating a generation of risk-averse guys who are unable (and unwilling) to navigate the complexities and risks inherent to real-life relationships, school and employment.

In the research, the satisfactions attained in the fantasy experiences were just substantial enough to drain away the impulses to take risks in real life, in either relationships or other challenging life situations.

### Conception and Birth Control

Many parents report that the moment of conception is consciously perceived, although the mechanism is not known. The key is to appreciate that larger forces are at work; the play is not just between the mother and father. The new being is also exerting an influence on the process. Understanding this may help the parents relax.

A new factor in conception is the effect of environmental problems such as the increase of estrogen-mimicking plastics that seem to be related to decreasing sperm counts. There is no simple solution to the problem, but would-be parents are well advised to become

---

[269] Philip G. Zimbardo, co-author, *The Demise of Guys*. TED, 2011. Quoted by CNN May 24, 2012. See also www.demiseofguys.com.

more studious about environmental exposures including pollution and radiation exposure such as air travel.

Birth control methods are fundamentally oppositional to biological design; they can be accommodated but there is not a simple solution. Understanding the side effects and disadvantages of each option is very helpful and a good topic for mutual discussion. Negotiation, compromise and a high level of attention are invaluable when two people are trying to figure out what form of birth control is appropriate. Many young people tend to deny the existence of the side effects just out of convenience or in order to continue promiscuous behaviors. It is a conundrum without a ready answer.

In Vitro Fertilization (IVF) and new strategies for "biotech" pregnancies are very complex, and not yet understood. Hopefully long-term scientific studies will be performed as new technologies are developed. In "biotech pregnancies" the Yin and Yang model expects that the same larger forces, the incarnation of a new soul, are still the basic theme, even though the circumstances are unusual in terms of natural design and the initial process was different from the biological blueprint. The interplay of the Three Principles and Five Elements is still present.

*Pregnancy*

In these hyper-important life events, education is everything. Many of the risks and complexities can be minimized with attentive learning and planning. This requires independent study and support from allies, and not necessarily relying on mainstream ideas and practices which seem to have lagged in terms of benefitting from modern scientific discoveries about the ANS, natural childbirth methods and the importance of successful maternal bonding. In any case, significant time invested in understanding basic concepts and preparations is likely to bring a great reward.

A key to the time of pregnancy is minimizing disturbing emotions, loud sounds and conflict. Extra attention is appropriate throughout the family, so that the prenate gains a strong foundation in ANS equanimity. Tranquility during pregnancy was emphasized by Mahatma Gandhi:

> And great is the responsibility that rests on the wife during the nine months that follow [conception]. She should be made to realize that the character of the child to be born will depend entirely on her life and conduct during this sacred period... It is also the husband's duty during this period to refrain from all wranglings with his wife, and to conduct himself in such a way as to make her cheerful and happy... There is no field of action in which the child does not imitate the actions of the parents.[270]

If disharmony does arise, the mother can help by "talking to the baby" and differentiating what is happening, emphasizing that the noise is not about the baby and that the underlying field is still secure. Using the Yin and Yang model, natural processes are the guiding orientation; when in doubt parents would be well advised to stay as close to nature as possible. The more we stray from biological design and nature, the higher will be the risk of complexity. When in doubt, partners can envision a primitive simple natural state, compare it to their current experience and seek ways of bringing the two closer together. This requires resistance to the economic forces of modern birthing; a couple going with the standard purchase of birthing services will pay far more (albeit through insurance), with more complex outcomes, than if they just stay close to nature. Many couples erroneously think that the "state-of-the-art" medicine and

---

[270] M. Gandhi, *Gandhi's Health Guide.* Crossing Press, 2000. pp. 168-172.

science leads to better outcomes, however statistics point in the opposite direction.[271]

Would-be parents need to be open for anything, including possible disappointments. Higher, invisible forces are at work, in addition to the more tangible attitudes and impulses that most people experience. The incoming baby is a consciousness of its own, with its own arc through life. Knowing this may help the parents relax and become observers of the process rather than attempting to micro-manage every detail.

In the Yin and Yang model, life begins at conception. The soul is a "unit of consciousness, from another sphere"[272] who is incarnating to learn particular lessons. The soul chooses parents, culture, time and a gender appropriate to the lessons to be learned. Nothing is random or accidental.

From this perspective, abortion is quite problematic. The embryo is a human being, from the very start, coming into the body for a noble and sacred purpose. However, such intimate experiences are not properly within the role of government, but rather a process to be closely held within the parents' own domain, assisted by their medical, spiritual and family support systems.

The net result of these considerations is to support education and avoidance of unwanted pregnancy, avoid abortion, and give women and their partners full authority to make choices for themselves in such extremely private and sensitive matters.

---

[271] In 2012, the USA was costliest in the world in birth expenditures, but only 34th among world countries in birth survival. See:
http://www.nytimes.com/2013/07/01/health/american-way-of-birth-costlie st-in-the-world.html

[272] R. Stone, *Polarity Therapy, Vol. 1.* CRCS, 1986. Book 1, p. 9.

### Birthing

When the time of birth approaches, parents will want to prepare to defend themselves and their baby from certain mainstream practices that do not acknowledge the existence of, or appreciate the importance of, the ANS. These practices are often sneaky and form a slippery slope: an early intervention can  lead to a string of unwanted additional interventions that become "necessary." For example, the high-tech desire for fetal heart monitoring, quite innocent and useful by itself, can require immobilization, which then can lead to a slower, more difficult labor, followed by induced labor, anesthesia, various extraction methods or cesarean delivery. In stories of complicated deliveries, it can be interesting to track the chain of events back to the start of the sequence, when a seemingly inconsequential decision often set the process on a different course.

As discussed before, the main problem is that the baby is not really regarded as a sentient being; this leaks out into numerous problematic practices in the birthing environment. It is useful to hold the questions, "How would we approach a highly-respected adult in this situation?" and "What would be happening in a more natural setting?" and act accordingly. A great failure of modern science and medicine is to think that babies are insentient and to treat them roughly as if they do not have feelings. Newborns are taken from their mothers, suctioned, pricked, left unattended, circumcised and talked over, all in a style that adults would not tolerate with each other. How far have we strayed from nature and common sense, to find ourselves in a place where "be nice to babies" is such a radical idea in health care?

French obstetrician Michel Odent has observed that mammals in the wild wait to give birth until two conditions

## Wilhelm Reich on Traumatizing Newborns (1950)

When a child is born, it comes out of a warm uterus, 37 degrees centigrade, into about 18 or 20 degrees centigrade. That's bad enough. The shock of birth... bad enough. But it could survive that if the following didn't happen: As it comes out, it is picked up by the legs and slapped on the buttocks. The first greeting is a slap.

The next greeting: Take it away from the mother. Right? I want you to listen here. It will sound incredible in a hundred years. Take it away from the mother. The mother must not touch or see the baby. The baby has no body contact after having had nine months of body contact at a very high temperature– what we call the "orgonotic body energy contact," the field action between them, the warmth and the heat.

Then, the Jews introduced something about six or seven thousand years ago. And that is circumcision. I don't know why they introduced it. It's still a riddle. Take that poor penis. Take a knife -- right? And start cutting. And everybody says, "It doesn't hurt." Get it? That's an excuse, of course, a subterfuge. They say the sheaths of the nerve are not yet developed. Therefore, the sensation in the nerves is not yet developed. Therefore, the child doesn't feel a thing. Now, that's murder! Circumcision is one of the worst treatments of children. And what happens to them? You just look at them. They can't talk to you. They just cry.

What they do is shrink. They contract, get away into the inside, away from that ugly world. I express it very crudely, but you understand what I mean. Now that's the greeting: Taking it away from the mother. Mother mustn't see it. Twenty-four or forty-eight hours, eat nothing. Right? Penis cut. And then comes the worst:

This poor child, poor infant, tries always to stretch out and to find some warmth, something to hold on to. It goes to the mother, puts it lips to the mother's nipple [bottle]. And what happens? The nipple is cold, or doesn't erect, or the milk doesn't come out, or the milk is bad. And that is quite general. That's average. So what does that infant do? How does it respond to that? How does it have to respond to that bioenergetically? It can't come to you and tell you, "Oh listen, I'm suffering so much, so much." It doesn't say "no" in words, you understand, but that is the emotional situation. And we orgonomists know it. We get it out of our patients. We get it out of their emotional structure, out of their behavior, not out of their words. Words can't express it.

Here, in the very beginning, the spite develops. Here, the "no" develops, the big "NO" of humanity. And then you ask why the world is in a mess.

are present: security and privacy. [273] These are unknown in many birthing environments, as the nurses come and go and

---

### Robert Fulford on Birth Trauma Effects

Another study from Sweden worth mentioning is one of 412 patients in six Stockholm hospitals, all born before 1940, who died of the effects of drug addiction and alcoholism or suicide between 1978 and 1984. The researchers found that, more than any other risk factor for which they tested, it was birth trauma that was most closely associated with suicide.

Even more persuasive is the work of Bertil Jacobson, head of the Department of Medical Engineering at Karolensha Institute in Sweden, who has spent a lifetime researching associations between prenatal experience and adolescent events.

According to Dr. Jacobson's studies, suicide was more closely associated with birth trauma than with any of the other eleven risk factors for which he tested (including such socioeconomic variables as parental alcoholism and broken homes). In addition, Dr. Jacobson's results indicate a strong correlation between the type of trauma suffered at birth and the method by which suicide or violent death occurred during adolescence. Two thousand nine hundred cases of suicide by asphyxiation were closely associated with some form of asphyxiation at birth. For those who killed themselves using some form of mechanical procedure, the researchers found many had experienced mechanical trauma at birth—for instance, the use of forceps or other metal instruments to help deliver the baby. And drug addiction among the suicide victims had a high correlation to administration of opiates and barbiturates during labor.

And, in a 1985 study published in the British medical journal Lances, psychologist Lee Salk of Cornell University Medical School also encountered strong links between birth trauma and suicide in adolescents. Three common denominators were detected in his study: (1) respiratory distress in excess of one hour at birth; (2) lack of proper prenatal care before the twentieth week of pregnancy; (3) chronic ill health of the mother during her pregnancy.

Robert Fulford, *Dr. Fulford's Touch of Life: The Healing Power of the Natural Life Force*. Gallery Books, 1997.

---

[273] Michel Odent, *Birth and Breastfeeding: Rediscovering the Needs of Women During Pregnancy and Childbirth*. Steiner Press, 2008.

the whole environment radiates the sights, sounds and smells of medical high-alert status.

During delivery, it is very helpful to "talk to the baby." Parents can appreciate that the baby is super-sentient from the very start, in ways that are not understood by modern science. In my view, many procedures can be accommodated if proper negotiation happens first. The theme is to treat the baby as a super-sentient, highly respected emissary from another dimension, and not do anything different from how we would treat such a very important person. If an adult needed suctioning or heel pricking, I would explain the procedure, the justification for it, and provide soothing reassurances before just charging ahead. These same considerations should be given to a baby.

Natural maternal bonding, which means leaving the baby on the mom, skin-to-skin, for the first twenty or more minutes and not cutting the umbilical cord until pulsing ceases, is the preeminent, most easily achieved strategy for lifelong autonomic wellness. Unfortunately, parents often have to fight for this all-important opportunity for nature to take its course.

Separation of mothers and their newborns became routine in the late 1800s under the banner of "infant hygiene." The impulse for this was valid, based on the discoveries of Semmelweis, Lister and Pasteur, but it was taken to extremes such as strict behaviorism in the early 1900s. The practice became so institutionalized that now it is almost impossible to break, despite abundant scientific evidence. Vast psycho-emotional suffering has resulted, but medical science lacks long-term tracking mechanisms to detect the effect. Scandinavian studies, made possible by having unified and nationwide health care systems, have been able to see the link between bonding problems at birth and negative adult psycho-emotional effects such as anxiety and depression.[274]

Circumcision is a major autonomic insult, predicated on the now-discredited belief that babies do not feel pain and do not form memories.[275] In fact the procedure is painful and is performed at a time when newborns are instinctually expecting safety and nurturance from their caregivers.[276] Trauma specialists Bessel van der Kolk has stated that the degree of trauma impact is a function of two factors: how early the event occurred and whether betrayal (threat or pain coming unexpectedly from a trusted person) was involved.[277]

Circumcision represents an extreme problem in both of these measures. Whatever tribal benefits are attained are more than offset by autonomic damage. If circumcision is so strongly desired for tribal or HIV prevention justifications, let it be done at the time of puberty and with full choice, not in infancy. In puberty the boy has much more psycho-emotional resources and the betrayal factor is less significant since presumably he is consenting to the procedure at that age, and very much wanting to become part of the tribe. In addition, at puberty, anesthesia could be used. The notion that circumcision has no detrimental autonomic impact is entirely wrong, another artifact of the medieval "babies are insentient" belief system.

---

[274] Many health care pioneers are heroically trying to overcome this problem, including David Chamberlain (www.birthpsychology.org), Thomas Verny, Michel Odent and others.

[275] Wilhelm Reich, *Children of the Future*. Farrar, Straus & Giroux, 1984. An excellent resource for the topic is http://www.circumcision.org/studies.htm.

[276] Benjamin Spock: *The Circumcision Question*. Wilbert Productions, 1994.

[277] Bessel van der Kolk, *Traumatic Stress, The Effects of Overwhelming Experience of Mind, Body and Society*, Guilford Press, 2006.

It can also be argued that circumcision is also unethical, since the foreskins are sold to burn clinics.[278] Sociological implications have also been noted. Nurse and activist Marilyn Milos describes circumcision as "where sex and violence meet for the first time."[279]

Along with interrupted bonding and circumcision, premature cord cutting is a third unnecessary practice that is also routine. This is probably an artifact of infant quarantine, as doctors sought efficiency in whisking the baby off to a germ-free environment. Premature cord-cutting has been thoroughly proven to be damaging due to the sudden unnatural drop in blood pressure and related complications.[280] Once again, the first question is to ask, what would happen in a natural setting? The umbilical cord naturally stops pulsing when the time is right.

Much suffering could be relieved if these three unnecessary practices were terminated. The autonomic wellness level of the whole planet would take a major step to increased resiliency and kindness.

Adoption has many benefits for all involved but will be strenuous because the child will inevitably have levels of abandonment/betrayal trauma as well as other factors. Adopting parents should be realistic with the process and the requirements, and fully understand the complex responsibility they are assuming. The two-chair process can help with re-establishing bonding.

---

278 Paul M. Fleiss, MD, *The Case Against Circumcision.* Mothering Magazine, November 1997.

279 George Denniston, Frederick Hodges, Marilyn Milos, Eds. *Circumcision and Human Rights.* Springer Science, 2009.

280 See Karen Strange, RN, http://www.newbornbreath.com.

## *Post-Birth and the Surrogate Spouse*

New parents are very susceptible to the surrogate spouse problem, also known as "husband lost in space." This phenomenon arises when there are young children and the mother feels very absorbed in her new life. The first child was a compelling experience; with a second child, full-scale overwhelm can set in.

The husband-wife pair is the primary polarized dyad in the family energy field. All fields depend for their stability on the existence of a primary dipole, to set the Yin and Yang tone of attraction and repulsion in the local "solar system." The archetype for the dipole in a family is sun and moon, played by husband/father and wife/mother. This dipole needs to be maintained with conscious effort, because it can easily slip away under the pressures of daily life and parenting. The children are dependent on the parental bond staying polarized and functional, with mother supplying nurturance and consistency, and father providing safety and respect. Parents can accomplish all this by using mindfulness, conscious intention and steady determination.

However it is very common for the mother to become absorbed in the new baby, especially if she is a first-time mom. Between breastfeeding and bedtime routines, she can subtly displace her husband with the baby as her intimate partner, without realizing what is happening. Her magnetic attraction with her blood-relative child is more forceful than her sexual bond with her husband, and the new relationship is so much easier because the child is totally compelling, dependent and initially compliant. The child can become her "surrogate spouse."

This can progress to an advanced degree, and soon the husband begins to feel that he has no place to plug in to the mother's system. What was a functional receptor site is now occupied by the baby. The shift can be gradual and sneaky.

After some time the husband feels unfulfilled and disoriented. He wonders what happened.

Meanwhile the wife is increasingly absorbed with the baby, and may become more critical of the husband, "Yin empty," without knowing why. The couple's sex life is likely to suffer as the field becomes de-polarized. The situation is compounded by the mother's physical and emotional fatigue as well as her body's need for recovery time.

In an advanced form, the Mom and child pair forms its own sun and moon unit, and the father feels "lost in space." The father will start to stay overtime at work or explore recreational activities, at the expense of time with the family. The Mother becomes the new Yang (sun) energy pole and the baby becomes the new Yin (moon) pole, with father increasingly lacking a sense of place. Only conscious effort can overcome the natural magnetic tendency for mom to enter into a special intimacy with the baby, replacing the husband as her primary gravitational orientation. The two-chair method is an excellent remedy, because the dynamic is made directly experiential and obvious.

The effect can be amplified when the baby is opposite-gender, as the gender difference compounds the natural magnetic intensity of maternal bonding. Less commonly, the father may bond with a daughter because the mother has become remote and he desperately needs a receptor site for his energy. The pattern can continue for decades, with the son becoming "mama's boy" and the daughter "daddy's girl." These kinds of patterns undermine the child's future ability to have a real relationship.

The surrogate spouse problem is most common with husbands who lose their position in the marriage. But it can also work the other way, when the child loses the bond and cannot regain the ability for intimacy because the mother can never be replaced with a watery bond. One client, age 60, had been devastated by the tragic death of his mother when he was 14. He was the oldest child, and throughout his childhood he was intensely bonded with her; their father/husband was always away at work. When she died, he went into relationship shock, subconsciously deciding never to love again at that depth to avoid the possible extreme pain of another loss. In subsequent relationships he was unable to be fully present with his wives: how could they possibly replace the departed mother in his subconscious process, especially in a Hollywood relationship? The marriages were unsatisfying for all and he tended to have extramarital affairs with minimal expectations or investment. Using the two-chair method, he was able to experience his grief with his departed mother, acquire some understanding about the nature of his wound, and subsequently he was able to reduce his alienation from his current wife by intentionally being more open to intimacy under the marriage triangle model.

In a surrogate spouse situation, the remedy is to use consciousness to recognize and address the problem. At least once a day, the husband and wife can take time to really focus with each other, with strong eye contact, physical connection such as hugging, sweet interpersonal sounds and refreshment of their archetypal Yin and Yang positioning.

---

### "Blood is Thicker Than Water"

The nature of water is to be slippery; $H_2O$ molecules easily flip from one molecular pair-bond to another, giving water its remarkable properties as the universal solvent. Energetically, this is seen in the frequent randomness of sexual attraction, a function of the Water Element, which easily flips from one bond to another. Again, water needs structure to be productive and safe, instead of destructive and chaotic. The husband-wife dyad is a watery bond held in a structure of intention and consciousness. Meanwhile the parent-child relationship is formed of blood, a much stronger energetic bond. The family benefits by the parents taking extra care to manage the water bond so that it is not displaced or obscured by the potentially stronger blood bond.

---

Ideally, these exercises are done in front of the children, so that everyone knows the priorities. Children will be insecure if their parents are not in harmony, so it can be very beneficial to "perform" or role play a polarized relationship for their benefit, such as by having husband make a balanced Yang comment and the wife respond with a balanced Yin comment. This can be done with pre-arranged intention, as actors prepare for a performance, and it can also be done with humor. As described in the Self-Help chapter, the husband might enter a room when the young children are present and firmly proclaim, "I am the benevolent King of this family." The wife then responds with a complementary statement, in a sweet sounding tone, "And I feel content and secure as the Queen." The statements are followed by a gesture of warmth and affection, such as a hug. Young children, even pre-verbal, will observe this "stage play" with great interest, even if they supposedly do not understand the words.

When this practice is introduced, some children may get upset and try to physically insert themselves between the parents, as if to try to maintain their now-familiar primary position in mom's field. If this happens, the parents can gently state what they are doing and why, as if the child understands adult language. The child can be gently moved to one side while the parents repeat the performance. Close observation will reveal the child becoming more secure once the newly-reorganized field has been tested a few times to make sure it is real.

### Parenting

"No growth without resistance"[281] is a guiding theme of parenting, as it is throughout life; parents can learn to embrace opportunities to say no, be consistent, set limits and

---

[281] Erich Blechschmidt, *The Ontogenetic Basis for Human Development: A Biodynamic Approach to Development from Conception to Birth.* North Atlantic, 2004.

create structure. This should all be done without violence or even excessive force or loud sounds. Giving the child consistent opportunities to push against the parents builds lifelong self-reliance and emotional intelligence.

Children are in the Yin role relative to their parents, but many anxious new parents enact a reversed positioning. For example, a mother or father might say, "It's time for bed, OK?" as if the child is actually in charge. Firm, gentle, consistent statements, not questions, are more likely to help children feel secure. Children do not actually know the answers to such questions, and subconsciously they know they don't know. An over-empowered child throwing tantrums may be feeling insecure due to a reversed Yin and Yang effect.

To repeat, the mother archetype is about providing nurturing and support; the father archetype is about creating safety and respect. Too often, the parents lose these archetypal roles, as mom becomes the disciplinarian and dad tries to be the child's buddy. These particular effects are clues that the surrogate spouse problem is manifesting. Once again, re-polarizing based on the Three Principles and the marriage triangle can be helpful.

Parents can benefit by becoming knowledgeable about the ANS, so that they can recognize its manifestations in the child's behavior. As stated earlier, the ANS is really the top health priority because safety is the child's pre-programmed, hardwired top biological imperative. Safety at the ANS level is first achieved through successful bonding, attunement and consistent safety. Accidents can be accommodated but betrayal leaves a deep mark.

The goal of parenting is not perfection; "Good enough" is more realistic. Coined by British pediatrician and psychoanalyst Donald Winnicott, this phrase is a great remedy for the idealism of full-term pregnancy, that can interfere with relaxed mothering due to need for everything to be perfect, a classic Yin dilemma.[282] Constancy, predictability and steadiness are the signatures of effective parenting. It is a great relief when parents are helped to be relieved of the desire for perfection, and begin to relax into "good enough" instead. Making minor errors is part of the normal process and repair can make the child stronger.

The more parents are unified the better; differences can be addressed and resolved in private, not in front of the children. Children should never be used for leverage in parental arguments; the parents can pre-agree to get help if this ever starts to arise. In front of the children, the parents can make clear statements and use body language to demonstrate their unity. If the parents are unable to do such strategies, the child will begin to exhibit symptoms of insecurity, because subconsciously children know that their well-being depends on having a functional sun and moon base of both father and mother.

Intoxication is fundamentally antithetical to healthy parenting, reducing constancy and safety. Without exception, children do not know what to make of altered behaviors that result from intoxication. The effects can be damaging to the child's ANS because the all-important social branch is compromised or disabled. This can lead to other autonomic problems later in life.

Unfortunately the intoxicated parent is likely to also deny that there is any problem, or try to normalize the behavior, often because it existed in previous generations. Parents thus repeat the errors of their parents, perpetuating destructive habits and creating a new generation of suffering.

---

[282] Frank Lake, *Clinical Theology, a Theological And Psychiatric Basis to Clinical Pastoral Care.* Emeth, 2006. See also G.V. Whitfield, *The Prenatal Psychology of Frank Lake and the Origins of Sin and Human Dysfunction.* Emeth, 2007.

Using the marriage triangle concept is protection against such rationalizations; viewed from that perspective, intoxication in the presence of children is indefensible.

Parents can benefit from the advice of veterans, however they should be wary of old-fashioned, now-discredited autonomic ideas that somehow persist out of long habit, such as "spare the rod and spoil the child" or "children should be seen and not heard." Just 200 years ago, the European pedagogical (expert child-raising advice) paradigm was extremely traumatizing.[283] It is no wonder we have so much suffering today.

Similarly caution should be used with traditional stories, songs and games, many of which have underlying trauma messages. For example, "Ring Around the Rosie" is actually an echo of the Great Plague of the Middle Ages and "Musical Chairs" teaches a fear of scarcity and competitive disadvantage. Ideally parents can review thoughtfully the activities that are so normal that they are taken for granted, and avoid unintentional hidden messages that can negatively affect a highly suggestible child.

Children are resilient, non-cognitive and self-centered, and unless there is a cause for concern, they are not overly focused on their parents. Parental fears are often exaggerated unnecessarily and can create an autonomic effect beyond the actual event. If a child stumbles and falls, a parent's over-reaction can be more impactful than the accident itself.

Children are in a receptive Yin role relative to their caregivers, with little choice but to adapt to the environment presented. Infancy and childhood, the springtime (most Yang)

---

[283] Alice Miller, *For Your Own Good: Hidden Cruelty in Child-Rearing and the Roots of Violence*. Noonday, 1983. Miller thoroughly refutes many of the pathologizing errors of early psychology, such as Freud's theory of infantile sexuality. Miller's other books (see Bibliography) are also excellent reading for re-framing the history of psychology.

phase of life, is couched in an extreme Yin relationship structure. This is another insight into the meaning of the Tao emblem: in the fullness of one is the seed of the other.

Parents can help children who are exceptional in some way, by maintaining a sense of normalcy and neutrality. In particular, girls who are extremely beautiful and boys who are extremely skilled in sports need special protection, because modern culture will tend to look past their essential qualities in over-emphasizing their surface qualities. These seemingly positive attributes can become a liability, skewing the child's sense of value and basic expectations about the world. Adults may value them for their appearance or skills, instead of their inner integrity, setting up a difficult adjustment when normal circumstances eventually arrive.

A protective parent will not buy in to the temptation about these children, and will maintain a gentle guiding intention about the inner qualities of integrity, self-esteem and confidence based on actual performance in life and relationships instead of constantly focusing on outward appearances. Popular events such as beauty pageants for young girls are actually a form of child abuse, with long-standing damage.

Similarly, over-emphasis on sports can be damaging, with overly pushy parents putting children in pressure situations that are not appropriate for their ages. The same can be true for intellectual prodigies, but the problem is not so difficult because social priorities often favor sports over intellect. The ideal is to have children enjoy physical activities and intellectual challenges in more natural settings, and also to have unstructured play time with peers so that imaginations and social skills develop. Unstructured play time is obviously a very different experience from a Little League championship game in which adult pressures are applied. The voracious appetite for content now has Little

League tournament games on national television, exploiting the young players with no sensitivity about the children's psychological wellness.

A similar potential "curse" for children is to be born into a family of extreme wealth. In this situation the parents can make a special effort to let the children have normal developmental sequences with other children, and minimize the impression of being special. Financial status is such a high priority and almost taboo; children can be ostracized or attract unexpected attention due to their parents' wealth instead of their innate natural qualities. The risk for these children is about being able to have successful personal relationships later in life.

The protective role of parents seems to be changing. In particular, the digital culture poses new challenges, because pervasive online entertainment and video games are real threats to young children. Electronic devices are the new babysitters. Keeping children involved with hands-on activities in real-life situations is more important than it was in the past, when children naturally stayed busy and grew up by participating in their parents' real lives.

Divorcing parents are consistently delusional about the breakup's negative effect on their children. Divorce has enormous impact on children, often more so for younger ones.[284] If divorce is unavoidable, extreme care and extra measures should be adopted to reduce the impact, using counselors and other resources who are not invested in divorce and who will not trivialize or minimize the effects. Desperate parents make many rationalizations about how the children will be better off, which has some truth in that they are less exposed to fighting. However the parents do not

---

[284] Andrew Root, *The Children of Divorce: The Loss of Family as the Loss of Being.* Baker Academic, 2010.

appreciate or comprehend the other side of the coin, that they were unable to step up to the challenges of making marriage and parenting work.

Sugar is particularly an under-appreciated issue for behavior, especially with children; in America, 43 percent of young children consume at least one sugar soda drink a day. "The more soda kids drank, the more likely their mothers were to report that the kids had problems with aggression, withdrawal and staying focused on a task."[285] Stone strongly advised against usage of what he called the white poisons (sugar, salt and white flour), and offered many comments about links between diet and mental-emotional wellness.

## Career

Career success revolves around the Yang principle; poor career progression suggests Yang imbalance and disability. In the modern era, everyone is wounded by Yang because modern history is such a tale of abuse, deception and exploitation. In millennial America, the grandparents lived through the great Depression and World War II and the parents lived through the Vietnam War and the betrayals and scandals of the late 1900s. These are all Yang disturbances that traumatized the whole planet.

If clients are having difficulty with career, I recommend that they explore Yang in their lives. Perhaps there are attitudes and expectations that are self-defeating or unrealistic. In a two-chair process, putting the father in the other chair (in order to invoke the Yang archetype) can be interesting and provide insight about binds and complications. Practices for healing the ANS, such as Body-Low-Slow-Loop, can be effective.

Another subtle factor in career frustration is the effect of cultural messages. The constant narrative from the media is

---

[285] Melissa Pandika, "Soda linked to behavioral problems in young children, study says." *Los Angeles Times*, August 16, 2013. See: http://www.fragilefamilies.princeton.edu.

that work is a drudgery, employment is scarce, the economy is fragile and that job satisfaction is not a realistic goal. The problem is compounded by the supposed split between work and play. Buying in to these beliefs is a blunting of Yang's inherent goal-oriented, highly mobilized nature. To awaken from these ingrained messages can be very liberating. Yang needs some field of action to exercise its natural impulses, or ANS difficulties will arise. Whatever niche the person finds in the overall economy, an attitude of curiosity, enthusiasm and sincere striving is essential for Yang to flourish.

"Retirement" is questionable in many situations, representing a disengagement from Yang energy fulfillment, with health problems often arising within a few years.[286] The longest-lived cultures have no concept of retirement. If retirement is desired, staying active and socially involved in some other way is a key to longevity. Being sequestered with just other elderly or disabled people is not natural. Staying involved in the give-and-take of daily life, adding value through service to others and receiving social interactions in common pursuits, is the key.

> Career choices can be classified elementally:
> **Earth**: Security, armed forces, crime, dense physical or purely monetary activities
> **Water**: Care-giving, nurturing including childhood education, nursing; Yin and Yang counseling is substantially located here and with Ether
> **Fire**: Business and commerce, including entrepreneurial activities and marketing/sales
> **Air**: Higher education, commercial art, some religious ministries, super-idealistic pursuits
> **Ether**: Art, spirituality

Within these possibilities, each person can gravitate toward the field of action that feels most compelling. The old adage, "Do what you love, the money will follow," has stood

---

[286] longevity.about.com/od/healthyagingandlongevity/a/retirement.htm

the test of time when contemplating a career path.[287] While career is low in the "hierarchy of action fields," achievements in career can greatly support the highest level, self-worth.

## Elder Care and "Deathing"

As with birthing, end-of-life care should also orient to nature. Elders today are often isolated, over-medicated, nutritionally neglected and not given an active role in society with interaction with other age groups. In the Yin and Yang model, the responsible caregiving child seeks ways to counter these tendencies for their elderly parents.

The dying process has similarities to birthing, together serving as bookends for the journey of the soul through an incarnation. In dying, the life currents withdraw up the body, step-by-step. The intention is to be as conscious of this process as possible, instead of the common approach of maximum medication. Medication has a value in helping reduce pain, anxiety and agitation, but the first orientation should be to maintain natural conditions and maximum awareness if possible.

The term "deathing" has been advanced in the hope that the end of life could receive the same amount of attention and education given to the beginning of life.[288] In the wisdom traditions, the dying process is seen as the way the soul departs from the material world and returns to the invisible realm to continue its journey. The Yin and Yang cosmology can be an enormous benefit, as can the literature on near-death experiences. If the big picture is really understood, the end will not be so feared by the person who is departing, or seem so sad for the people who are being left behind.

---

[287] Marsha Sinetar, *Do What You Love, The Money Will Follow: Discovering Your Right Livelihood.* Dell, 1989.

[288] Anya Foos-Graber, *Deathing.* Nicholas-Hays, 1989. Foos-Graber wrote this book after a near-death experience in a car crash; she was a student of Paul Twitchell (founder of Eckankar meditation), who crossed paths with Randolph Stone in India in the 1950s. *Deathing* is packed with Three Principles/Five Elements references.

Buddhism advises that the body should not be whisked away abruptly, as is often done. The soul's transfer is so momentous that a gentle gradual transition is preferred. The situation has some similarities to birthing in that transitions are better when they are soft and the pace of nature is allowed. It is an interesting commentary that the beginning and end of life should both be so rushed, often unnecessarily.

## Notes for Caregivers

The supportive caregiver should take care to not cling energetically or emotionally, or in any way cause the departing soul to be pulled back against the current. As with birthing, the veil between realms can be felt to grow thin, giving end of life mystical dimensions for the conscious privileged observer who is not pulled off center by emotions.

As one's parents age, a point is reached at which the traditional Sun-Moon relationship is flipped, and the now-adult child takes over the Yang position in the dyad. Eventually one or both parents begin to decline and the children assume increasing responsibilities. The same values that applied for very young children now apply for the elderly. The intention is about steadiness and consistency.

A child caring for a declining parent may encounter the disruption of Sun and Moon within his or her marriage, and this must be kept in consciousness to avoid the unrelated partner losing a receptor site for the primary relational flow that is the foundation of the marriage. The effect is similar to the "husband lost in space" danger of having very young children. This can be very difficult, not least because of the emotions surrounding the impending or actual loss, but it can be managed with focused attention and adequate support. When the duties are complete with the parent at the end of the day, the related spouse can return to the marriage and re-establish the primary dyad with attentive interactions.

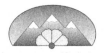

## Chapter 12

# How Involution and Evolution
# Create the Emotions

In Randolph Stone's view, the mind, feelings and body are linked in a chain of cause and effect, constantly cycling from the subtle to the dense and back, from the mind down to the body and the body back up to the mind. The many manifestations of this cycle are reflections of the larger cosmic process of involution and evolution, by which a soul travels into creation and ultimately returns to its source.

Esoterically, the Journey of the Soul implies the creation of emotions. The individual came from the invisible world, where the larger meaning of life seems to be fully known.[289] Moving into an incarnation in a new body is like squeezing the vast potential of the soul into a tight, constraining box.

In the Yang descent-into-form sequence, the inevitable discomfort of constraint is accompanied by the first emotion, *grief*, at being separated from the spirit world. Soon after, an impulse arises to assuage the grief by occupying the senses, leading to the second emotion, *desire*. Desire works to some degree, but inevitably it falls short of the real desire, which is reunion with the Source, and the third emotion, *anger*, begins to manifest. We get frustrated that we are still separate from our source, realizing that worldly desires are no substitute for the real experience of unity with spirit. In time, the frustration

---

[289] Michael Newton, *Journey of Souls.* Llewellyn, 1994.

begets *attachment,* as we cling to the fragile, temporary comforts of sense pleasures and family love. But even this can only work to a certain extent, and in time the last emotion, *fear* of losing the material pleasures of life, comes into play. The five-step process describes a sequence of descent from spirit to matter in emotional terms.

For example, imagine that I receive a gift of special chocolate, from Zurich, Switzerland (where chocolate is serious business!). I have loved chocolate ever since I visited my grandmother as a small child, and this reminds me of that wonderful time in my childhood, in addition to being delicious right now. I savor each bite and have a blissful moment with my chocolate (ether element), but with a wistful edge because I miss my departed grandmother. Soon I notice there are not so many pieces left, and I want more (air element). I try to shop for it but the stores don't have the same kind (for this purpose let's say the Internet is down as well). I can feel myself getting anxious and trying harder (more air) to get some. Then as the supply is getting seriously low, I become frustrated (fire) at the unsuccessful search, and right then my wife discovers my stash and eats one of the remaining pieces; I try to stay cool, but inside I am more than a little upset (more fire). Now I am clinging (water element) to the few remaining pieces, and not feeling exactly affectionate with my wife (more water). Soon I am hunkered down (earth element), protecting the last pieces and afraid (more earth) that someone might take another one.

The sequence with my chocolate is the same as Stone's descent sequence. One emotion leads to the next, all the way down to fear and immobilization. It is also parallel to the ANS sequence, with high activity (sympathetic) devolving to immobility (parasympathetic) especially after my relationship with my wife is disturbed (social).

Stone also described the Yin return journey back to the Source in terms of the emotions. From the fear state of the earth element, in time there arises its complement, *courage*. We start to re-mobilize, regaining a sense of purpose and direction. This leads to the appearance of *discipline*, by which we begin to become immune to excessive focus on pleasure and create order in our personal lives, the realm of the water element. In the upward process, discipline is like having secure channels for managing water flow and avoiding floods. From this base a third emotional level can be attained, *responsibility*, in the fire element. Here we gain increasing capacity to be responsible in life and use willpower to manage worldly activities in a coherent way organized around self-realization and service to others more than fear. In time, this elevated state engenders a fourth level in the air element, generating *hope* and *idealism*. Here higher consciousness and more profound expression and sensitivity can be manifest. This leads to the fifth element, experienced in the emotions of *love, inspiration* and *devotion*. Again a sequential emotional process is described, this time as an ascent from matter back toward spirit.

| Emotions and the Five Elemental Stages | | |
|---|---|---|
| **Element** | **Descending** | **Ascending** |
| Ether | Grief | Devotion |
| Air | Desire | Idealism |
| Fire | Anger | Responsibility |
| Water | Attachment | Discipline |
| Earth | Fear | Courage |

We can complete the chocolate analogy with the reverse sequence. Luckily, in time, I recover my senses and start the upward path again. I snap out of immobility, realize that chocolate is not all that important, reconcile with my wife, become very industrious, get a great idea for making a chocolate business, and become a global chocolate tycoon and philanthropist supporting worthy idealistic causes.

The downward and upward sequence of the emotions has unfortunately occasionally been misinterpreted to imply a condemnation of Yang. Again, involution and evolution are equally essential for the "Journey of the Soul."

## Sensory and Motor in the Emotions

Stone used the words "sensory" and "motor," normally applied to nerve action, to also describe the two sides of Yin and Yang in the emotions. The motor function is the movement from blueprint through motivation into materialization. The sensory function is the information feedback movement from materialization through feelings back to blueprint. These cycles can also be described in psychological terms.

The feedback from the Yin sensory function is the primary way for the motor function to know if its action is successful. Ever fond of aphorisms, Stone said, "The senses open the way, and the motor impulses obey." [290] Therefore the Yin aspect has the real power, although it is more subtle when compared to the obvious force of the muscles. Without the moon, the sun cannot know itself. If the feedback is painful, the next impulse of the motor current will be adapted to seek a more successful result.

The act of eating provides a simple example, using nerve action as the familiar base. Our blueprint (mind) is preprogrammed to act to satisfy hunger. When we feel

---

[290] R. Stone, *Polarity Therapy, Vol. 1.* CRCS, 1986. Book 1, p. 70

hungry (sensory), we seek food (motor) and find it (more sensory). Our hands reach (motor again) out and touch the food, but perhaps it is too hot (sensory) and we pull back our hands (motor). The whole sequence is a recurrent feedback loop, experienced constantly in all aspects of life.

The situation is similar, but more complex, for emotional issues. Similar to biological needs, all children are "programmed" with basic subtle emotional needs. As in the food example, the motor currents initiate action to fulfill the needs, and the sensory currents guide adaptation by giving feedback on those actions. When the need is not met, the feedback loop tries an alternative action.

Using the Polarity hierarchy of needs based on the Five Elements (Chapter 5), the emotional necessities are the needs for security (earth), belonging (water), warmth (fire), inspiration (air), and expression (ether). All of these are given and received to varying degrees through parental love for the child.

Pia Mellody offers a model which fits nicely: the child is (and has a right to be) vulnerable (earth), dependent (water), imperfect (fire), immature (air) and valuable (ether).[291]

## Pia Mellody's "Inalienable Rights of the Child"

| The child has a right to be... | Symptom if denied | Element affected | Emotion |
|---|---|---|---|
| Vulnerable | Boundaries | Earth/Security | Fear |
| Dependent | Needs | Water/Belonging | Attachment |
| Imperfect | Reality | Fire/Warmth | Anger |
| Immature | Moderation | Air/Hope | Desire |
| Valuable | Self-esteem | Ether/Expression | Grief |

[291] Pia Mellody, *Facing Codependence*. Harper & Row, 2003. p. 113.

Young children spontaneously initiate motor activity to have their needs met, manifesting the five innate "rights" as they do. For example, babies spontaneously use facial and vocal expression to attract their mothers' attention and secure the emotional warmth and neurochemistry of "love." Actions for all the five levels of needs are undertaken in this way in a developmental progression. The nature of these actions is a function of the child's blueprint, which combines traits from that family and culture with traits common to all others of that gender and age-specific neurochemistry.

Immediately after conception, even long before birth, sensory messages begin to flow to the child. Motor actions go out and sensory feedback comes back in a continuous loop of Yang and Yin action and reaction. In theory, this will go on indefinitely in a smooth progression of ever-widening experience. Even under the best circumstances, resistance is inevitably encountered, and adaptations begin. In an optimum scenario, the resistance is always manageable; the longer a feeling of being overwhelmed can be delayed, the better, so the child's base of confidence will have time to solidify. Inevitably there will be frustration (after all, in the words of British poets Mick Jagger and Keith Richards, "You can't always get what you want") and modest resistance is essential for growth. Ideally the frustration should be in a manageable range and it should not include betrayal.

### Search for Love

In the child's pre-programmed motor-branch search for love in the five elemental categories, disappointments and traumas occur. Perhaps the parents do not feel secure themselves, so the sensory feedback indicates danger. Perhaps the child's innate qualities are denied, due to parental inability to function in a mature way and a lack of being reflected healthfully. Perhaps external factors intrude on the process. In a dysfunctional scenario, the sensory feedback is painful or unsatisfying, so a new adapted motor action is attempted. The process continues, motor and sensory constantly attempting to fulfill the inherent blueprint for love, but getting ever further from the expected experience with its profound ANS value.

Adapted strategies soon become habits. We form habits to at least make our lives more predictable. In laboratory experiments described by trauma expert Robert Scaer, animals will choose scheduled expected painful stimuli over random pains that may never happen.[292] Strategies that lead to love set the stage for successful emotional navigation later in life. Conversely, adaptive strategies that are unsuccessful in gaining love set the stage for lives of psychological pain. Mellody specifically identifies the types of adaptation that result from frustration of each of the five original motives, complete with the adult dysfunctional symptoms that inevitably result. Again, the symptoms appear as problems with: boundaries (earth), needs (water), knowing and expressing one's reality (fire), moderation (air) and self-esteem (ether).

Once we have established an adaptation, we don't analyze new situations on their own merits. Instead we use the skewed perspective of a now-distorted expectation. Our judgment may not mature past this moment of childhood emotional injury, as we become fixated and unable to move developmentally past that point, like the hypnotized patient left to cope after the hypnotist has gone, or like a needle stuck on an LP record track.

Accessing and reprogramming these subconscious blueprint level mental attitudes and expectations is a central goal of emotional therapy. The two-chair method is effective

---

[292] Robert Scaer, *8 Keys to Brain-Body Balance*. Norton, 2012. Scaer's books describe all these parasympathetic research items.

because the overall inertia of fixation is reduced. The specific times, people and situations that caused the fixation can be safely put in the other chair to re-establish flow.

### "Energy Blocks"

Adaptation also interrupts the cycle of involution and evolution. In the presence of pain, we block the reception of sensory feedback or withhold the expression of motor action. This can occur at four points in the cycle described in Chapter 3: the Yang side can withhold action or resist feedback, while the Yin side can block the receiving of action or distort the feedback. These problems can appear physically in the body as "energy blocks."

Overcoming the inertia of habitual patterns is a great challenge in healing the emotions. We deny the sensory input as part of our pain-management strategy. Because we are immersed in dysfunctional patterns, our patterns are largely invisible and difficulties seem to be just random events. We settle into an emotional range that is far short of our true potential for love, as we display when we answer the inquiry "How are you?" with a quick, "I'm fine," when sometimes we are not fine at all.

Thus the first priority in therapy is to become aware of how we are feeling, and to accept the reality of those feelings. Becoming aware, or "waking up" in Buddhist terms, is a way to get access to the blueprint, and lasting changes can then be made. The therapeutic process for the emotions is parallel to the larger "Journey of the Soul." Just as the soul eventually awakens to its plight of separation from its Source, the healing of emotional problems requires an awakening to their presence, and a restoration of movement instead of fixation. As we become aware of the pain of our dysfunctional family histories and regain a sense of movement, the quest for self-understanding can resume.

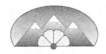

# Chapter 13

# Body Reading

The capacity to recognize the links between physical, emotional, and mental levels is extremely valuable from a Yin and Yang perspective. The general importance of the practitioner skill of recognition was discussed in Chapter 7. If you have no background in subtle anatomy, the material in this chapter is not essential, but the potential importance of body reading is clear. As author Deepak Chopra explains:

> Now we know that the mind and body are like parallel Universes. Anything that happens in the mental universe must leave tracks in the physical one. As you see it right now, your body is the physical picture, in 3-D, of what you are thinking.[293]

Body reading is well known and widely practiced in psychology, with attention being given mainly to useful interpretations about posture, authenticity and ANS states.[294] Body reading is also highly valued in Oriental medicine[295] and many alternative health care systems.

---

[293] Deepak Chopra, *Quantum Healing*. Bantam, 1990. p. 69

[294] For a concise summary, see: Pat Ogden, Kikuni Minton, Clare Pain, *Trauma and the Body: A Sensorimotor Approach to Psychotherapy*. Norton, 2008. pp. 189-190.

[295] Michio Kushi, *Your Face Never Lies: What Your Face Reveals About Your Health, An Introduction to Oriental Diagnosis*. Red Moon, 1976. Also see Lillian Bridges, *Face Reading in Chinese Medicine*. Churchill Livingstone, 2004.

Looking beyond the field of psychology, attorney Max Fulfer is highly valued in the legal field for his ability to predict potential jurors' dispositions; his book *Amazing Face Reading* is one of the best on the subject and its long bibliography covers the topic superbly. He notes, "Our faces provide a clear and accurate mirror of our life experiences."[296]

This chapter offers a different approach, body reading based on the Three Principles and Five Elements.

Body reading is a way to bypass a common problem, which is that a client's verbal reporting may be flawed or off-point. While the words coming from clients may lack self-awareness or be delusional, the body never lies. The verbal commentary from the mind may be confused or even intentionally misleading, but the body is almost incapable of deception.[297]

Through decades of testing, body reading has only continued to be validated. In a Yin and Yang approach, clients often express surprise at how quickly deep material is discovered. The efficiency is due to the fact that close observation of shapes and micro-movements reliably indicates how the Three Principles and Five Elements are in play, enabling the Yin and Yang practitioner to pose better questions and also to validate a client's answers.

The body reading method described here is used as a gentle indicator. Its goal is the prompting of self-understanding, not the diagnosis of disease. In India and China, however, body reading has a higher place. Virtually all traditional Asian health systems use some form of body reading involving some or all of many factors: blood or energy pulses, face, eye, ear, breath, voice quality, torso,

---

[296] Max Fulfer, *Amazing Face Reading*. Max Fulfer, 1996.

[297] Paul Ekman, *Telling Lies: Clues to Deceit in the Marketplace, Politics and Marriage*. Norton, 1985.

hands and feet. In some cases, these are very difficult for the Westerner to penetrate, as author and doctor John Thie noted:

> The Chinese physician can detect imbalances in meridians by feeling the pulses, but this is a sensitive touch, and it may take 10 to 20 years to develop proficiency with it.[298]

Similarly, Stone sought clear information from his patients by combining psychological and physical information. He called the resulting subject matter "psycho-physiology."

> Our research in Psychiatry would benefit greatly if we could reduce this jumble of man's mental-emotional impulses to an exact science of mental-emotional anatomy, coordinated with the physical one. Then a sound Psycho-physiology and even a Pathology of these finer energy fields could be established. This would be a great step forward in the science of understanding the mystery of man's complex being, which defies all present man-made rules and findings.[299]

Clearly, Stone advocated a psychology that can recognize subtle signals arising from clients "mental-emotional anatomy." Body reading is an excellent method for this purpose. Linking emotions and physicality supplies a way to connect obvious and physical information to its hidden and subtle origins. Thus, body reading can be seen as a "missing link" between physiology and psychology.

Polarity Therapy makes extensive use of body reading.[300] Stone's system is a composite of several traditions, and these do not always entirely agree with each other. The

---

[298] John Thie, *Touch for Health*. DeVorss, 1979. p. 17.

[299] R. Stone, *Polarity Therapy, Vol. 1*. CRCS, 1986. Book 3, p. 14.

[300] Julius Fast, *Body Language*. Evans, 2002. p. 151.

polarity model offers an umbrella to unify many different systems. Stone's work is an answer for the problems faced by earlier Western commentators on body reading. "What must be found is one common system that will work for all cultures and all ethnic groups."[301] There is enough confirmation by experience, to allow us to move forward. Body reading is not a be-all and end-all, the aim is more modest: to acquire useful and reliable information to move the therapy session forward efficiently.

The Three Principles archetypes can often be identified physically. Sun/tyrant/wimp and moon/doormat/critic have characteristic postures, voice tone, pacing and similar attributes.

### Yin and Yang in the Whole Body

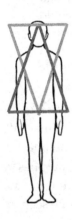

Human body shapes also reflect the great duality of Yin and Yang, with male characteristics (wider shoulders, external genitals) reflecting the Yang attributes, and female characteristics (wider hips, internal genitals) reflecting the Yin attributes.[302] The six-pointed star [303]has been used to represent the great duality of all phenomena, with the downward-pointing triangle used to describe the journey of Yang and the upward- pointing triangle used to describe the journey of Yin.

---

[301] Julius Fast, *Body Language*. Pocket Books, 1970.

[302] Michio Kushi, *The Book of Macrobiotics*, pp. 86-87, 9. Also see Naboru Muramoto's *Healing Ourselves*, pp. 8-9, 21-37.

[303] The topic of which triangle reflects which principle is a long-term curiosity: either direction could be justified. Medieval alchemists had Yin pointing down to Mother Earth and Yang pointing up to Father Sky. Macrobiotics uses the same directions. Similarly, Taoism sources note that fire (Yang) flows up and water (Yin) flows down. The description here reflects Stone's Polarity Therapy understanding, which highlights anatomy and the consciousness continuum of spirit and matter.

The upward and downward triangles suggest the basis of perception as well as the direction of focus and attention. Yang has a base in cerebral objectivity, and is moving toward physicalization, whereas Yin has its base in emotional sympathy in the pelvis and is moving upward toward awareness of larger forces through consciousness expansion in the head.

A five-pointed star has also been used to describe Yin. In this view, which is also a reflexology map of the torso, the upper point is at the throat, highlighting the importance of expression. At the south end is space, suggesting the power of attraction, as in the vacuum attraction of emptiness. Yin is therefore a story of empty space constantly being filled and then emptied by verbalization and expression of feelings.

Both five- and six-pointed star designs are packed with therapeutic applications and sacred geometry information and symbolism. These are worthy topics but beyond the scope of this book.

## Body Reading as a Small Town Grid

Polarity body reading is about identifying which Principle and Element might be used for connecting with the client. An analogy is figuring out where to meet a friend in a small town with a grid as its basic layout. To find the friend, we need an address, which consists of two coordinates, an avenue name and a number; the number tells us the cross street. There are three avenues in one direction (the Three Principles) and five streets (The Five Elements) in the other.

We use any of several cues to determine the "address." For example, male gender, loud voice, fast pace, forward lean, right-sided gestures, "hyper" states, concerns about money or actions relating to Yang roles (husband, father, boss, teacher) would all suggest Yang. Conversely, female gender, soft voice, rearward lean, left-sided gestures, "hypo" states, concerns about feelings or actions relating to Yin roles (wife, employee, student) would all suggest Yin. Now we have the avenue!

Next we need to know what street. The location of an injury, the level of hand gestures around the torso, the topic of conversation and related cues supply a starting point. To do this we need to be familiar with the Five Elements in more detail than we have attempted to describe so far in this book.

Body reading is an intuitive art, not a precise science. There are no "right" answers; the process is more about making an educated guess and then experimenting to verify whether it is correct. "All roads lead to Rome;" even a wrong answer will nudge us closer to the right answer. The point is not about a medical diagnosis; it is more about synchronizing

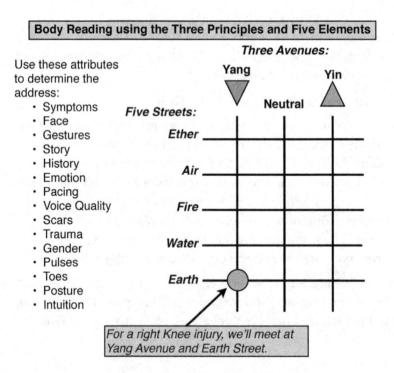

**Body Reading using the Three Principles and Five Elements**

Use these attributes to determine the address:
- Symptoms
- Face
- Gestures
- Story
- History
- Emotion
- Pacing
- Voice Quality
- Scars
- Trauma
- Gender
- Pulses
- Toes
- Posture
- Intuition

*Three Avenues:* Yang, Neutral, Yin

*Five Streets:* Ether, Air, Fire, Water, Earth

For a right Knee injury, we'll meet at Yang Avenue and Earth Street.

our perceptual process with our clients' reality so that they will feel heard, and in the company of a friend who appreciates them, rather than just a tourist.

For example, a person with an injury to the right knee might be considered to be at the intersection of Yang Avenue (because the injury is on the right side) and Earth Street (because the knee is an Earth Element location). The suspected emotions are something about tyrant/wimp for Yang and security/fear for Earth. With the two-chair method, this starting hypothesis could be investigated to efficiently get to what is happening for the client.

Numerous cues can be used, as listed on the left side of the chart. Symptoms, facial expressions, gestures and other indicators are reliable pointers to the underlying processes at work.

The first level of assessment is about symmetry and visible signs. For symmetry, the three dimensions are observed: right/left, back/front, top/bottom. Of these three, the right/left is often most obvious.

**Body Zones:** Like a bar magnet divided into pieces, the body's polarity relationships are maintained in subsections of the whole, with the Yang end at the north pole, Yin at the south pole and Neutral in the middle.

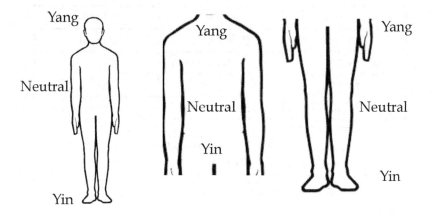

...the left is the side with which we take things in. It is receptive [Yin]. The right side is outgoing, expressive, the side with which we act [Yang].... The left side of the body (which is controlled primarily by the right side of the brain) is associated with feelings, emotions, and the relations to the mother. The right side is associated with the father, reason, thinking, logic. [304]

Which side of which dimension draws one's attention, and for what reason? A client may use the right hand when talking about one topic, then the left will become active when the subject changes. Similarly a client may gesture to touch one body area, left or right, when expressing a particular feeling. It is also common for the client to lean one way or the other, when a particular situation is being described.

For example, during a two-chair session, a client reported that her sensations were predominantly in the upper right (Yang) quadrant around the shoulder (Air Element), and she felt that her contact with the chair was more on the right.

|  | *Yang* | *Yin* |
|---|---|---|
| **Posture** | Lean forward | Lean rearward |
| **Voice** | Loud | Soft |
| **Tone** | Hyper | Hypo |
| **Gestures** | Right | Left |
| **Gender** | Male | Female |
| **Injuries, scars** | Right | Left |
| **Parental focus** | Father | Mother |
| **Topic** | Active, Career | Reflective, Spirit |

[304] Ron Kurtz and Hector Prestera, *The Body Reveals*. HarperCollins, 1984. p. 47. R. Stone, *Polarity Therapy., Vol. 1.* CRCS, 1986. Book 3, p. 29 and Ken Dychtwald, *Bodymind.* Tarcher Putman, 1986. p. 27. All these agree with this left-right categorization.

Using this observation, I suggested putting her father in the other chair and moved the conversation into a curiosity about "what she wanted," (the emotion of the Air Element) and what he wanted, in their relationship. Rather quickly, rich material was discovered and the session was beneficial. Later the client asked how I "knew" to have a dialogue with her father and about "wants," because she had not said anything about him. My answer was, "through body reading."

It is important to repeatedly emphasize that there are no right or wrong answers with body reading. In this case, the curiosity was about the client's own Yang energy just because of the rightward signals, and father is an archetypal representation of Yang. The session could have easily gone a different direction, and the value would still be present because the simple act of changing chairs begins pendulation no matter who is in the other chair.

---

### "The Outside reflects the Inside"
### and the Body reflects the Mind

According to Stone, physical signs are not accidental. Outward events reflect inner experiences. In this view there is no such thing as a random event. With body reading, we assume that all injuries, illnesses, gestures, shapes, lines and events have a significance, even though we are limited in the degree to which these may be understood.

> Life is from within, out. External trauma and effects are in the fields of the external nature, of mechanical skill and principles. *But the within rules the without.* All external happenings are precipitated by unperceived, internal (mental-emotional) causes. (R. Stone, *Polarity Therapy Vol. 1,* Book 3, p. 5).

It is a central premise of this approach that all events have a place and meaning. Using body reading gives a great advantage for therapists because inner issues are revealed much more efficiently.

---

Body reading is also about visible marks such as scars, injuries, distortions and decorations (such as tattoos). The fundamental question is about which area draws our attention.

Clients can be assessed when they are relatively still, but even more information becomes available when they move and speak. As described in the two-chair chapter, each autonomic state has a signature configuration that can be recognized by close observation. During conversation, the body is constantly in motion: which hand is used to express a feeling, where does it touch the body and what Principle-Element "intersection" is being indicated?

Similarly, Ron Kurtz and Pat Ogden have well-developed interpretations of posture, gesture and related systems.[305] Even without a Three Principles and Five Elements "energy anatomy," many psychotherapy systems use the basic approach.

### Body Reading for the Face

The face reflects current-time autonomic activity and is invaluable as a window into the client's true inner experience. As Kurtz put it:

> Of all the parts of the body, none is so directly
> expressive of a person as that complex unity of
> structure we call a face.[306]

In Yin and Yang-based therapy, we observe the client's face closely. Micro-movements and gestures can be subtle and easily missed, but they are entirely reliable. The "Truth

---

[305] Pat Ogden, Kikuni Minton and Clare Pain, *Trauma and the Body: A Sensorimotor Approach to Psychotherapy*. Norton, 2008. p. 167.

[306] Ron Kurtz and Hector Prestera, *The Body Reveals*. HarperCollins, 1984. p. 89

Wizards" research of Paul Ekman and colleagues[307] has advanced the study of micro-movements enormously. I greatly enjoyed the television series *Lie to Me* (2009, starring Tim Roth), especially the first few episodes, which were packed with educational examples of Ekman's method. However, I found myself wishing that Roth's character had known about energy anatomy, in addition to the muscles and facial expressions involved in truth detection. It was another "I wish I had been there" moment for me.

To interpret the face at an introductory level, we first look at left/right symmetry and at visible marks. The left/right comparison may be facilitated by covering one side of the client's face, then the other. Which side is contracted, as measured from corner of the mouth to the eye? Does one side

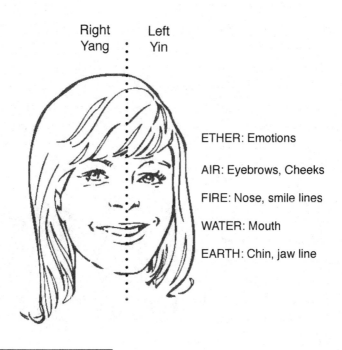

Right Left
Yang Yin

ETHER: Emotions

AIR: Eyebrows, Cheeks

FIRE: Nose, smile lines

WATER: Mouth

EARTH: Chin, jaw line

---

[307] Paul Ekman, *Emotions Revealed: Recognizing Faces and Feelings to Improve Communication and Emotional Life*. Holt, 2007.

convey a specific feeling more than the other? Very few faces are symmetrical, and the emotions expressed can be dramatically different when one side is hidden.

Horizontal zones (top to bottom) may be viewed generally or individually. What is the overall image? Which horizontal zone shows marks, scars, discoloration, loss of tone, creases or other unusual signs?

For specific zones, begin at the top. The area including the cheeks and higher to the eyebrows indicates the air element; its analogue in the body is the chest. The eyebrows reflect the shoulders and the upper cheeks reflect the breast/lung area. Dark circles under the eyes suggest kidney stress because the kidneys are the neutral pole of the air element. Air is manifested emotionally as desire, including hope and ambition. Thus, indicators in these areas of the face suggest desire (including hope or hopelessness) as an active area of interest.

Lower, across the nose and lower cheeks and the area above the mouth, is the zone for fire element; its analogue in the body is the solar plexus. The lines from the nostrils around the mouth reflect the line of the respiratory diaphragm at the lower ribs. The nostrils and tip of the nose are heart indicators; images of J. P. Morgan or W. C. Fields show dramatic heart/fire Element indicators. Emotionally unbalanced or stressed fire manifests as anger or "coldness," so deep lines or a swollen nose suggest these as active emotional issues.

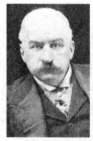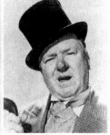

The mouth area and upper jaw reflect the status of the water element. The analogue for this area is the pelvis, including reproductive and digestive functions. The lips show the condition of the lower abdominal and genital area, with the upper lip related to Yang (outgoing, paternal) and lower lip related to Yin (receiving, maternal). The tip of the tongue also indicates sexuality and genital conditions. These may be observed closely when bodywork or emotional process therapy is underway. The mouth area may indicate activation of old emotions relating to attachment or sexuality.

Identification of the lips and tip of the tongue as genital reflexes has been described in several sources. Michio Kushi describes kissing as a reflexology substitute for sexual contact. Similarly, painting the lips bright red makes sense as a use of subliminal reflexology to stimulate sexual interest.

Reference to lipstick leads to other interpretations of makeup practices for subliminal signaling. Blue and green eye shadow on the eyelids are the elemental colors for ether and air (reflecting the emotions of loneliness and desire, respectively); rouge on the cheeks signals a reflex to the breast area, and so on. Similarly, the choices and locations of jewelry, piercings, tattoos and other ornamentation may be interpreted as subliminal statements. For example, the custom of wearing a gold wedding band on the left "ring" finger makes sense as an subconscious intention to stimulate the receptive Yin and the water element and its emotional aspect, attachment. Deployment of the middle finger on the right hand as a road rage gesture makes sense as expressing the Yang Principle and the Fire Element (anger). Full treatment of the whole topic of subliminal signaling is beyond the scope of this book, but endlessly fascinating.

The lower chin and jaw line is an analogue for the area at base of the spine and pelvic floor. Lines or marks here suggest tension relating to security or fear, the emotions managed by the Earth Element. Marks, loss of tone, different skin color and other cues indicate distress in this zone.

Putting these observations of the face together with the earlier left/right comparison enables us to make educated guesses about the individual. These can be developed as a basis for recognition, while being careful to avoid pathologizing. Which element (and therefore emotion) is indicated, and in which style or from what parent? Which areas in the torso are likely to be involved?

The eyes deserve special attention. Stone's commentary on the eyes identifies them as the positive poles of the Yang principle, "to give external direction for the internal impulses..."[308] More recent research has provided useful additional information on eye interpretation. Observing the eyes can reveal which part of the brain is activated,[309] how the person processes information and the level of stress that is present.

*Sanpaku*[310] is a Japanese term meaning "three whites," a condition in which the white sclera is visible below the iris (eye is rolled up, a Yin condition) or above the iris (eye is rolled down, a Yang condition), in addition to normal white showing on the two sides. Either of these suggests imbalance subsequent to trauma; extreme sanpaku suggests danger (Yin being danger to self, Yang being danger to others). Sanpaku also changes naturally with age, as the person moves from Yang to Yin position (Yang at the start in newborns, Yin at the

---

[308] R. Stone, *Polarity Therapy, Vol. 1.* CRCS, 1986. Book 1, p. 77.

[309] References for eye movement's relationship to brain activity include Tony Robbins (1997), Paul Dennison (1992), Gordon Stokes and Daniel Whiteside (1987). Reading the eyes is a major specialty in bodyreading, giving accurate information about unconscious or hidden feelings and brain function. The field of hypnotism has great understanding in this area. Stage hypnotism is a grass roots form of psychology and an early source for body reading information.

[310] Lillian Bridges, *Face Reading in Chinese Medicine.* Churchill Livingstone, 2004. p. 121. Also, see Michio Kushi, *Your Face Never Lies.* Red Moon, 1976.

end as death approaches). Babies are more Yin relationally but more Yang in terms of physical vitality: again, in the fullness of one is the seed of the other.

Eye flickering or twitching and poor eyesight suggest imbalance (excess or deficiency) of Yang energy. If the flickering is more on the right, it indicates stress relating to applying force and creativity to a situation and, more remotely, to Father. If on the left, it suggests stress relating to receiving creative energy or authority and experiences of mother.

### Body Reading for the Torso

"Reading" the language of the torso repeats the basic approach described for the face. However, the torso also has additional variables including posture, breathing and expressive movements.

One of the best ways to access this information is to imitate the body posture, to get an internal felt-sense of what the client is experiencing. As Moshe Feldenkrais observed,

> If one assumes the bodily attitude of another person, one can sense the meaning, have the feeling of, that body expression.[311]

The general guiding concept of looking at the right side for Yang indicators, and the left for Yin, continues to apply. In the torso, which hip is higher? Usually, the high hip indicates the side with greater stress. Similarly, which shoulder is lower? The diaphragm area can reveal signs of contraction, swelling or rigidity. Scars may be visible.

The idea of horizontal zones for each element, and of elements being associated with specific emotions can be applied again. Look at each horizontal zone and characterize its appearance with a few words. Is it expanded or

---

[311] M. Feldenkrais, *Body and Mature Behavior.* Frog Books, 2005. p. 93.

# Body Reading Head to Toe

*Watch closely when a person talks, to detect their authentic process. The body never lies! Hand gestures often point to the relevant area.*

| Body Area | Emotions & Notes |
|---|---|
| Face | The best, most accessible, most present tense area. Use reflexology, ANS and "Truth Wizards" (Paul Ekman) approaches. Tip of nose relates to heart, lips to sexuality. |
| Head | Mental processes, vision, "me-first" attitude; headaches often mean digestive trouble or lack of downward flow. |
| Eyes | Yang Principle; flickering eyelids means sympathetic ANS activation; poor eye contact means social ANS limitation. |
| Throat | The Ether Element, gateway to the emotions. Watch for grief, choice, discrimination, expression. Swallowing suggests managing the flow of feelings. |
| Neck | Stubbornness, dependability, forceful determination. |
| Shoulders | "Carrying the load" for self and others, communication skills. |
| Arms, hands, fingers | Defensive responses, non-verbal expressions, which elements |
| Chest | Love, desire, hope, inspiration; heart is the center of "I am" identity; breathing shift means ANS is active. |
| Solar Plexus | Will-power, frustration, irritability. |
| Abdomen | Digestion of life experiences, protection against vulnerability. |
| Kidneys | Ambivalence, managing binds: simultaneous "green light/red light." |
| Liver & Gall Bladder | Anger, resentment, bitterness. |
| Genitals | Sexuality, regeneration, secrecy. |
| Thighs | Muscular action including flight impulses, risk-taking. |
| Knees | Surrender, yielding, humility. |
| Calves | Reflex to abdomen and pelvis including colon. |
| Ankles | Linking mysteries with practicality. |
| Feet | Deep mysteries, connection to earth. |
| Toes | Each toe relates to a Three Principles/Five Elements address. |

contracted? What is the tone of skin and muscles? Are there unusual marks or distortions? Are there scars or injuries? Then, refer to the table of emotional correlates of the Elements to recall what emotion relates to the area. With this information, we can formulate an hypothesis which combines the descriptive words with the relevant emotions, possibly also in terms of Yang (right side) or Yin (left side).

For example, a caved-in chest (air) might reflect sunken hopes and lost desire. A rigid or swollen solar plexus (fire) could indicate withheld or chronic anger. A swollen pelvis (water) can suggest excessive enmeshment and holding on. Tightened buttocks with locked knees, and tight walk (earth) could reflect chronic anxiety or fear.

Torso body reading can be combined with the earlier observation of the face. A good way to do this is to look in a mirror at one's own face, then look at the torso, with a curiosity about whether the patterning is similar or different. There may be correlations between the face and torso, indicating more evidence for a particular hypothesis.

Observing the torso in motion offers additional information. When asking a probing question, the classic being, "Give three adjectives describing your mother," the

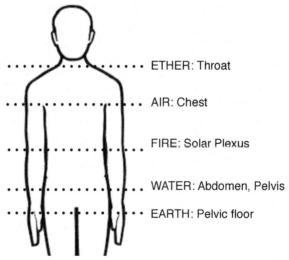

ETHER: Throat

AIR: Chest

FIRE: Solar Plexus

WATER: Abdomen, Pelvis

EARTH: Pelvic floor

client might spontaneously and involuntarily touch the solar plexus, throat or any other torso location, signaling which Element is relevant emotionally.

In addition to the left/right and horizontal zone analysis described for the face, the whole person is considered. Author Tony Robbins identifies eight main areas to watch in body reading: breathing, eye movement, lower lip size, posture, muscle tone, pupil dilation, skin color/reflection and voice.[312] Breathing, eye movement, posture and voice are particularly easy to observe, giving accurate and useful signals.

**Breathing** indicates the measure of participation in life and whether a person is "holding back" (over- or under-expansion, a Yang stress condition) or "holding on" (over- or under- contraction, a Yin stress condition). Some effective therapies dwell entirely on the expansion and balancing of breath. Spontaneous (involuntary) shifts of breathing, such as a sudden sigh or abrupt exhalation, indicate that the ANS has just changed in its regulatory activity.

**Posture** is a major area. The unique upright stance of humans allows a delicate blending of gravitational response and subtle "moving toward" vs. "moving away from" positioning, expressing a person's psychological attitude. This idea has been developed in great detail by Stanley Keleman,[313] Ron Kurtz, Pat Ogden and others. The use of the arms and hands, the carriage of the shoulders, spine and pelvis, the style of gait and postural cues can all be interpreted valuably. Alexander Lowen classifies posture in two general categories that mesh well with Yin and Yang theory. He characterizes mankind as having two general styles of motivation, aggression (to push, Yang) and longing

---

[312] Tony Robbins, *Unlimited Power.* Free Press, 1997. p. 328.

[313] Stanley Keleman, *Emotional Anatomy.* Center Press, 1989.

(to pull, Yin). He found a direct reflection in the spine: those too insecure to act (a Yang stress indicator) have locked knees and rigid pelvis; those unable to successfully adapt to life's pressures (a Yin stress indicator) have rounded shoulders and a slumping neck, the "dowager's hump."[314]

Building on the theme of the duality of pulsation (expansion and contraction, or Yang and Yin) Keleman shows a continuum of postural change from resistance to exhaustion, from youthful ambition to elderly fatigue.

**Hand placement** is an important part of postural body reading. The hands will move naturally to the zones where emotions are activated, either to suppress or release expression. When the hands are crossed over the solar plexus, a diaphragm stress (fire/anger) is indicated; when touching the hips (water), enmeshment or abandonment; when touching the mouth, sexuality and clinging; when at the throat, expression or grief. Again, insight may be bolstered by replicating the posture, especially with the hands.

With the **Voice**, we can differentiate qualities of sound by tone and loudness. Lower tones indicate lower elements, greater loudness suggests more Yang. Furthermore, important cues for identifying elements involved can be found in pitch, speed and timbre: Beaulieu and Robbins, among others, offer detail in this area. Lowen emphasizes the therapeutic significance of voice quality:

> If a person is to recover his full potential for self-expression, it is important he gain the full use of his voice in all its registers and in all its nuances of feeling.[315]

---

[314] Alexander Lowen, *Bioenergetics*. Penguin, 1976. pp. 236, 250, 299.
[315] R. Stone. Polarity Therapy, Vol 2, p. 271.

## *Body Reading for the Feet*

Body reading of the feet is very interesting and rewarding. According to Stone, the feet and particularly the toes represent the oldest shapes in the system, and therefore they can be indicators of ancestral legacies and early years with mother and father. The shape of each toe indicates the chronic condition of the corresponding element, including related emotions, with left for the maternal legacy and right for the paternal.

> These living current areas divide the body into five zones or fields of receptivity, like the use of the five senses over the five fingers and toes on each side of the body, over which they actually flow. This is a vertical classification of areas of response of the five energy currents operating in the body.[316]

> The bones and the joints of the fingers and toes often give a hint in diagnosis, where everything else is obscure and indefinite, and the patient merely exists and suffers. This is nature's own finger of diagnosis and indication, and not mere theory. It reveals the disrupted relationship of the extremities on the surface with the centers of energy within, in the particular region specified by the finger or toe.[317]

Correspondences depicted by Stone[318] show earth, water, fire, air and ether centers represented by toes in sequence, from small to large. In this context, "shape" means tone (circulation, flexibility, presence of calluses or bunions), alignment (location, direction, whether one toe is parallel to other toes), and symmetry (size and shape compared to other toes). "Chronic" in this situation refers to long-term family patterns inherited both genetically and emotionally.

---

[316] R. Stone, *Polarity Therapy Vol. 2.* CRCS, 1986. p. 33.

[317] R. Stone, *Polarity Therapy. Vol. 1.* Book 3, CRCS, 1986. p. 39.

[318] *Ibid.*, p. 37. The arrangement is repeated concisely in the chart on pages 9 and 127 of Book 2.

## Sample Toe Reading

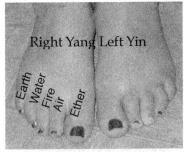

Water toe is the most curved, slightly more on the left: meet at Yin Ave. & Water St.

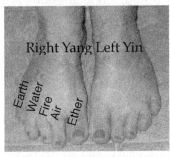

Fire toe is most curved, on the right: meet at Yang Ave. & Fire St.

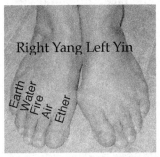

Ether toe on the left is most curved: meet at Yin Ave. and Ether St. Note there was an ankle injury on the right

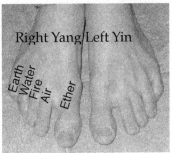

Earth toe on the left is more curved: meet at Yin Ave. and Earth St. Note the space between big toe and the rest, slightly more on the left, suggests separation of feelings from conscious awareness.

Precipitation [the coalescence into density from subtlety] occurs most often here [the foot] because of its great distance from the invigorating center.[319]

The body suffers as an innocent bystander, not as the causative factor. But it gets all the blame because effects and end products accumulate there as precipitates of highly emotional chemical action.[320]

As indicated in preceding chapters, emotions are identified by Stone in his "Enquiry into the Gross Body" charts;[321] Earth/Fear, Water/Attachment, Fire/Anger, Air/Desire and Ether/Grief. In addition, Stone goes much further with the Elements, describing how each element has three "personalities" and related three-part body locations. These additional archetypal attributes of the Elements are beyond the scope of this book, but well worth study for readers who want more energy anatomy.

Of course, most psychotherapists never see the toes, unless the client is wearing sandals. Some useful information is therefore not available, but the face, torso and gestures are likely to be sufficient to enable a Three Principles/Five Elements interpretation.

For those seeking more, other resources are available in print[322] and online.[323]

---

[319] *ibid.*, p. 38.

[320] *Ibid.*, p. 33.

[321] Stone, *Polarity Therapy, Vol. 2*, CRCS, 1986. pp. 222-223.

[322] John Chitty and Mary Louise Muller, *Energy Exercises*. Polarity Press, 1988; also, Bruce Berger, *Esoteric Anatomy*. North Atlantic, 1998.

[323] See www.energyschool.com.

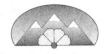

# Conclusion

Psychology has made great strides in understanding the material processes of disease, with a steady stream of new discoveries in neuroscience, genetics, technologies, pharmaceuticals and techniques. If the Yin and Yang model is valid, the holistic mental health care of the future will add important new tools to its arsenal. Each perspective offers extraordinarily useful approaches.

• **Yin:** Allowing health to emerge from the inside-out offers ways to restore the ANS to its original functioning. Resilience increases, recovery times are faster, and the physical body functions better when Yin is brought into the foreground. The centerpiece of the Yin health care strategies will be supporting movement as the basis for health instead of fixation: "Running water clears itself."[324]

• **Yang:** Intervening to correct fundamental errors, a Yang understanding offers specific methods for restoring the ANS, particularly in the area of relationships. Yang approaches use conscious intention and studious reference to the principles of Yin, Yang and Neutral. Instead of wandering around in the dark, randomly bumping into obstacles in a vast experiment, a sense of direction becomes possible and stress levels go down naturally. When disturbances arise, there can be at least a point of reference to start to understand what happened.

---

[324] R. Stone, *Polarity Therapy, Vol. 1.* CRCS, 1986. Book 1, pp. 60, 85.

• **Neutral:** Restoring flexibility and graceful ease in adapting to daily challenges, Neutral offers liberation from fixation, the root cause of disease. Neutral includes taking some time each day for quiet contemplation of the circumstances, feelings and impulses of life. Ideally, the quiet time includes appreciation of some aspect of experience: beauty, nature, kindness, authenticity, service and love are good places to start. Adding this practice to daily life will help re-set the ANS in preparation for the inevitable next swings of the dynamic flow of Yin and Yang.

> The secret to learn here is for man's consciousness to remain still in the CENTER OF BEING, in its eternal Essence. Then things will right themselves. The Holy Bible states this in simple terms: "Be still, and know that I am God." (Psalm 46:10).
>
> The whole body recuperates when life's Central Energy is permitted to flow naturally, without interference by our own mind's desires, etc. Faith, based upon this understanding, holds the mind in check and tunes it into the field of Power and Reality. All things are possible to such a belief of REALITY within us.
>
> Paracelsus, the great alchemist, observed this also when he stated that man is ill because he is never still. He said there was great healing in the quiet depths of space, but man never tuned into it by being quiet himself![325]

---

[325] R. Stone, *Polarity Therapy, Vol. 1.* CRCS, 1986. Book 1, p. 47.

# Epilogue

## "How I Got Here"

I grew up on a college campus, the University of the South in Sewanee, Tennessee, where my parents were administrators. They were notable for their open-minded intellectual curiosity and dedication to their social and educational causes. As a child, I experienced my parents hosting visitors from Europe, Africa, Korea, India and other faraway places, and our living room was often a salon for multi-cultural conversations. My parents' home was deeply religious (Sewanee is an institution of the Episcopal Church) and my parents were ardently pro-civil rights, so pro- and anti-establishment ideas were always present, often simultaneously; in national elections my parents often voted for opposite candidates. During my years in high school (my high school was military, church, all-male, all-Caucasian), the Vietnam War was flaring up. It was openly debated as to its moral, political and economic justifications, so my perspective started to widen beyond just the small pond of Sewanee.

I attended college in the peak years of counter-cultural fervor, Princeton University in 1967-1971. It was a magical time of seemingly unlimited possibilities, mixed with experimental pushing of boundaries in all directions; I consider myself lucky to have survived some of the experiments. I met my life partner, Anna, in college; she arrived in the first wave of coeducation when, after 200 years of being all-male, my first two years, Princeton opened its doors to women, my second two years. My senior thesis was about Marshall McLuhan and how perception/consciousness is affected by media; my wife's thesis was about Zen Art and

Surrealist Art, studying consciousness from two complementary, vastly different angles. Her thesis was a brilliant comparison of disparate thinkers coming to similar conclusions, foreshadowing what was to follow for both of us.

At the time of graduation, I was at a loss about what to do next. I acquired a teaching certificate, interned for a summer at a law office and tried my hand at journalism, but I was too immature to make a go at any of these. In the words of biologist Jos Verhulst in *Developmental Dynamics*, I "avoided specialization" for an unusually long time. In evolution theory, postponing specialization has many advantages.

After college, contemplating society from a distance (now married, we lived on a remote island off the coast of British Columbia for seven years), my explorations in mysticism continued expansively, based on books such as *Be Here Now* by Ram Dass, *Autobiography of a Yogi* by Paramahansa Yogananda and *Foundations of Tibetan Mysticism* by Lama Anagarika Govinda. I was entranced by the *I Ching* and even had the audacity to create a hexagram in public at our wedding ceremony in 1973; what was I thinking? Luckily it yielded something auspicious, hexagram 14. I dabbled in hatha yoga and shiatsu, and studied Macrobiotics with Michio Kushi. I sampled the fields of anomalous science (such as *Chariots of the Gods* by Erich von Däniken and *Biological Transmutations* by C. Lewis Kevran) and the most far-out of psychic phenomena literature (such as *The Third Eye* series by Lobsang Rampa). I lived in three different Utopian intentional communities, for 18 years. I was gifted with a meditation practice; it found Anna, who conveyed it to me.

All these diverse strands came together for me in 1979 when, at Anna's instigation, we took a weekend seminar in Polarity Therapy, featuring the two-chair process: Fritz Perls'

Gestalt Therapy combined with Dr. Stone's cosmology and energy anatomy. Polarity combined all my interests in one package; we stayed for the full practitioner training spanning eleven months residential, full-time six days a week, an extended immersion education that is unheard-of nowadays. Dr. Stone had already retired to India, so I never met him in person; he died in 1981, at the age of 91. We experienced Polarity Therapy's amazing effectiveness first-hand as groups of 10 to 20 people rotated through for seven-week programs. Complex personal challenges were explored and resolved rather efficiently in the two-chair method of "Polarity Counseling," the name that gradually stuck for me.

I spent 10 years as a close observer of the four Polarity methods (bodywork, diet, exercise, counseling) in action especially at Murrieta Hot Springs Resort where Anna was director of educational and therapeutic programs. As the years progressed I kept studying and adding more ideas. I worked for natural health pioneer Dr. Evarts Loomis (1910-2003), "father of holistic medicine," at his Meadowlark Center, immersing myself in psychology, the interconnections of mind and body, dream interpretation, homeopathy and naturopathy. "Miracle healing" became commonplace.

In 1989, I met Franklyn Sills, who illuminated the profound, paradigm-busting "inherent treatment plan" indirect approach of biodynamic craniosacral therapy. In the 1990s I became involved in the American Polarity Therapy Association, serving five terms as president. I heard about Peter Levine in 1993 and created a slide presentation of his ideas, still used today, to fill the void before his debut book *Waking the Tiger*. In 2003 I met Jaap van der Wal, with his deep insight into the meaning of life as demonstrated by embryological development.

As I added more sources, I kept looking for more information; if a modality is out there I have probably tried it at least a little. However after all these decades of gathering, I still have yet to find a model so all-encompassing as Dr. Stone's Polarity Therapy.

From a historian's perspective, Stone's achievement is astonishing. He cast such a wide net, recognizing that the ancient wisdom traditions really were on to something with their Yin and Yang model, at a time when these ideas were unknown in the America of the 1940s and 1950s. If anything, the breadth of Stone's multi-cultural findings has always been daunting for students, who struggle to wrap their heads around such vast and comprehensive explanations. The scope of his vision reminds me of how Sleeping Beauty was surrounded by a thorny hedge, as if to separate the deeply inquisitive from the mildly curious.

Throughout these years, I taught Polarity to small groups, maintained a private practice, and continued my research. I also held several day jobs, to support my family. Being a husband and father was a preeminent learning experience, providing a never-ending laboratory for application of theories and refinement of methods. I wish I had known at the beginning what I had learned by the end, but that is not the way of nature.

In more recent years, I also observed that my lineage of Polarity Therapy ("Alive Polarity") was gradually fading as my generation aged and the handful of still-active teachers moved on to more specialized interests. At this time, I am not aware of any of the old Alive Polarity teachers still conducting educational events about the two-chair method, so it has become an endangered species.

Then in 2010, I was pronounced to have a serious medical situation, asymptomatic "stage 4 d2" prostate cancer with metastatic infection of lungs and bones. Both of my grandmothers died of hormone-driven cancer of a similar category, and both my parents also had episodes of cancer. I was not eligible for the normal treatment including surgery, radiation or chemotherapy due to lack of a clear target, and I was therefore pushed to an intensive alternative regimen including strict anti-cancer nutrition (Stone's purifying diet, no sugar, low carbohydrates and related naturopathic practices), oxygen therapy, supplements and treatments, hormone therapy and the invisible world treatments of Tao Master and Doctor Zhi Gang Sha, to whom I am especially grateful. Having such a diagnosis is like a near-death experience, but in slow motion.

This book is partially a result of that process. I had always thought that someday I might try to record what I had learned, "later." Under these conditions it appeared that there might not be a "later." My hand was forced by events to face facts and "just do it" even though I still do not feel qualified. With the phrase "bucket list" now having more meaning, I felt motivated to at least try to pass along the knowledge of my lineage and experience in case it might be useful for future travelers.

So there you have it, "in a nutshell," as Robert Fulford, DO, champion of being nice to babies, used to say. At the time of this writing I feel well and the medical emergency seems to be reduced. My wish is that young people might somehow catch the spark that illuminated my life experience and carry it into the future where its full potential might be realized: Stone's vision of a truly full-spectrum health care including both *treatment* as we have today but also *prevention* based on a deep understanding of the laws of nature and the purpose of life.

# Appendix A

## Considerations for Polarity Therapists

Randolph Stone spent decades seeking the common ground among the wisdom traditions and brought that multi-cultural synthesis into modern medicine, with excellent results. His Polarity Therapy effectively addresses the need for a big-picture umbrella to create a health care perspective that is unified, secular and multi-cultural.

In addition to his medical training, Stone was a lifelong, avid student of mysticism and esoteric philosophies. His writings are a collection of ideas and experience, following his motto, "Whatever works, works!" He backed up his theoretical studies with practical applications, operating a successful general medicine practice in Chicago for over 50 years, in the period 1924-1974. As stated at the beginning, he even advertised to his medical colleagues in the region, "Send me your hopeless cases."

Polarity Therapy provides a useful support for applying Yin and Yang to psychology, but polarity is not a necessity; the concepts and methods stand on their own merits and can be called whatever seems appropriate in any setting. Polarity is used here as a framework, but the value is bigger than the professional category. This distinction has been termed "Big Polarity" (the universal principles) vs. "Small Polarity" (the specialized modality) by polarity teachers such as John Beaulieu, Jim Feil, Phil Young and Urs Honauer. Any health care system can benefit by adding the Yin and Yang perspective, whether or not Stone's work is involved or even known.

Polarity Therapy has esoteric ideas that may be problematic for people who are not receptive to mysticism and "energy medicine." However, these ideas also do not need to be adopted for the methods to work. The methods have stood the test of time and deserve recognition and at least experimental consideration.

## *The need for "Polarity Counseling"*

For those who approach the topic of counseling from a background in Polarity Therapy, this book has a specialized intention: to raise counseling to its rightful place in the field. The four knowledge areas in the Stone's system, or "four legs of the polarity chair," encompass a wide range of skills and applications. Best known is bodywork, with hands-on methods to balance and restore energy's natural flow. Exercise and diet are the second and third methods, less well known but alive and well in the Polarity Therapy world with books and videos to support their continued growth.

But Polarity's implications for psychology and the practice of counseling have languished, in spite of Stone's firm assertion that the mind, feelings and body are inseparable and that mental/emotional experiences often develop into physical manifestations. Stone clearly knew the importance of mental/emotional support: "…40 to 60 percent of all diseases have a psychosomatic origin…"[326] He wrote extensively about the causes of human suffering, the power of the mind, mind-body interdependence and related topics. Based on the sheer volume of information offered, a Polarity Therapy practice should include ways to address psychological and emotional dimensions of health conditions.

Despite its central place in the theory, psychotherapy is the least known polarity skill set and is relatively absent in print or any other media. The Polarity literature, including about 20 books, barely mentions mental-emotional therapy at all. Similarly, "communication and facilitation" make only a small appearance in the *Standards for Practice and Education* of

---

[326] R. Stone, *Polarity Therapy, Vol. 1*, CRCS, 1986. Book 2, Chart 44.

the American Polarity Therapy Association,[327] when practitioner skills of empathy and resonance are discussed. The profound psychological applications of Stone's legacy deserve a better fate.

### Reasons for the Absence of Counseling from the Literature

Stone did not write much about applying his energy principles to psychotherapy. He definitely used counseling methods, both direct and indirect, but he did not give much in the way of solid instructions. Among several factors, his work took place before the full significance of trauma was understood; in 1950 trauma resolution had not been much developed.[328] Psychotherapy was considered to be a process of analyzing subconscious factors, strengthening will power, clarifying goals and creating more functional habits. These are all worthy aims and effective to varying degrees, but major discoveries that came later have transformed the profession. Stone's relative lack of practical commentary about psychology and psychiatry reflects the limited knowledge of his time.

Meanwhile, two modern trends in health care have complicated the situation: increasing regulation of all therapy and increasing specialization.

**Regulation:** The eminently worthwhile purpose of consumer protection comes with a high price. In some jurisdictions, practitioners who touch their clients cannot talk to them and practitioners who talk cannot touch. In effect the separation of mind and body, so contrary to common sense and antithetical to Stone's holistic vision, is systematized by some aspects of professional regulation.

---

[327] See www.polaritytherapy.org.

[328] The American Psychiatric Association formally recognized "trauma neurosis" for the first time in 1952, in its DSM-1, thereby creating the first formal pathway for treatment.

**Specialization:** The world has moved toward increased specialization, even though it is not necessarily conducive to effectiveness or innovation. Clients see one practitioner for help with structure, another for circulatory problems, another for emotional stress relief, another for nutritional advice. Aside from the added expense and trouble of having to find and deal with different practitioners, an obvious shortcoming with this approach is that information acquired by one specialist is unlikely to be fully shared with the others due to time and other constraints. In addition, the treatments might not all be supportive of each other. Obviously specialization is needed to keep up with the constant expansion of information, but again something important is being lost.

Specialization has also led to a parallel trend: the increasing disempowerment of clients. Stone's vision was the opposite: a grassroots, common-sense health care that all people could comprehend and practice for themselves. In his words,

> Is it not possible for man to keep well by doing a
> few simple things daily and by living less
> strenuously? The answer is yes.[329]

Polarity Therapy goes against the grain of the modern trends, valuing general, multi-dimensional knowledge over specialization. Stone himself held at least eight different professional certifications; he was a generalist in the fullest sense of the word.

This book is therefore intended to be helpful for the layman, in addition to healthcare professionals of all categories and modalities, in the hope that psycho-emotional wellness need not always require complex strategies and expenditures. Support from skilled professionals will always have major significance, especially in extreme dysfunctions,

---

[329] R. Stone, *Health Building*. CRCS, 1985. p. 101.

but in this approach the client can "own" more of his or her wellness. Prevention can be raised to a status that is equal with treatment. Personal responsibility can offer a real solution to the enormous complexity of modern health care, with its ever-increasing costs, technological-pharmaceutical dominance and socio-economic injustices due to unevenly distributed access.[330]

This book seeks to explore Yin and Yang principles in counseling, assuming that the trends of regulatory environment and specialization are separate issues. Polarity Therapy practitioners can figure out for themselves how to accommodate these trends in their own specific professional situations. For Polarity practitioners, the primary concern here is that the concept of a Yin and Yang-based psycho-emotional therapy, that can add value to a holistic general practice, should not be lost just because the trends are flowing in the other direction. The counseling ideas in this book are safe and effective for addressing and resolving a host of conditions and problems, while also being very low-risk for both practitioner and client, and often less difficult for the practitioner compared to some other psychotherapy models.

---

[330] For a thorough analysis of the cost problem, see *Time Magazine*, "The Bitter Pill." March 2013.

# Appendix B

## Embryology and Morphology
## Confirm the Three Principles

According to anatomist Jaap van der Wal, living form and structure arise from motion and process. In closely observing the movements of development, we find clear support for the Three Principles as the foundation of form and function. Embryology is particularly valuable for the purpose because the body is in its most simplified state.[331] The earliest origins of what will later become systems, organs and tissues show Yin, Yang and Neutral in their most essential nature. Because these three are present at the start, and everything that follows is built from them, we can expect to find them later, at all scales of size and complexity of organization, including psychology.

The developmental process begins with the most polarized cells in the body, male sperm and female egg. We have discussed these as defining principles in their own right, as embodiments of Yang and Yin, respectively. After union, there is a 24-hour pause, a time of stillness, that can be interpreted to represent the Neutral Principle. Already, in the first moment and day of existence, the Three Principles are the essence of our organization and anatomical development.

The next step is cell multiplication. This phase is not cell division or mitosis, but rather metameric cell division,

---

[331] Jaap van der Wal, *Embryology: Where Biology Meets Biography.* 8-disk DVD set. CSES, 2005. Also, see van der Wal's chapters (8 and 9, p. 137 ff.) in *Biodynamic Craniosacral Therapy, Vol. 1,* by Michael Shea. CRCS, 2007. Also, van der Wal wrote Chapter 4 (*Dynamic Morphology and Embryology* (p. 87) ) in G. van der Bie and M. Huber, Editors, *Foundations of Anthroposophical Medicine* (Floris, 2010). van der Wal's web site www.embryo.nl is also an excellent resource.

involving unspecialized duplication. The zygote does not actually expand, it self-organizes into a multi-cellular body. This continues through the first week as we are moved through the fallopian tube down to the uterus for implantation. Implantation is a mutual process between our mothers and ourselves (called the zygote at this stage), and it brings us to finding a nest embedded in our mother. Once we are in position, another Three Principles miracle ensues, the first differentiation of cells.

Embryologically, all cells in the body derive from three basic "germ layer" groups, and these align perfectly with the Three Principles:

**Ectodermal** cells orient to the outside world, using the senses and thinking to perceive and comprehend external factors. These cells give form to the Yang functions.

**Endodermal** cells orient to the inner world, including digesting and metabolizing nutrients. These cells give form to the Yin functions.

**Meso-**[332] cells provide the filling between the inner and outer worlds, and the bulk of the body. Two tissue groups in particular, the heart and fascia, epitomize the principle of Neutral. The heart manages inward and outward circulation, (discussed next). The fascia simultaneously connects and separates space throughout the body.

### Origins of the Three Germ Layers

For more detail about the origins of the three germ layers, a step-by-step description is helpful. The cells that are closest to mom's blood supply grow more quickly because of closer proximity to nourishment, and cells on the other side grow more slowly. Out of this differentiation arise two of the

---

[332] The common term "mesoderm,"meaning "middle skin" is not correct because there is no skin, or defining inside-outside surface.

three great tissue groups, epiblast and hypoblast, layers that will later become known as *ectoderm* and *endoderm*. Ectoderm will specialize further to become the nervous system, sense organs and skin representing the principle of the "outside" or parietal body wall. These Yang tissues are about our relationship with the outside world. Endoderm will specialize further to become the inner lining of the digestive and respiratory tracts, representing the principle of the "inside" or visceral body wall. Yin tissues are about one's relationship with the inside world. Where these two polarized principles are present, Neutral is also present, in the form of meso-tissue. Meso-tissues form the bulk of the body: bones, muscles, fascia and blood, the in-between of the body, balancing and managing outside and inside factors.

These two tissue groups continue to cell-divide for the next weeks, leading to a form that looks like two soap bubbles joined together, one for ectodermal cells and one for endodermal cells. Then the Neutral principle reappears. Newly-specializing cells arise in the periphery and flow to the core: these new cells will become the *meso-* tissues, beginning with the blood and heart and continuing to form the majority of our tissues including bones, muscles and fascia. The first appearance of meso- is the mesenchyme, primitive connective tissue with the dual capacity to connect as well as shape (separate or define) space. The symbolism of our being mainly composed of Neutral is inspiring, elevating the importance of gracefully managed and balanced flow between two complementary poles as the central theme of functionality. What is true physically is also true psychologically.

Each step in the sequence lends itself to profound interpretations. Gradually the three axial dimensions become visible: first to appear is front-back (Yang, according to Stone), and next is bottom-top (Yin). Last is left-right

(Neutral), on about the 14th day, as the primitive streak forms bulges on either side of the midline.

Interestingly, the first three tissue organs to appear are the heart, (Neutral, meso-, on about the 18th day), then next the beginning of the nervous system as the neural tube closes (Yang, ecto-) and finally the liver and primeval gut (Yin, endo-), a few days later. The primacy of the Three Principles arrangement is confirmed again and a new sequence is implied. First is the Neutral field of action, then the first Yang push of the pendulum, then the Yin return swing. van der Wal teaches that there are three "heads:" heart, brain and gut, in that order, and they are formed by three toroidal tubes (vascular tube of the heart loop, neural tube and gut tube).

## *Morphology also Demonstrates the Three Principles*

Another anatomical perspective is derived from the interpretation of body shapes, a field of study known as morphology. Jaap van der Wal uses a fist to differentiate morphology from anatomy. Anatomically, a fist is a list of tissues and relationships; morphologically it is a gesture that could mean determination, defiance, anger or other emotional states.

Many authors have contributed insights in this field,[333] and the Three Principles are often observed in the descriptions.

A fundamental observation about human form is that it is substantially composed of "Radials" and "Spheres." This appearance is seen at the start with sperm and egg, respectively, as essence of Yang and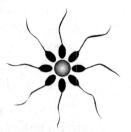

---

[333] Johannes Rohen, *Functional Morphology, the Dynamic Wholeness of the Human Organism*. Adonis, 2007. Also: Jos Verhulst, *Development Dynamics in Humans and Other Primates: Discovering Evolutionary Principles through Comparative Morphology*. Adonis, 2003.

Yin. Later in life, the cranium has the appearance of a sphere, and the limbs are radials or rods. These two interact, with rods becoming spheres (the rod-like ribs together creating the sphere-shaped thorax) and spheres becoming rods (the vertebrae each with a circle for the spinal canal together form the spinal column). Meanwhile Neutral can be observed in the center of spheres, such as the center of the spinal vertebral bodies, the brain's core and the heart.

The point of all this is to add more evidence that Yin, Yang and Neutral are at the very foundation of human organization. Projecting Yin and Yang to mental and emotional experience is just a further extension of the underlying basic design. All life exists in a matrix of cyclic expansion and contraction, out from the core to the periphery and then back. "Yin and Yang" describes not just momentary phenomena such as personality or behavior, it is an understanding of the whole ebb and flow of life, the "breath of life" celebrated by teachers from throughout the medical arts, sciences and wisdom traditions.

Jaap van der Wal is fond of a particular image[334] (shown below) for the Three Principles manifesting in human form. Radials are fundamentally Yang and spheres are fundamentally Yin, but their appearances in the human body are often blends. Beginning with the general view that the bottom is Yin and the top is Yang, we find the fullness of one holding the seed of the other, repeatedly.

• **Yin:** The legs at the bottom are pronation-only radials pushing against the earth in order to walk.

• **Neutral:** The arms are adaptable for both supination and pronation. They also form the circle of a hug centered on the heart, and the gesture of prayer, for reunion with spirit.

---

[334] LFC Mees, *Secrets of the Skeleton: Form in Metamorphosis.* Steiner Books, 1984.

• **Yang:** The sphere-shaped cranium at the top has an inward (supination only) morphology but accommodates the outward sensory functions. The two mandibles (which are appendages like the arms and legs) turn inward, the mouth draws food inward and the brain spirals in on itself.

The result is a complete summary comparable to the Tao symbol of Yin and Yang. Leonardo Da Vinci, who speculated deeply about these ideas and came to similar conclusions in his famous "Vitruvian Man" sketch, would be proud!

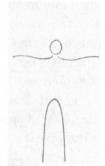

Vitruvian Man adaptation: Image from Jaap van der Wal, www.embryo.nl, based on Mees.

## Yin and Yang in Morphology

**Sphere**: Yin Principle
Examples of perfect spheres in nature:
Egg, Electron

**Radial**: Yang Principle
Examples: Sperm, Neurons & most bones

Radials (ribs) "performing" as a sphere to create the thoracic cavity

*Spheres & Rods in Ancient Yin/Yang Symbolism*

Above, the Egyptian Ankh; A frequent symbol in Egyptian hieroglyphics, it is translated as "fruitful union" and "eternal life."

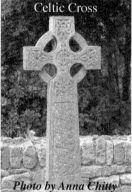

Celtic Cross

*Photo by Anna Chitty*

Spheres (vertebrae) "performing" as a rod to create the spine

# Appendix C
## The Heart Balances Yin and Yang

The heart plays a key role in the whole process of emotional experience. Esoterically, the heart manages the balance of Yin and Yang, including the ascending and descending cycles of the emotions and the involution-evolution process of the Journey of the Soul. The heart serves as the neutral midpoint between mind and body, Father Sky and Mother Earth.

The importance of the heart is well-understood in popular culture. We intuitively know what is meant with the dozens of heart references, all suggesting feelings: "hearty, heart-touching, heart-sick, disheartened, heart-to-heart." A further language clue appears in how "heart" is often used in emotional opposites, such as warm- or cold-hearted, soft- or hard-hearted, heartfelt or heartless and others. No other organ appears in language with even a fraction of the frequency of "heart."

Popular common sense knows something that science has a hard time quantifying. Modern medicine's materialistic view of the heart as only a physiological pumping machine is a serious error, and a reason that conventional treatment of heart disease (the top cause of death) remains incomplete. For example, the risk factors for heart problems[335] fail to account for over half of the cardiac cases,[336] but mainstream science has not yet come up with a theory to accommodate the data.

---

[335] http://www.nhlbi.nih.gov/educational/hearttruth/lower-risk/risk-factors.htm

[336] Paul Pearsall, *The Heart's Code: Tapping the Wisdom and Power of Our Heart Energy.* Broadway Books, 1999. Also, see: Dean Ornish, *Dr. Dean Ornish's Program for Reversing Heart Disease: The Only System Scientifically Proven to Reverse Heart Disease Without Drugs or Surgery.* Ivy Books, 1995.

## *The first problem: the heart is not just a pump*

Look up "circulatory system" or "heart" in any textbook and the first sentence is likely to describe the heart as a pump that pushes blood through the arteries, capillaries and veins to deliver oxygen- and nutrient-rich blood and evacuate waste products to and from the tissues of the body.

However, even a basic analysis of the mechanical requirements for this function lead to the conclusion that the supposed pumping is not possible. Numerous experts have pointed out the problem, to no avail.

> "Nowhere else in nature or in mechanics is manifested such a miracle of a pump the size of the owner's fist to circulate a semi-heavy fluid through miles and miles of the finest vessels and tubes, as the heart is supposed to do."[337]

> Modern analysis of the heart has shown that in spite of the fact that the most powerful ventricle of the heart can shoot water six feet into the air, the amount of pressure actually needed to force the blood through the entire length of the body's blood vessels would have to be able to lift a one hundred pound weight one mile high. The heart is simply incapable of producing the pressure actually needed to circulate the blood."[338]

The pump description prevails against overwhelming evidence to the contrary. What a commentary on modern culture's coexisting knowledge and ignorance, that so basic a situation is so misunderstood.

Significant problems with the "heart is a pump" model include:

---

[337] R. Stone, *Polarity Therapy, Vol. 2*, CRCS, 1986. Book 4, p. 30.

[338] Stephen Buhner, *The Secret Teaching of Plants: The Intelligence of the Heart in the Direct Perception of Nature*. Bear and Co., 2004. p. 75.

• Again, not nearly enough force is applied to accomplish the task. Moving a viscous fluid though more than 40,000 km of vessels requires a pushing force much greater than the measurable 1.5 watts exerted by the heart; to move the blood a force strong enough to lift 4,000 tons one meter annually has been estimated.[339]

• A pump works efficiently with a closed system. But the entire non-corpuscular volume of the blood is replaced 80 times each day. With this "leakage," the return flow in the veins is entirely unexplained since there would be no fluid pressure left after the capillaries that open into the tissues. Furthermore, there is more blood volume in the veins than the arteries, by a wide (65% to 12%) margin; an efficient pump design would operate on the larger volume directly.

• The relationship between flow and pressure is opposite what would be expected of a heart pump, with highest pressure and lowest volume throughout the system (including the veins) when the heart's pumping action is highest. However, the volume of blood and venous pressure increase when the heart's pumping action weakens.

• The aorta bends under systole, when it should straighten under the higher pressure.

• Heart problems and circulatory problems do not necessarily coincide.

• Replacement by a mechanical pump only works for a limited time.

• The location of the heart in the upper third of the body makes no sense if efficient pumping action is the functional goal; ask any farmer whether to put a pump at the top (suction action) or bottom (push action) of a hill.

---

[339] Callum Coates, *Living Energies: An Exposition of Concepts Related to the Theories of Viktor Schauberger.* Gateway, 1995. p. 192.

## *If not the heart, what moves the blood?*

The cells and tissues of the body are churning engines of metabolic activity, taking in and expelling materials to accomplish their tasks of growth, replacement, energy conversion, mobility and defense. To find a force capable of moving the blood through the circulatory system, the capillary side of the equation is a far better candidate. In effect, each cell is microscopically pulsating and replacing the blood constantly. This is the consensus explanation for the real force behind circulation in the body. Substantial evidence supports this explanation, as many writers have discussed:

> "The force that causes the blood to flow into the heart is the result of work performed by the tissues continually replenishing the fluid volume of the blood... The function of the heart is to regulate resistance."[340]

> "Osmotic pressure, in the form of the production of water from food and oxygen, is the pump... The heart does not pump, what it does is listen. This amazing organ senses what is in the blood and then calls forth the necessary hormones so that homeostasis is maintained and the cells can function optimally... The heart is not a mechanical pump but actually a sensitive integrator of all our experience."[341]

Viktor Schauberger offers additional insights: the spiral shape on the inner surface of the blood vessels, the temperature differential between core and extremities and the electromagnetic charge differential between arterial (oxygen-rich) and venous ($CO_2$-rich) blood also seem to

---

[340] Craig Holdrege, *The Dynamic Heart & Circulation*, AWSNA, 2002. p. 70.

[341] Thomas Cowan, *The Fourfold Path to Healing: Working with the Laws of Nutrition, Therapeutics, Movement and Meditation in the Art of Medicine.* Newtrends, 2004.

support the conclusion that the heart is not the main source of circulatory action.[342]

## *If not a pump, what is the heart's primary function?*

At a mechanical level, the heart's rhythmic beating is its most obvious characteristic. The forceful expulsion of the blood sets a basic cadence for bodily functioning, and forceful delivery of blood to the nearby (and appropriately uphill) brain is a cornerstone of health. The cadence itself seems to serve as a sort of metronome to which many other functions orient.

> Our heart is the metronome of our body's biorhythm and health happens when we are in rhythm with ourselves, synchronized with other living systems, and moving to our pre-set beat.[343]

> The heart wave is the body's master wave that reflects and organizes the degree of synchronization of all behavioral waves from those of the whole organism through molecular biological and genetic oscillations.[344]

But a greater interest arises as our inquiry into the heart's functions turns to more subtle levels.

From the perspective of Polarity Therapy, the true function of the heart is to regulate the dualistic action (cycles of inward Yin and outward Yang pulsation) of the primary energy field of the body. Furthermore, this polarity action is the foundation of physical, emotional and psychological

---

[342] Callum Coates, *Living Energies: An Exposition of Concepts Related to the Theories of Viktor Schauberger.* Gateway, 1995. pp. 188-190.

[343] Paul Pearsall, *Heart's Code: Tapping the Wisdom and Power of Our Heart Energy.* Broadway, 1999. p. 222

[344] Irving Dardik, "The Origin of Disease and Health Heart Waves," *Cycles Magazine,* Vol. 46, No. 3, 1996.

well-being, therefore the heart's role is a central, perhaps *the* central, esoteric function at the foundation of health.

For Randolph Stone, the true function of the heart was its dynamic management of inward and outward reciprocal action throughout the whole system. This view is presented in one of Stone's most famous charts, shown again here for convenience.

Because the polarized cycle of expansion and contraction is the fundamental engine for all phenomena, the "glue of the universe,"[345] the heart's activity can be characterized as the subtle basis for all health. According to Stone:

CHART NO. 2. OPPOSITES POLARIZED. DIAGRAM OF THE PATTERN OF LIFE FORCE AND THE TISSUE CELL.

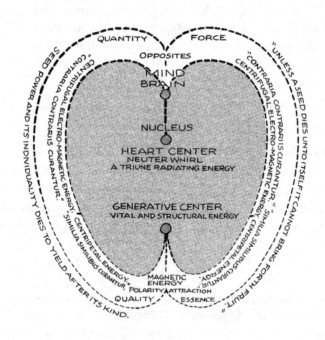

---

[345] Gary Zukav, *The Dancing Wu Li Masters: An Overview of the New Physics*. Bantam, 1984. p. 206.

The outward and inward currents must move in all fields if there is to be health and happiness... The heart center is the pivot for the circulation of these energies through the blood... and becomes the control center for these energies. [346]

This concept has not found acceptance in medicine and science.[347]

Compelling confirmation of the heart's esoteric properties comes from the literature relating to heart transplant recipients and research by the Institute of HeartMath.[348] Many other resources also explore this topic thoroughly; use the footnotes in this appendix as a starting bibliography.

The arising of the early heart in the embryo offers additional possible insights into its subtle function. This theme has been beautifully developed in the anthroposophical literature inspired by Rudolph Steiner and others. In a developing embryo, the precursor of the heart appears as a horseshoe-shaped group of specialized cells at the cranial end of the primitive streak. These cells act as if they are catching the streak's midline-defining directional impulse (symbolically a key gesture of the soul's incarnation) and pivoting the energetic signal back toward its source, in a spiral flow pattern. The spiral is preserved in the form, as revealed in the spectacular research of Spanish doctor Francisco Torrent Guasp (1931-2005).[349] Metaphorically, the

---

[346] R. Stone, *Polarity Therapy, Vol. 1*, CRCS, 1986. Book 3, p. 36.

[347] "It's just a stupid pump!" –Transplant recipient Claire Sylvia's cardiologist, reported in her book *A Change of Heart: A Memoir*. Grand Central, 1998.

[348] www.nexusmagazine.com/articles/CellularMemories.html has excellent accounts of transplant phenomena. For HeartMath Institute, see www.heartmath.org.

[349] http://www.youtube.com/watch?v=Mih37LLv6IQ

heart is describing the experience of self-awareness, which in turn reminds us of Stone's purpose of life, "the fulfillment of consciousness," described earlier in the book.

Following this line of thinking, the heart might be considered the first and foremost instrument for self-awareness in the body. This identity of the heart suggests the key attribute of the Ether Element. The heart's migration past and fascial connection to the throat via the pericardium also supports this link to the Ether Element. In this context, the heart is the organ of "I am," a notion that can be supported easily by asking anyone, "Where are you, in the body?" Invariably the response is a gesture pointing at the heart.

The heart also shows the earliest formal expression of meso-tissue in the body. Energetically, the neutral principle complements the Yang ectodermal (central nervous system) and Yin endodermal (digestive) factors. This idea of the heart as the key neutral organ matches Stone's ideas of it being the pivot between outward (Yang) and inward (Yin) expressions. The firm attachment of its container, the pericardium, to the respiratory diaphragm, the midpoint in the body, also supports this interpretation. Stone highlighted this relationship with one of his more famous statements, "When the diaphragm is free, the heart is free, to act without fear or apprehension."[350]

---

[350] R. Stone, *Polarity Therapy, Vol. 2.* CRCS, 1986. p. 46.

# Bibliography

ACE Study, summarized,
http://www.psychotherapynetworker.org/magazine/recentissues
/1107-as-the-twig-is-bent.

Alexander, Eben, Proof of Heaven: A Neurosurgeon's Journey into the
Afterlife (Simon & Schuster, 2012)

Almaas, A.H., The Unfolding Now: Realizing Your True Nature through
the Practice of Presence. Shambhala, 2012

Almaas, A.H. & Johnson, Karen, The Power of Divine Eros: The
Illuminating Force of Love in Everyday Life. Diamond Heart, 2013.

Amen, Daniel, Change Your Brain, Change Your Life. Three Rivers
Press, 1998.

American Polarity Therapy Association, www.PolarityTherapy.org.

Andrulis, Erik, Theory of the Origin, Evolution, and Nature of Life. Life
Journal, 2012. www.mdpi.com/journal/life

Aposhyan, Susan, Body-Mind Psychotherapy: Principles, Techniques,
and Practical Applications. Norton, 2004.

Barash, David & Lipton, Judith Eve, The Myth of Monogamy: Fidelity
and Infidelity in Animals and People. Holt, 2002.

Beaulieu, John, Human Tuning: Sound Healing with Tuning Forks.
Biosonic, 2010.

Becker, Rollin, Life In Motion, Stillness Press, 1997.

Becker, Rollin, Stillness of Life, Stillness Press, 2000.

Bell, Taunjah, Vagus Nerve Stimulation and Anxiety. iUniverse, 2010.

Berceli, David, The Revolutionary Trauma Release Process. Namaste,
2008.

Blasband, Richard, (Book Review) of Adventures in the Orgasmatron by
Christopher Turner, published in the Journal of Scientific
Exploration. Winter 2012, Volume 26, Number 4, page 895.

Blechschmidt, Erich, The Ontogenetic Basis for Human Development: A
Biodynamic Approach to Development from Conception to Birth.
North Atlantic, 2004.

Bly, Robert, The Third Body. From the collection, "Ten Poems to Open
your Heart" by Robert Housden. Harmony, 2003.

Boucher, Sandy, Opening the Lotus: A Woman's Guide to Buddhism.
Beacon, 1997.

Bower, Sniffle-busting personalities: positive mood guards against
colds. Science News, Vol. 170, p. 387.

Brennan, Barbara, Hands of Light, Bantam, New York, 1987.

Brill, Steven, The Bitter Pill: Why Medical Bills are Killing Us, Time
Magazine, March 2013.

Brinkley, Dannion, Saved by the Light, HarperOne, 2008.

Brown, Michael, The Presence Process: A Journey into Present Moment
Awareness. Namaste, 2010.

Burger, Bruce, Esoteric Anatomy, North Atlantic, 1989.

Campbell, Morag, Sink the Relation Ship: Transform the Way You Relate. Masterworks, 2010.

Campbell, Morag, Quinta Essentia: The Five Elements. Masterworks, 2003.

Capra, The Tao of Physics. Shambala, 1975.

Castellino, Ray, www.raycastellino.com

Chamberlain, David, The Mind of Your Newborn Baby. North Atlantic Press, 1998.

Chamberlain, David, www.birthpsychology.org

Chitty, Anna, Man and Woman DVD. Alive Polarity, 1988.

Chitty, John, Gifts: How Polarity and Craniosacral Complement Each Other. www.energyschool.com, 2008.

Chitty, John, The Heart is Not (Just) a Pump, www.energyschool.com.

Chitty, John, Origins of Polarity Therapy, www.energyschool.com

Chitty, John & Muller, Mary Louise, Energy Exercises, Polarity Press, 1988.

Chopra, Deepak, Quantum Healing, Bantam, 1990.

Corsi, J., 232 J. Corsi, Healing From Trauma, Marlowe & Co., 2007.

Cozolino, Louis, The Neuroscience of Psychotherapy: Building and Rebuilding the Human Brain. Norton, 2002.

Dalai Lama, Destructive Emotions: How Can We Overcome Them? Bantam, 2003. Narrated by Daniel Goleman.

Damasio, Antonio, The Feeling of What Happens: Body and Emotion in the Making of Consciousness.Harcourt, 1999.

Dardik, Irving, The Origin of Health and Disease, Heart Waves. The Center for Frontier Sciences Vol. 6 No. 2, 1997.

Deida, David, Intimate Communion. HCI,1995.

Dennison, Paul, Brain Gym, EduKinesthetics, 1992.

Denniston, George, Hodges, F., Milos, M., Circumcision and Human Rights, Springer Science: 2009.

Diamond, Marian, The Brain: Use It or Lose It. Mindshift Connection (vol. 1, no.1), Zephyr Press, edited by Dee Dickinson.

Dreeke, Robin, It's Not All About Me: The Top Ten Techniques for Building Rapport with Anyone. Robin Dreeke, 2011.

Duffy, William, The Sugar Blues, Grand Central, 1986.

Eadie Betty, Embraced by the Light (Bantam, 2002; 1st edition 1992.

Eagleman, Dan, Ten Unsolved Mysteries of the Brain. Discover Magazine, Aug. 2007.

Eagleman, Dan, Incognito: the Secret Lives of the Brain. Vintage, 2011

Eisler, Riane, The Chalice and the Blade. HarperOne, 1988.

Eckberg, Maryanna, Victims of Cruelty: Somatic Psychotherapy in the Treatment of Posttraumatic Stress Disorder.North Atlantic, 2000.

Ekman, Paul, Telling Lies: Clues to Deceit in the Marketplace, Politics and Marriage. Norton, 1985.

Ekman, Paul, Emotions Revealed: Recognizing Faces and Feelings to Improve Communication and Emotional Life. Holt, 2007.

Emerson, William, http://emersonbirthrx.com

Erikson, Erik, Identity and the Life Cycle. Norton, 1994.

Fehmi, Les & Robbins, Jim, The Open-Focus Brain: Harnessing the Power of Attention to Heal Mind and Body. Trumpeter Press, Boston, 2007.

Feldenkrais, Body and Mature Behavior. Frog Books, 2005.

Feldenkrais, Moshe, Master Moves. Meta, 1985.

Feldenkrais, Moshe with Mark Reese, The Potent Self: A Study of Spontaneity and Compulsion. Frog Books, 2002.

Fields, Rick, Chop Wood, Carry Water: A Guide to Finding Spiritual Fulfillment in Everyday Life. Tarcher, 1984.

Fine, Cordelia, Delusions of Gender. Norton, 2011.

Fleiss, Paul, The Case Against Circumcision. Mothering Magazine, November 1997.

Foos-Graber, Anya, Deathing. Nicholas-Hays, 1989.

Forrest, Lynne, Which Child Were You? Roles by Birth. http://www.lynneforrest.com.

Freyd, Jennifer, Betrayal Trauma. Harvard, 1998.

Gandhi, Mohandas, Gandhi's Health Guide. Crossing Press, 2000.

Goddard, Philip, www.clarity-of-being.org/

Goulding, Mary & Goulding, Robert, Changing Lives through Redecision Therapy. Grove Press, 1997.

Gray, John, Men are from Mars, Women are from Venus. Harper, 2003.

Greenwald, J.A., 53 J.A. Greenwald, The Ground Rules in Gestalt Therapy, in The Handbook of Gestalt Therapy, by Hatcher and Himmelstein (Eds.). Aronson, 1976.

Grossman, Dave, On Killing: The Psychological Cost of Learning to Kill in War and Society. Back Bay Books, 2009.

Hamer. G., The New Medicine, Amici de Dirk Publishing, Spain, 2000.

Hanson, Rick, Buddha's Brain: The Practical Neuroscience of Happiness, Love and Wisdom. New Harbinger, 2009.

Haramein, Nassim, Crossing the Event Horizon DVD. The Resonance Project, 2009. www.resonanceproject.org.

Haramein, Nassim, Black Whole DVD. The Resonance Project, 2011

Heller, Diane, Crash Course: A Self-Healing Guide to Auto Accident Trauma and Recovery. North Atlantic, 2001.

Herman, Judith, Trauma and Recovery. BasicBooks, 1992.

Iacoboni, Marco, Mirroring People: The New Science of How We Connect With Others. Farrar, Strauss and Girouz, 2008.

Jealous, James, The Biodynamics of Osteopathy, Audio CD Lecture, 2004. wwwjamesjealous.com.

Johnson, Julian, The Path of the Masters (Abridged). RSSB, 1940.

Johnson, Steven, Mind Wide Open: Your Brain and the Neuroscience of Everyday Life. Scribner, 2004.

Johnson, Wendell, People in Quandaries: The Semantics of Personal Adjustment. IGS, 1995.

Jones, Joshua, Behavior and Learning Using Inferred But Not Cached Values. Science, Vol. 338, p. 953. Nov. 16, 2012.

Joseph, Peter, Zeitgeist: The Movie. DVD, 2007.

Kaptchuk, Ted, The Web That Has No Weaver, McGraw-Hill, 2000

Keeney, Bradford, Shaking Medicine: The Healing Power of Ecstatic Movement. Guilford, 2007.

Keleman, Stanley, Emotional Anatomy. Center Press, 1989.

Kern, Michael, Wisdom in the Body. North Atlantic, 2005.

Korn, Leslie, Rhythms of Recovery: Trauma, Nature and the Body. Routledge, 2013.

Korzybski, Alfred, Science and Sanity: An Introduction to Non-Aristotelian Systems and General Semantics. IGS, 1996; first published in 1933

Korpiun, Olaf, Cranio-Sacral-S.E.L.F.-Waves: A Scientific Approach to Craniosacral Therapy. North Atlantic, 2011.

Kurtz, Ron & Prestera, H., The Body Reveals, HarperCollins, 1984.

Kushi, Michio, The Book of Macrobiotics. Square One, 2012.

Kushi, Michio & Jannetta, P., Macrobiotics and Oriental Medicine: An Introduction to Holistic Health. Japan Publications, 1991.

Laing, R.D., The Politics of Experience. Pantheon, 1967.

Lair, Jess, I Ain't Much Baby But I'm All I've Got. Fawcett, 1995.

Lake, Frank, Clinical Theology, a Theological And Psychiatric Basis to Clinical Pastoral Care, Emeth, 2006. ).

Lawlor, Robert, Sacred Geometry: Philosophy and Practice. Thames and Hudson, 1982.

Ledoux, Joseph, Synaptic Self: How Our Brains Become Who We Are. Viking Penguin, 2002.

Lee, Paul, 52 Paul Lee, Interface, Stillness Press, 2003. p. 103

Lerner, Eric, The Big Bang Never Happened. Vintage, 1992.

Levine, Barbara Hoberman, Your Body Believes Every Word You Say. Aslan, 1991.

Levine, Peter, In an Unspoken Voice. North Atlantic, 2010.

Levine, Peter, It Won't Hurt Forever. Sounds True Audio, 2004.

Levine, Peter, Waking the Tiger. North Atlantic, 1998.

Levine, Peter, Ray Iraq Vet TBI (DVD). FHE, 2009.

Lewin, Roger, Is Your Brain Really Necessary? Science Magazine, Dec. 1980.

Lipton, Bruce, 21 B. Lipton, The Biology of Belief. Hay House Publishing, 2008.

Lipton, Bruce, 169 Bruce Lipton, The Honeymoon Effect. Hay House, 2013.

Lowen, Alexander, Bioenergetics: The Revolutionary Therapy That Uses the Language of the Body to Heal the Problems of the Mind. Penguin, 1994.

Manne, Joy & Hellinger, Bert, Family Constellations: A Practical Guide to Uncovering the Origins of Family Conflict. North Atlantic, 2009.

Marcher, Lisbeth, Body Encyclopedia: A Guide to the Psychological Functions of the Muscular System. North Atlantic, 2010.

Maslow, Abraham, A Theory of Human Motivation. CreateSpace, 2013. Originally published in 1943.

McEwan, Bruce, The End of Stress as We Know It. Joseph Henry Press, 2002.

Mellody, Pia & Freundlich, L., The Intimacy Factor. HarperOne, 2003.

Mellody, Pia & Freundlich, L., Facing Codependence, Harper & Row, 2003. p. 113.

Mellody, Pia & Freundlich, L., Permission to be Precious, Audio CD set. Encore, 1987.

Meredith, Mukara, www.matrixworkslivingsystems.com.

Miller, Alice, For Your Own Good: Hidden Cruelty in Child-Rearing and the Roots of Violence. FSG, 1983.

Mitchell, William, Bye Bye Big Bang, Hello Reality (Cosmic Sense Books, 2002.

Morrison, Jaydean, I'm Not Sick. Society Is!: ADD/ADHD is an Adaptation to Society - Not an Illness. AuthorHouse, 2006.

Muramoto, Naboru, Healing Ourselves. Avon, 1973.

Narby, Jeremy, The Cosmic Serpent. Tarcher/Putnam, 1998.

Newton, Michael, Journey of Souls. Llewellyn, 1994.

Odent, Michel, Birth and Breastfeeding: Rediscovering the Needs of Women During Pregnancy and Childbirth. Steiner Press, 2008.

Odent, Michel, The Scientification of Love, Free Association Books, 2001.

Ogden, Pat, Minton, K. and Pain, C., Trauma and the Body: A Sensorimotor Approach to Psychotherapy. Norton, 2008.

Ornish, Dean, Love & Survival, William Morrow, 1999.

Peaceful Societies, www.peacefulsocieties.org/

Pearsall, Paul, Schwartz, G. & Russak, L., Organ Transplants and Cellular Memories. Nexus Magazine, April-May 2005. Also see http://www.namahjournal.com/doc/Actual/Memory-transferenc e-in-organ-transplant-recipients-vol-19-iss-1.html

Porges, Stephen, The Polyvagal Theory: Neurophysiological Foundations of Emotions, Attachment, Communication, and Self-Regulation. Norton, 2011.

Rabagliati, Andrea, Initis: Congestion of the Connective Tissue. Masterworks, 2012.

Rama, Swami, Ajaya, S. & Ballentine, R., Yoga and Psychotherapy: The Evolution of Consciousness. Himalayan Institute, 1976.

Ramachandran, V.S., Phantoms in the Brain: Probing the Mysteries of the Human Mind. William Morrow Paperbacks, 1999.

Reich, Wilhelm, Children of the Future. Farrar, Straus & Giroux, 1984.

Robbins, John, Diet for a New America (Kramer, 2012; first published in 1988)

Robbins, Tony, Unlimited Power. Free Press, 1997.

Rohen, Johannes, Functional Morphology, the Dynamic Wholeness of the Human Organism. Adonis, 2007.

Root, Andrew, The Children of Divorce: The Loss of Family as the Loss of Being. Baker Academic, 2010.

Roots of Empathy, www.rootsofempathy.org

Rosenberg, Marshall, Nonviolent Communication, Puddledancer Press, 2003.

Rushkof, Douglas, Present Shock: When Everything Happens Now. Current, 2013.

Russell, James, Psychosemantic Parenthetics. IHTR, 1988.

Satir, Virgina, The New Peoplemaking. Science and Behavior Books, 1988.

Scaer, Robert, 8 Keys to Brain-Body Balance. Norton, 2012.

Schlain, Leonard, The Alphabet Versus the Goddess. Penguin, 1999.

Schneider, Michael, A Beginner's Guide to Constructing the Universe: Mathematical Archetypes of Nature, Art, and Science. HarperPerennial, 1995.

Schwartz, Gary, Simon, W. & Chopra, D., The Afterlife Experiments: Breakthrough Scientific Evidence of Life After Death. Atria, 2003.

Seppa, Nathan, (Book review of Present Shock: When Everything Happens Now, by Douglas Rushkof (Current, 2013). Science News, June 15, 2013.

Sha, Zhi Gang, Divine Soul Song of Yin Yang. Institute of Soul Healing and Enlightenment, 2009.

Sha, Zhi Gang, www.DrSha.com

Sha, Zhi Gang, Soul Mind Body Medicine: A Complete Soul Healing System for Optimum Health and Vitality. New World Library, 2006.

Sheldrake, Rupert, The Science Delusion: 10 Paths to New Discovery. Coronet, 2012.

Sheldrake, Rupert, www.sheldrake.org/Research/morphic/

Sheldrake, Rupert, The Sense of Being Stared At and Other Unexplained Powers of Human Minds. Park Street Press, 2013.

Sheldrake, Rupert, Science Set Free. Deepak Chopra Books, 2012.

Siegel, Daniel, Mindsight: The New Science of Personal Transformation. Bantam, 2011.

Sills, Franklyn, The Polarity Process. North Atlantic, 1986.

Sills, Franklyn, Being and Becoming: Psychodynamics, Buddhism and the Origins of Selfhood. North Atlantic, 2009.

Sills, Franklyn, Foundations in Craniosacral Biodynamics. North Atlantic, 2012.

Sills, Franklyn, Craniosacral Biodynamics, North Atlantic 2001.

Sinetar, Marsha, Do What You Love, The Money Will Follow: Discovering Your Right Livelihood. Dell, 1989.

Singh, Sawan, Tales of the Mystic East. RSSB, 1961. p. 51.

Smail, David, Power, Interest and Psychology - Elements of a Social Materialist Understanding of Distress. PCCS Books, 2005.

Soloman, Marion & Tatkin, S., Love and War in Intimate Relationships: Connection, Disconnection, and Mutual Regulation in Couple Therapy (Norton, 2011.

Still, Andrew Taylor, Philosophy and Mechanical Principles of Osteopathy. Forgotten Books, 2012. First published in 1902.

Still, Andrew Taylor, Philosophy of Osteopathy. Forgotten Books, 2012. First published in 1899.

Strenberg, Esther, The Balance Within: The Science Connecting Health and Emotions. Freeman, 200o.

Stokes, Gordon & Whiteside, Daniel, One Brain. Three in One Concepts, 1987.

Stone, Randolph, Polarity Therapy, Vol. 1 & 2. CRCS, 1986.

Stone, Randolph, Health-Building. CRCS, 1986.

Stone, Randolph, Mystic Bible. RSSB, 1956.

Szalavitz, Maia & Perry, Bruce, Born for Love. Morrow, 2010.

Szasz, Thomas, The Second Sin. Doubleday, 1973.

Tannen, Deborah, You Just Don't Understand. William Morris, 2001.

Tarrant, John, The Light Inside the Dark: Zen, Soul and the Spiritual Life. Harper, 1999.

Tatkin, Stan and Hendrix, Harville, Wired for Love: How Understanding Your Partner's Brain and Attachment Style Can Help You Defuse Conflict and Build a Secure Relationship. New Harbinger, 2012.

The Listening Project, www.education.umd.edu/EDHD/faculty2/Porges/tlp/tlp.html

Thie, John, Touch for Health. Devorrs, 1979.

Treffert, Darold, Extraordinary People: Understanding Savant Syndrome. Backinprint, 2006.

Tuffey, David, The Four Sublime States: The Brahmaviharas. Altiora, 2012.

van der Bie, G. & Huber, M., Foundations of Anthroposophical Medicine. Floris, 2010.

van der Kolk, Bessel, McFarlane, A. & Weiseith, L., Traumatic Stress, The Effects of Overwhelming Experience of Mind, Body and Society, Guilford Press, 2006.

van der Wal, Jaap, Dynamic Morphology and Embryology in Foundations of Anthroposophical Medicine (Floris, 2010).

van der Wal, Jaap, Embryology: Where Biology Meets Biography. DVD set. CSES, 2005.

Varona, Verne, A Guide to the Macrobiotic Principles. www.macrobiotics.co.uk/articles/principles.htm.

Verhulst, Jos. Developmental Dynamics in Humans and Other Primates: Discovering Evolutionary Principles through Comparative Morphology. Adonis, 2003.

Verny, Thomas, The Secret Life of the Unborn Child. Dell, 1982.

Wake, Lisa, NLP: Principles in Practice. Ecademy, 2012.

Wallace, B. Alan, The Four Immeasurables: Practices To Open The Heart. Snow Lion, 2010.

Watts, Alan, The Two Hands of God. Collier Books, New York, 1963.

Wehrli, Katharina, The Why in the Road - Soul Healing for Changing Times. Earthlit, 2005.

Weil, Andrew, Spontaneous Healing. Ballantine, 2000.

Whitfield, G.V., The Prenatal Psychology of Frank Lake and the Origins of Sin and Human Dysfunction. Emeth, 2007.

Wilhelm, R. & Baynes, C., translators, I Ching. Princeton Univ. Press, 1967.

Wilson, Robert Anton, Quantum Psychology: How Brain Software Programs You and Your World. New Falcon, 1990.

Wylie, Mary Sykes, As the Twig is Bent. PsychotherapyNetworker. http://www.psychotherapynetworker.org/magazine/recentissues/1107-as-the-twig-is-bent.

Young, The Art of Polarity Therapy, A Practitioner's Perspective. Prism Press, 2000.

Zimbardo, Philip, The Demise of Guys. TED Conferences, 2011. See also www.demiseofguys.com.

Zukav, Gary, The Dancing Wu Li Masters. Bantam, 1979.

Zur, Ofer, The Conversation Continues... Notable Shifts in the Debate of Therapeutic Boundaries, in California Psychologist, 2008. 41 (1), 6-9.

# Index

Bold indicates the primary reference

# Also from Polarity Press

## *To Order: www.energyschool.com*

### Energy Exercises: Easy Exercises for Health and Vitality
by John Chitty
and Mary Louise Muller

$17.95

This "Polarity Yoga" book gathers all Randolph Stone's self-help exercises in one place, including clear directions, benefits, documentation and references to related modalities. Every posture and movement is illustrated by Mark Allison. Additional supportive material summarizes Polarity Therapy and energy-based exercises from other teachers.

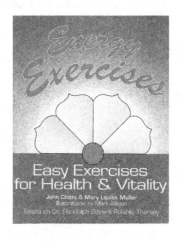

### The Triune Autonomic Nervous System Wall Poster
by John Chitty

$24

This 18x24 color poster combines seven diagrams in one view to fully summarize the Polyvagal Theory. The diagrams are the same as those that illustrate Chapter 6 in *Dancing with Yin and Yang*. Additional commentary is added to discuss implications of the theory.

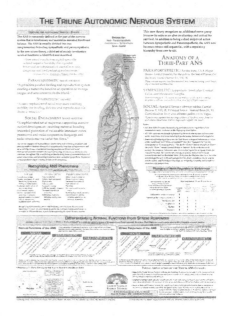

## Polarity Therapy Wall Charts
Text by John Chitty, art by Mark Allison

$10 each

These black and white 18x24 wall posters are based on some of Randolph Stone's most information-rich charts from *Polarity Therapy: The Complete Collected Works*. Art is by Mark Allison.

## *To Order: www.energyschool.com*

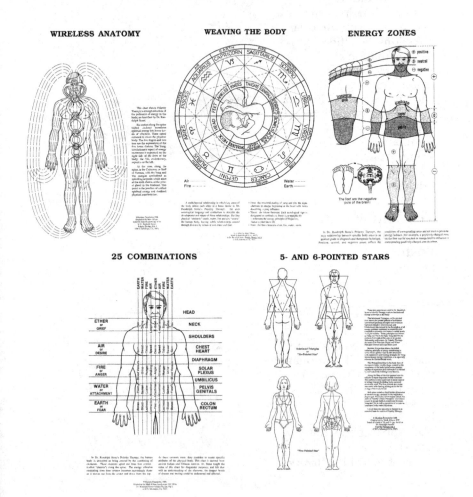

WIRELESS ANATOMY

WEAVING THE BODY

ENERGY ZONES

25 COMBINATIONS

5- AND 6-POINTED STARS

CPSIA information can be obtained
at www.ICGtesting.com
Printed in the USA
FSOW04n0522021017
39181FS